FOODSERVICE MANAGEMENT— BY DESIGN

THIRD EDITION

FOODSERVICE MANAGEMENT—BY DESIGN

Dee Legvold, MPH, RD
Kristi Salisbury, CDM, CFPP, RD
Soniya Perl, MS, RDN

Association of Nutrition & Foodservice Professionals

Association of Nutrition & Foodservice Professionals
PO Box 3610
St. Charles, IL 60174
800.323.1908
www.ANFPonline.org

978-0-578-78561-5

Copyright © 2020, 2018, 2015 Association of Nutrition & Foodservice Professionals. Copyright © 1992, 1985 Purdue Research Foundation. All rights reserved. No part of this publication may be reproduced, stored in a retrieval system, or transmitted, in any form or by any means, electronic, mechanical, photocopying, recording, or otherwise, without the prior written permission of the copyright owner. Material within this publication retained from the 1992 and 1985 editions are used with the permission of Purdue Research Foundation.

Printed in the United States of America

Dedication

We dedicate this book to all those dietary managers who strive to better themselves through increased education. We have met many Certified Dietary Managers®, Certified Food Protection Professionals® (CDM®, CFPP®) throughout our careers who have inspired us to learn and improve our own skills.

This book is written as a textbook for students and as a future reference for working managers. We are proud of how it turned out and look forward to seeing more CDM, CFPPs meet the evolving needs of our senior living, hospitals, schools and other creative foodservice careers.

We thank the authors of the past editions who laid the groundwork for us. It was our goal to build upon the foundation they established and to provide operators with a hands-on working resource.

Finally, we thank our families who have supported our time over the last year of writing, discussing the best options, talking about the book and finally completing the book. We appreciate the opportunity provided by the Association of Nutrition & Foodservice Professionals to share our experiences as operators and management consultants with you.

Table of Contents

The chapters are color coded based on CDM, CFPP competencies. This book includes four areas; Foodservice, Personnel and Communications, Sanitation and Safety, and Business Operations.

CHAPTER

Foodservice

1. The Foodservice Operation 1
2. Menus—The Foundation of the Department 17
3. Prepare Standardized Recipes for Food Production 35
4. Standards and Procedures for Purchasing and Preparing Food 57
5. Food Production Systems 81
6. Preparation and Delivery of Between-Meal Snacks and Supplements ... 91
7. Evaluate Food Acceptance and Satisfaction 101
8. The Quality Process 113

Personnel and Communications

9. Labor Analysis and Staffing Needs 133
10. The Employment Process 145
11. Ongoing Employee Education 161
12. Employee Scheduling and Assignments 175
13. Manage Department Personnel 189
14. Policies and Goal Setting in the Workplace 211
15. Communications and Managing Change 227
16. Professional Development and Ethics 243

Sanitation and Safety

17. Safe Food Handling: Personnel 249
18. Safe Food Handling: Purchasing, Receiving, and Storage 271
19. Safe Food Handling: Food Preparation 281
20. Safe Food Handling: The Physical Plant 307

Business Operations

21. Manage the Operating Budget 337
22. Manage the Capital Budget 355
23. Department Design and Layout 361
24. The Purchasing Process 381
25. Revenue and Cash Handling 411
26. Financial Reports and Cost Control 429

APPENDIX

A. Focus on Formulas 431
B. Commonly Referenced Food Temperatures 449
   Index 452

Preface

Non-commercial food service is changing rapidly. The lines between commercial and non-commercial food service are blurring as hospitals, schools, and long-term care facilities provide more choice for their clientele. In hospitals, retail sales are becoming an increasingly important part of the overall foodservice budget. In schools, more options are available to students. Long-term care facilities are preparing for the next generation resident that is demanding more choices than ever before.

Today, Certified Dietary Managers®, Certified Food Protection Professionals® (CDM®, CFPP®) are responsible for the daily operations of their department while helping the facility fulfill its mission and goals. They coordinate the service of food and nourishments among various departments, such as dining services and nursing. CDM, CFPPs ensure that clients are satisfied with their dining experience and that the meals meet their nutritional and emotional needs. In addition, they oversee food safety, the inventory and ordering of food, equipment, and supplies, and arrange for the routine maintenance and upkeep of the foodservice equipment and facilities. CDM, CFPPs are generally responsible for all administrative and human resource functions of the foodservice department, including recruiting new employees and monitoring employee performance and training.

The authors' design in writing this textbook is based on tasks that a team of CDM, CFPPs has identified as common to most foodservice operations. These tasks represent current practice in the United States. As the driving force of any foodservice department, "The Menu" is the starting point of the *Foodservice Management—By Design* textbook. The authors have structured the content and flow of material to build from that central concept. This book is intended to be both a student's textbook and a reference for working managers in operating a foodservice department. The textbook is based upon and integrates the 2021 Detailed Content Outline.

In addition, *Supplemental Materials—Foodservice* is included as an online resource for the student. The supplement offers supporting documents, articles, and forms to assist in learning to become a CDM, CFPP.

Foodservice is referenced in the Preface, however within the body of the book, foodservice may be interchanged with Dining Services. Foodservice is used primarily as a generic term including all types of meal and food preparation, from fast food and food trucks to white linen fine dining and room service. The term Dining Services generally refers more to quantity food production and meal service in care centers, schools, correctional facilities, hospitals and employee feeding venues. All terms are correct. Dining Services, however, is more specific to the segments of the foodservice departments that many Certified Dietary Managers are employed.

Acknowledgements

We would like to recognize the contribution of the review team who generously invested their professional expertise and valuable time in this book:

Christina Derbes, BS, DTR
Dr. Beth Gankofskie, RD
Joann Gruner, MBA, RD, LD
Kristin Klinefelter, MS, RDN, LD
Barbara Thomsen, CDM, CFPP, RAC, QCP

Content Editor: Beatriz U. Dykes, PhD, RDN, LDN, FADA, FAND
Technical Editor: Diane Everett
ANFP Staff: Cindy Zemko, BS, CDM, CFPP
Art Direction/Graphic Design: Mercy Ehrler

A Personal Invitation

As a student enrolled in the Nutrition & Foodservice Professional Training Program, we invite you to join the Association of Nutrition & Foodservice Professionals (ANFP) as a Pre-Professional member.

ANFP is the premier resource for foodservice managers, directors, and those aspiring towards careers in foodservice management, with more than 14,000 professionals dedicated to the mission of providing optimum nutritional care through foodservice management and food safety.

> **Pre-Professional membership is a stepping stone for professional growth. Network and connect with members in all practice areas, understand the profession, and gain valuable tools and resources at your fingertips.**

Enjoy benefits such as:

- 24/7 Members-only access to website, online community, and social media
- An electronic version of *Nutrition & Foodservice Edge* magazine
- Scholarship opportunities
- eNews monthly online newsletter
- Special discounted member pricing for ANFP products and services
- Network nationally, locally, and even globally with peers

You are the future of our profession. Take the first step in nourishing your career. Join ANFP today! For more information, visit www.ANFPonline.org or call 800-323-1908.

ANFP | Association of Nutrition & Foodservice Professionals

The Foodservice Operation

Overview and Objectives

How do you provide meals to your clients? The decision depends upon the dining venues, equipment available, and needs of the clientele. This chapter will take you through the steps of assessing your options and recognizing that no one style is always best for the clientele. After completing this chapter, you should be able to:

- Identify types of food service
- Discuss some trends in food service and their impact on the foodservice industry
- Describe the different styles of meal service and menus
- Understand the role of the Certified Dietary Manager®, Certified Food Protection Professional® (CDM®, CFPP®) in foodservice operations

Types of Food Service

Food services is an ever growing, ever changing industry and operations are commonly categorized as either **commercial** or **onsite** (noncommercial) food services. A commercial food service can be a full-service restaurant, a fast food outlet, a caterer, or simply kiosks at recreational facilities and convenience stores. Any place that prepares, serves, and sells food to the general public for a profit would fall under commercial food service. These for-profit restaurants may also be found at hotels, country clubs, airports, cruise ships, zoos, museums, and sports venues. The onsite foodservice industry, on the other hand, includes long-term care facilities, hospitals, and healthcare centers; schools, colleges, and universities; correctional facilities; congregate feeding programs; and military operations.

It is important to recognize foodservice trends for both commercial and onsite services as they influence the way food is purchased, prepared, and served. For example, the elderly are choosing to live in continuing care retirement communities (**CCRC**s). CCRCs are a combination of independent living, assisted living, and nursing home. Health care now includes CCRCs with country club-style dining rooms and steakhouse concepts. Dining services in senior living communities range from the traditional large dining room to the smaller "neighborhood" concept, with room service meals offered to patients in the transitional care unit. In hospitals, meal services can range from the typical tray-line and cart delivery, to high-end room service and specialty dining options.

Culture Change in Healthcare Dining Services

The choices for healthcare communities for older Americans are expanding and the type of food and nutrition care will need to expand as well. With 2017 CMS regulations, F561, "the facility honors the resident's right to make choices about aspects of his/her life in the facility that are significant to the resident." At the same time, it is important to tailor a menu to the dietary requirements of the client. How do we accomplish this? This section will describe the culture change movement around the dining experience and the menu options to support the change.

The culture change movement in dining is driven, in part, by the large numbers of Americans who are aging and who will be entering the various healthcare communities as they age. It is also being driven by the change in regulations to implement more person-centered, resident-driven dining programs. This is indeed an opportune time to showcase dining services and your ability to enhance the quality of life through food and dining choices. One service option change is to offer restaurant or in-dining room tableside service instead of the traditional trayline.

As with any change, there is resistance based on concerns about cost, staffing, and coordinating the changes with regulations. As you begin to adopt a new culture, there are many questions that need to be answered. Start with questioning clients to help decide what they want for dining services. You might ask questions such as:

- What time of day do you like to eat your meals?
- Do you snack regularly?
- How frequently during the day do you want coffee, tea, or water?
- Where do you prefer to eat your meals?
- What foods do you usually eat at breakfast, lunch, and dinner?
- Where should you begin with the culture change? (expanded snack program, restaurant services, selective menu)

GLOSSARY

CCRC
Continuing Care Retirement Communities offer a continuum of care as a person ages

Next, you will want to choose appropriate resources for changing your dining and/or menu options. You could survey other facilities in your area to determine how/if they have begun to implement a culture change in their dining services. Also, in August 2011, Pioneer Network announced the New Dining Practice Standards. The Pioneer Network promotes culture change in long-term care to meet the needs of clients. The New Dairy Practice Standards were established by convening a group of stakeholders/organizations with a vested interest in this topic.

Once you have data for what you want to do and why, the next step is to work with all departments in your facility. This will be a change for them as well, and you want them to support your efforts. Other departments that are likely to be affected are maintenance and nursing. You will want to develop a policy and procedure that outlines every department's responsibility for each type of change you initiate. Communication and training will be key steps. It is important to note that a culture change is a process that takes some time to implement.

While the changes outlined in Person-Directed Dining are directed at the healthcare field, they apply to any dining service. Dignity in dining is a concern in all marketplaces. Providing customer choice, quality products, and trained staff are hallmarks of good management.

Your **menu** and the **style of the service** are major components in developing a new dining culture. The equipment available defines many of the meal delivery options available to you. Decisions to transition away from a set trayline/no choice meal system, to a more accommodating meal service, and options, take planning and forethought. Let's discuss style of service and service options and then talk about menus.

Updates to revised Pioneer Network Dining Standards can be found in the Supplemental Material when available.

Style of Service

How you provide food in your facility is considered your style of service. There are many different methods for delivering meals to your clientele. A CDM, CFPP needs to use judgment to design and/or revise systems. In addition to the needs of clients, the manager must consider:

- The physical design of the kitchen
- Locations of dining rooms or service areas
- Requirements for off-site service (if any)
- Mission and goals of the organization
- Staffing resources
- Budget and operating costs
- Timing requirements for service

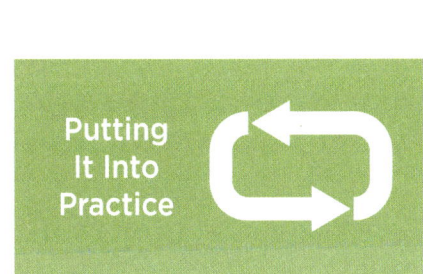

1. List at least three steps you would take to implement a culture change in your facility.

Service Options—The Traditional Trayline and Beyond

Trayline Service

A trayline, or the modified version **POD system**, is still the most common meal assembly process in acute care and many senior living communities. Trayline systems are also common in correctional facilities.

A trayline system moves trays through an assembly line where employees place items on trays. During this process, trays may move along a straight line or a circular platform, often with the help of a conveyor belt. Some conveyor belt systems are powered by electric motors with speeds that can be regulated. Other facilities operate skate wheel systems where trays are manually slid along the wheels. In a POD system, all of the serving stations are compressed into a small wrap-around space so everything is within easy reach of the server.

Centralized Versus Decentralized Meal Service

Centralized meal service means that food is portioned onto trays in a central location, such as the dining services department. An alternative is **decentralized meal service**, in which food is distributed to other locations for plating at the point of service, such as tableside service in senior living. In both centralized and decentralized systems, the equipment used must support the service and delivery model. Temperature control from the time of assembly to actual delivery is of paramount concern. To help ensure food safety, as well as quality, food must be kept out of the danger zone (41°-135°F). Let's look at the flow of food through a typical trayline service and the equipment used for transport.

The individual trays are typically transported by carts and delivered to clients. Serving meals through a trayline system involves a number of steps that are tightly integrated with the diet order system and a menu management process. How these steps are implemented varies from one operation to another. Figure 1.1 provides a sample flow for a traditional trayline service.

Figure 1.1
Sample Flow for a Traditional Trayline Service

1. Prior to the meal service time, either an individual meal ticket or tray identification card is prepared for each client.
2. The meal tickets are grouped by unit or dining room location.
3. Staff send the Meal tickets or Tray identification cards down the trayline for assembly.
4. Food items and supplies are organized by stations on the trayline.
5. Items selected or appropriate for the diet are added to the tray.
6. Staff place the tray on a cart or traveyor (an elevator belt with platforms for transporting trays to higher floors).
7. Nursing or dining services staff deliver trays to the client.

GLOSSARY

POD System
A small serving station with all items within reach of the server

Centralized Meal Service
Foods are prepared and portioned onto trays or plates at a central location or adjacent to the main kitchen

Decentralized (Delivery) Meal Service
Bulk quantities of prepared foods are sent hot or cold to other locations for finishing and service

Tray Delivery Options

Typically meal trays are transported throughout the facility in enclosed "food only" carts. Tray transport carts are designed to securely hold the trays while going up ramps, over bumps in the flooring, etc. Some carts are designed to provide thermostatically maintained heat, while others include a refrigeration section.

- **Insulated trays:** Each compartment is separated and insulated, keeps hot foods hot and cold foods cold. The tray on the left in Figure 1.2 illustrates a typical insulated tray.
- **Heated based systems:** Wax filled bases are pre-heated prior to meal plating. The tray on the right in Figure 1.2 illustrates a heated base tray.
- An instant heating system is available from some manufacturers. It transfers heat into a base plate while keeping the edges cool. Figure 1.3 illustrates a Heat-On-Demand base heater.
- **Insulated transportation carts:** In this type of system, the cart is insulated and may even be heated to help maintain hot food temperatures. Figure 1.4 shows an insulated cart for transportation of completed trays.

Not all meals are served from pre-plated meal trays. In today's marketplace, tableside meal selection is fairly common in senior dining where the client is served a meal from a hot-cart located within the dining room. Typically heated bases, transport carts, and insulated trays are not viewed by CMS (Centers for Medicare & Medicaid Services) as part of the home-like dining experience.

See Figure 1.5 for a temperature-controlled cart system. During assembly, employees place hot foods on the hot side of the tray and cold foods on the cold side. A dividing seal helps maintain temperature control. Some units can plug into a controller unit to rethermalize hot foods on trays immediately prior to service. Although this system can be very successful in maintaining temperatures, the "high tech" appearance of the tray becomes visually institutional looking

Figure 1.2
Insulated Tray and Dinnerware

Source: Aladdin-Temp-Rite®. Reprinted with permission.

Figure 1.3
Heat-On-Demand

Source: Carter-Hoffmann. Reprinted with permission.

Figure 1.4
Insulated Cart for Transporting Completed Trays

Figure 1.5
Temperature-Controlled Cart System

Source: Aladdin-Temp-Rite®. Reprinted with permission.

If an operation is using a cook-chill pre-plated tray system, in which foods are delivered cold and rethermalized just before service, trays are pre-assembled and delivered in carts. The carts and related technologies are designed to heat the food quickly using induction or convection heat. Figure 1.6 illustrates some rethermalization systems. Note that tray rethermalization can occur in a centralized location (in the dining services department just before tray distribution), or in a decentralized location (on the nursing units).

Also, specialized rethermalization systems generally require specialized dinnerware to integrate with the systems. In selecting equipment, it is important to review related needs and costs for dinnerware. Many are available in a range of colors and designs.

With today's service equipment, a manager can use software support for meal delivery systems to track temperature data, program rethermalization features, control and monitor remote delivery systems and generate reports through a desktop computer. Each style of service has its benefits and its compromises.

Pantry Service—Made to Order

In an effort to better meet client expectations, some facilities have implemented a **pantry** mini service on the unit. Typically food is prepared in a central kitchen and supplied to kitchenettes or pantries on the unit for plating and service to the clients. The pantry servery can support any menu format, from non-select to room service meal on demand, with what is expected to be hotter and fresher meal service.

Room Service

Many definitions of **room service** have been brought forward over the past 10-15 years. Originally conceived as a hotel style of room service, the process has evolved to reflect the needs of the healthcare setting and delivery of meals in a business account. Menus are often altered to provide options that are known to function better on a room service format.

GLOSSARY

Pantry
A small serving station or kitchenette where items can be plated and served to clients

Room Service
Meals selected and served upon request

Figure 1.6
Rethermalization Systems

Bulk Rethermalization System

Tray Rethermalization System

Source: Dinex. Reprinted with permission.

In hotels and commercial dining locations, a service or delivery charge is typically added to the bill to cover the cost of labor related to special delivery of the meal. In health care, although the added cost of labor is a factor, implementing a service charge is not an option.

Room service, or some variation of the concept, is now a common element in healthcare from the large metropolitan acute care hospital to the transitional care unit services in a community health center. Typically the room service concept is one of several styles of service within a given facility from:

- A non-select meal served at a defined time for clients unable or unwilling to select their meal; to
- Menus selected by the client served from a traditional trayline at defined meal times in some units; to
- A "meals-on-demand" room service concept

Tableside In-Dining Room Service

In an effort to provide a more "homelike" atmosphere in the senior living and congregate dining setting, many communities have turned to a **Tableside Service** using a hot well service station in the dining room. Plating and delivery of the meal to the client is completed in front of the clients. The meal served is often a select menu with two or more choices for the entrées and side-dishes.

GLOSSARY

Tableside Service
Serving clients from a hot well cart present in the dining venue

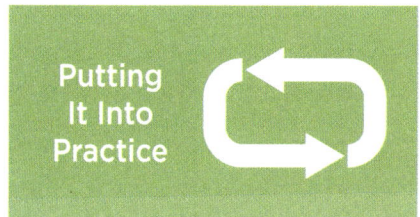

Putting It Into Practice

2. Your facility uses tray service where trays are plated in the kitchen and transported to the clients. What steps would you take to ensure that the trays are plated correctly, and the temperature is maintained?

A number of communities have established the "neighborhood" concept for the senior living environment. Typically, in this setting, the clients live within a small group and share their meals around a family style dining table. Meals supplied from dining services are plated and served to the clients from a home or residential looking kitchen. Often special services, such as eggs made to order or sandwiches prepared upon request, are offered in the neighborhood dining room.

Buffet Style Service

Buffet style service is offered in some long-term care facilities as a way to create an atmosphere of choice. Facilities offer the same number of choices as with restaurant style service (further discussed below), only clients can serve themselves. Be prepared to offer extra help for those clients who may not be able to manage walking a buffet line, handle their tray/plate, serve themselves, and carry the meal to the table. The buffet style of service is commonly used at a catered function whether in health care or the business setting. Catered events can be anything from coffee and donuts for a staff meeting of six to a full holiday meal for the board of directors.

Restaurant Style Service

Restaurant style is another way of implementing a new culture in residential dining. Your regular menu cycle entrée can be the daily special with an option of sandwiches, grilled items, vegetables, and salads. Restaurant style dining might include the following:

- Dining service staff waiting on tables
- Food ordered and delivered in courses
- Food plated in the dining room
- Specials such as sandwiches, salads, or desserts offered tableside from a cart

In many CCRC and corporate dining rooms, a high-end or white linen dining service is the norm. Meal options are more extensive and also upscaled with an emphasis on presentation. Training of staff on the correct service techniques in formal dining is essential to completing the fine dining experience.

Cafeteria Service

School or dormitory food service, employee dining rooms, commercial feeding, and correctional facilities all use a variation of the **cafeteria model**. Whether the straight-line tray slides or the more popular scramble concept, the cafeteria is designed to move a large number of customers through the meal selection process quickly.

Typically the actual plating of the food is provided by a cafeteria server with some self-serve or "grab-and-go" items available. Often the cafeteria includes a grill and some made-to-order items like sandwiches and specialty salads. Other than the correctional or dormitory setting, cafeterias are a cash-based operation.

C-Store—Sandwich Counters and Kiosks

Many of the CCRCs and independent senior living communities offer a c-store (convenience store) with frequently needed staples and supplies. Often a sandwich counter is an added service for a simple lunch meal when the main dining room is not available. A coffee kiosk or sandwich counter may be available in the lobby of an office complex, hospital out-patient surgery unit, or campus walkway.

GLOSSARY

Buffet Style
Meals selected by the client from buffet style serving line

Restaurant Style
A set menu of multiple options that does not change from day to day

Cafeteria Model
Straight-line or scramble system offers cafeteria style options

Multiple Venues

Dining services are being offered in more locations and with different "personalities" all within a single facility. Senior living communities may have a traditional dining room seating 50-100 residents, plus a wellness smoothie bar, a coffee kiosk with fresh bakery items and sandwiches, a white linen steakhouse, and a lounge with a full-service bar and appetizers—all on the same campus.

Satelliting Foodservice

Equipping and staffing a food production kitchen is expensive and requires a lot of space and utilities support. Sometimes organizations decide to obtain their food items from a production center. Whether the food is delivered in bulk for reheating and service in a dining room, such as congregate dining, or pre-plated meals for individual clients in a school or care center, satelliting of meals is becoming more common.

One type of satellited meal that has been employed across the country is home-delivered meals for the homebound and the elderly.

Service Concerns and Issues

Even with well-designed equipment and well-planned systems, foodservice departments sometimes face challenges with delivery of trays. For example, in a healthcare facility, if trays reach their destinations through a cart service, staff then need to distribute trays to clients. This task may be the responsibility of either nursing or dining services staff.

Staff who deliver trays need to accomplish several things:

- Be available as trays arrive and distribute trays promptly.
- Verify that each tray is reaching the right client.
  > Two "patient identifiers" is a guideline by The Joint Commission and recommended by World Health Organization (WHO) and Centers for Medicare & Medicaid Services (CMS).
  > Verify a client name and medical record number or date of birth against the name on the menu or ticket on the tray. Some tray tickets include client photos for easier verification.
- Be alert to any diet changes that have just occurred.
- Help the client set up the tray and open any packaging.
- Obtain substitutes or make adjustments if a client has any difficulties with the meal.
- Make sure food is arriving to the client at the appropriate temperature and accurate to the menu ticket.

These tasks require training. In addition, they can take a lot of time. When nursing staff members are required to assist, there can be time conflicts. A nurse may be involved in another clinical task at the time that trays arrive and this can cause delays. Furthermore, the CDM, CFPP needs to review schedules carefully to assure that they are reasonable and feasible with respect to client schedules. An effective staffing plan takes into account the skills and time requirements of the job. In addition, it involves coordination between nursing, rehab, and dining services departments.

Delays in the distribution process are a common reason for complaints about food temperature and/or quality. In addition, there is a food safety concern with trays that sit at room temperature too long. How can a CDM, CFPP tackle this challenge?

There is no single best answer. Some healthcare organizations have begun using additional auxiliary staff to assist with tray distribution and client feeding. Some have begun switching tray distribution from nursing to dining services staff to avoid timing conflicts. In addition, some of the rethermalization systems described earlier allow staff to control temperature much closer to the time of service. A temperature control cart that holds food temps may help provide a longer window of time in which to accomplish the job without sacrificing safety and quality. Also, to facilitate delivery, sequence the menus or tray tickets to ensure that trays are assembled and grouped in a meaningful order.

Meal delivery schedules must also comply with additional regulations to assure that frequency and timing fit prescribed needs. For example, in health care, the time frame between supper and breakfast cannot be more than 14 hours (i.e., 5:30 supper and 7:30 breakfast).

If delivery problems arise, it is up to the CDM, CFPP to review them with a nursing supervisor or administrator to help ensure that the entire meal delivery system functions effectively.

The Menu

The menu, a list of food items, is a key component of the food service and can impact all aspects of the operation. It dictates production, equipment purchased, staffing needs, as well as reflects the culture of the foodservice operation. Two of the most common options are selective and nonselective. Whether you have a select or non-select format, you need to have a defined number of days over which the menu is used. This is referred to as the **menu cycle**—how fast you return to day one of the cycle. You do not want to write a new menu every week and end up with a cycle 365 days long.

In the acute care setting, the average length of stay is now around four days. Many hospitals have gone to a cycle of five to eight days so that the same items do not always fall on a Tuesday.

In the residential segment of business (senior living, rehab, and group homes) the cycle is more likely going to be three–six weeks. Often using an odd number of weeks works better for these communities and employee cafeterias. Typically staff work every other weekend and when the menu is set to a two or four week cycle the staff see the same thing every weekend. By using a five week cycle a nurse will work 10 weeks before they see the Oven Roasted Turkey and Dressing on Sunday again.

Business and industry dining rooms and school food service also benefit from a longer menu cycle of three to five weeks just to avoid the repetition of items on the serving line. The presence of the daily standard items in the grill, sandwich service, and salad bars allow for an ever-present and popular set of alternatives.

Selective Menus

A **selective menu** is the way to implement current federal regulations, and, more importantly, enhance the quality of life and quality of care for your clients. A selective menu is one in which clients have the opportunity to make choices or selections in advance of meal service. For example, it usually offers at least two choices for an entrée and multiple choices for most items.

GLOSSARY

Menu Cycle
The number of days over which a menu is used

Selective Menu
A menu designed with multiple choices

Computer-based selective menu systems may use handheld computers and/or telephone systems for entry of choices into an automated system. Typically, a selective menu is distributed to clients in advance of the meal.

Select menus generally fit one of the following types:

Preselect

- Typically a printed menu with choices for breakfast, lunch, and dinner.
- Often distributed to the client the morning of or the day before service for selection and return to the meal preparation area.
- The selection may be limited to two entrées with the same side dishes or, more commonly, offer two to three entrées, two to three starches, and vegetables.
- Family members may preselect the meals for a week in advance knowing the client's preferences.
- No matter how many options are offered, a defined menu is set for each day as the non-select meal for those who choose not to make their selections.
  > The defined menu ensures nutritional adequacy of the default meal being provided.

Tableside Select

- This may be the same base menu designed for the Preselect with a selection made in the dining room at the time of service.
- The menu is typically posted in and around the dining room so clients can see in advance what the choices will be for the meal.
- There is also a non-select menu for those who choose not to make their selections.

Spoken

- This may be the same base menu designed for the Preselect.
- The menu is presented to the client by a dining services staff member by speaking. For example: "Good morning Mrs. Jones, today for lunch we have a garden salad, spaghetti with meat sauce, green beans, and lemon sorbet for dessert. How does that sound to you?"… "I did not realize that you don't like green beans, would you prefer broccoli or chopped spinach?"
- By placing the first or non-select default item as "today for lunch we have…" leads the client to the preferred choice, but leaves them with the option to request an alternative.
- The printed version of the menu may be available to clients to see in advance what the choices will be for the meal.
- There is also a non-select option for those who choose not to select their menu.

Restaurant Variation

- Typically this menu format is set up with a list of items that are always available as standard choices.
- Additionally a daily feature or chef's choice is presented as the preferred or default option for the meal.
- Standard items tend to be a short order type that can be finished quickly, such as baked fish or chicken stir-fry.
- The featured selection is often one that takes more time to prepare and would not be available every day, such as pot roast or pork chops.

- The printed version of the restaurant menu is available to clients to see in advance what the choices will be for the meal and the daily features may be printed for the day or the week for client review.
- There is also a non-select meal (typically the daily feature item) for those who choose not to make their selection.

Cafeteria

- Typically this menu format is set up with a list of items that are always available as a set or standard choices.
- Additionally, a daily feature or chef's choice is presented.
- Standard items tend to be a short order type that can be finished quickly, such as baked fish or chicken stir-fry.
- Featured menu selections are often ones that take more time to prepare and would not be available every day, such as pot roast or pork chops.

Buffet

- Generally a buffet menu is planned for a self-serve line.
- This style is often centered around single-serve or portion-controlled items like baked chicken breast or lower-cost products where over-portioning does not negatively impact financial performance.

Menus can be printed in a number of formats but typically start out as a Week-At-A-Glance (WAG) layout with breakfast, lunch, and dinner (or supper) planned for the week. This allows the manager and coordinator of the meal services to see in one place all of the meals planned for several days. Problems with repeating food items are easier to spot when looking at the WAG version. The WAG meets the needs of the "back of the house" production team but does not market well to your customers. For the "front of the house" or customer-facing menu, most organizations prefer to jazz up the appearance and highlight the specials. Examples that demonstrate the typical WAG for a healthcare facility and a sample select menu for the day may be found in the Supplemental Material for this chapter.

View the Supplemental Material for this chapter for typical WAG layouts for a healthcare facility and a sample select menu for the day. See Figures 1.7 and 1.8.

In healthcare facilities, or in any environment where the dining services department is responsible for honoring therapeutic diets, it is standard practice to review meal choices before they are served. If clients make choices on a selective menu, a member of the dining services team then reviews these choices against the medical diet of record and the nutrition guidelines for the diet. Common adjustments that may need to be made are:

- Portion sizes of products that count as fluid, for a fluid-restricted diet.
- Portion sizes of high-carbohydrate foods, for a carbohydrate counting diet.
- Consistency of foods and liquids, for specific dysphagia diets.
- Special adjustments for diets with multiple restrictions.
- Adjustments to incorporate a standing order, such as the addition of a liquid nutritional supplement to meals.

3. Using Figure 1.8 as an example, develop a Select Menu for a Wednesday for a hospital patient meal service. Explain your choices for each meal in ensuring its nutritional adequacy.

What happens if the client does not request enough food on a selective menu? What if the client selects food that is not on his/her diet? Dining Services staff should be trained to address a client's diet when they drop off the menu, for example:

- "Good morning Mrs. Smith. I know that you are on a sodium restricted diet and here are your menu selections for today." This helps remind the client of their diet and sets the stage for their choices.
- If they see that the client has not selected very much food, the dining services staff might say, "Oh, Mrs. Smith, our roast chicken is very tender and moist today. May I add that to your selection?"
- If the client insists on selecting something that is not on their menu, such as bacon on a salt-restricted diet, gently remind the client that bacon does not support their salt-restricted diet.

Always treat clients with respect and respond in such a way that they don't become defensive. Keep in mind that you need to educate clients on the limits of their medically-ordered diet, however, their resident/patient rights may overrule the dietary restrictions. Refer diet conflicts like these to the clinical nutrition staff for intervention and documentation in the medical record.

On a selective menu, there may also be items a client writes in as a special request. How this is handled depends on the facility policy. In general, health facilities attempt to honor write-in requests when practical. Many facilities develop a standardized list of write-in options to provide greater choice for clients.

Non-Selective Menus

A **non-selective menu** is one in which clients do not have the opportunity to make choices. Instead, they receive a standard, predefined menu. This is more common in a group dining experience such as a nursing home or assisted living facility. Even with a non-select format, you can focus on the clients by following their individualized food preferences with appropriate substitutions.

In a non-selective menu system, it is also important to review and modify standard choices to accommodate specific diet orders. You still want to follow individual food preferences, which may mean changing a food item. Substitutions must be of equal nutritional value. For instance, if someone doesn't like cabbage, the replacement should be a food that has similar Vitamin C, such as tomatoes. Since menus are planned to incorporate color, try to replace a food with a similar or a complementary color. Your facility should have a list of approved substitutes for your menu cycle. When making adjustments, always document the change and keep a record. This helps to prove during surveys that you are meeting client needs and preferences. A table with suitable vegetable substitutions is provided in Figure 1.9.

Late Trays

In a healthcare setting, it is essential to have a system for providing meals to clients who have just been admitted, whose diet orders have changed, or who have missed a meal due to testing or special procedures. Trays delivered between meal times are called **late trays**. Particularly in an acute care environment, diet-related information can change quickly.

In many situations, late trays are cumbersome and expensive to produce and deliver. Obtaining required adjustments just before tray assembly can sometimes reduce the

> **GLOSSARY**
>
> **Non-Selective Menu**
> A menu with no defined alternatives—a predefined menu plan
>
> **Late Trays**
> Trays delivered between meal times

volume of added trays. Many healthcare operations strive to reduce out of sequence requests through their meal system design. Room service is an example of a service model that can virtually eliminate late trays, because all meals are provided on demand.

The Role of the Certified Dietary Manager, Certified Food Protection Professional in Food Services

A **Certified Dietary Manager, Certified Food Protection Professional (CDM, CFPP)*** works in a variety of service venues today. Both onsite and commercial food services recognize the value of trained CDM, CFPPs as part of their supervisory and management team. The CDM, CFPP has the education, training, and experience to competently manage a foodservice operation and ensure its food safety. They are responsible for implementation of menus, foodservice purchasing, and food preparation. They apply nutrition principles, document nutrition information, manage work teams, and much more.

Most CDM, CFPPs work in long-term care facilities, healthcare centers, schools, universities, correctional facilities, congregate feeding programs, restaurants, and other work settings. The population or audience served by a CDM, CFPP may include patients, seniors, students, toddlers, prisoners, restaurant patrons, and attendees at catered events (all known as clients in this book).

The CBDM (Certifying Board for Dietary Managers) has a formal policy, the Code of Ethics for CDM, CFPPs, and procedures which incorporate due process for discipline. Code of Ethics reflect the ethical principles guiding the CDM, CFPP in their professional practice and conduct. This will be discussed in detail in Chapter 16.

Summary

There are many different foodservice operations. As new trends emerge, the style of meal delivery service and menu you provide to your clients may be modified to implement a culture change. Whatever menu or service style you use in your foodservice process, make sure there are adequate policies, staff training, and oversight to be able to provide the quality of service expected. You also need to establish policies for working with clients who choose foods that are contrary to the therapeutic diet that was ordered for them. In addition, a facility needs to implement procedures and provide adequate staffing to assist with person-centered dining. The CDM, CFPP is equipped with information and skills in 10 areas of food services and is instrumental in ensuring the success of the foodservice facility.

GLOSSARY

CDM, CFPP
Certified Dietary Manager, Certified Food Protection Professional (CDM, CFPP) has achieved defined competencies in 5 key areas:
- Nutrition
- Foodservice
- Personnel & Communication
- Sanitation & Safety
- Business Operations

Figure 1.9
Examples of Food Substitutions*

FOOD ITEM	FOOD CHOICES	VITAMIN A CONTENT (per 1/2 cup serving)	VITAMIN C CONTENT (per 1/2 cup serving)
Dark Green Vegetables	Asparagus, boiled	905 IU	7 mg
	Broccoli, frozen, boiled	1,208 IU	50 mg
	Brussels sprouts, frozen, boiled	1435 IU	70 mg
	Green beans, canned	54 IU	8 mg
	Green peppers, boiled	194 IU	28 mg
	Kale (use in soups)	8853 IU	265 mg
	Mixed vegetables, frozen	1944 IU	1.5 mg
	Pea pods, boiled	532 IU	17 mg
	Peas, frozen and boiled	824 IU	38 mg
	Romaine lettuce, 1 cup	2098 IU	1 mg
Bright Orange Vegetables	Carrots, frozen	9094 IU	1.6 mg
	Sweet potatoes, boiled and mashed	1444 IU	8 mg
	Winter squash, baked	793 IU	7 mg
White Vegetables	Cabbage, boiled	60 IU	28 mg
	Cauliflower	7 IU	27 mg
	Celery	226 IU	1.5 mg
	Rutabaga	1.5 IU	16 mg
	Turnips	0 IU	10 mg

Source: U.S. Department of Agriculture—National Nutrient Database for Standard Reference

* Vegetables are often the foods that clients will have an aversion to. Remember that substitutions have to be equivalent in nutritional value, so choose another vegetable(s) that is roughly equivalent to the content of the leader nutrients, vitamin A and vitamin C.

Chapter References

RESOURCES	
Aladdin Temp-Rite®	aladdintemprite.com
Bowman, Carmen (2010). The Food and Dining Side of the Culture Change Movement: Identifying Barriers and Potential Solutions to furthering Innovation in Nursing Homes: https://www.pioneernetwork.net/wp-content/uploads/2016/10/The-Food-and-Dining-Side-of-the-Culture-Change-Movement-Symposium-Background-Paper.pdf	
Carter-Hoffmann®	carter-hoffmann.com
Centers for Medicare & Medicaid Services (CMS)	cms.gov
Dinex®	https://www.carlislefsp.com/heathcare
The Joint Commission	jointcommission.org
World Health Organization (WHO)	who.int

Menus—The Foundation of the Department

Overview and Objectives

The menu is the starting point for many decisions involving purchasing, production, and service of food. You will examine the basics of menu planning and utilize techniques to provide satisfying meals for your clients. You will identify standard food weights and measures related to the meal service and portioning. You will also review both your legal and ethical responsibilities for providing nutritious food to your clients. After completing this chapter, you should be able to:

- Identify factors affecting menu planning
- List resources available for menu planning and development
- Identify how cultures can impact the menu
- Describe how management decisions affect the menu
- Evaluate the quality and accuracy of each meal service

By now, it is clear that a menu is a strong force in achieving client satisfaction. It has been said that the menu drives everything in the kitchen. It is also a means of communicating with clients—and even marketing your fare to future clientele. However, it's more than that; a menu governs the series of events that define the department's overall workflow. Figure 2.1 identifies this process in a simplified format.

As you can see, recipe specifications, the products you need to carry in inventory, production information for the prep staff, and the final food presentation all hinge on the menu plan. In addition, the menu may define the requirements for staffing, equipment, physical layout, and design of the department. Figure 2.1 displays the basic steps in the workflow, starting with menu planning through to meal delivery.

Ultimately, the financial performance of your operation rests heavily on your menu. What it costs to produce and serve meals impacts your expenses. What you sell in cafeterias and retail venues impacts your revenues. In short, the menu is a critical and dominant force in your operation. As such, it merits special attention and careful planning.

As you learned in Chapter 1 there are several styles and types of menus used in Dining Services. Each one is designed to meet the needs of the individual facility. In this chapter, we will focus on the various factors that impact menu planning. We will also learn how menu substitutions and revisions are made after careful monitoring and evaluation.

Figure 2.1
Simple Flow of Work in a Foodservice Operation

Menu Planning Considerations

Whether a menu is written in the facility or purchased from a third party, several points need to be considered to ensure a quality menu is offered to the clients.

Key Points

Customer/Client Satisfaction

The most important consideration in menu planning is satisfying your customers/clients. Chapter 7 will address the many ways to monitor and track customer satisfaction. Audits to evaluate "plate waste," client surveys or "menu scorecards" help identify opportunities for menu edits.

In an effort to improve client satisfaction and meal consumption, many senior living facilities have moved to a more liberalized menu, allowing more options for all modified diets. However, it is still important to include special needs such as cultural factors, food habits, and especially food preferences and diets when planning your menus.

Facilities often use a menu developed by their corporate office or a third party. It is essential to adapt this menu to the needs, wants, and regional preferences of your clients.

Nutritional Considerations

Nutrition considerations should also be a primary goal of menu planning. It is important to maintain adequate nutritional status, to the highest extent possible. There are a number of resources to help; some of those include the **Dietary Guidelines for Americans** (refer to the most current at www.DietaryGuidelines.gov as these guidelines are updated every five years), the USDA DRI (Daily Reference Intakes), MyPlate (www.ChooseMyPlate.gov), facility diet manual, and Recommended Dietary Allowances (RDAs). Note that these resources are updated on a regular basis and the Certified Dietary Manager®, Certified Food Protection Professional® (CDM,®, CFPP®) should look periodically for the most current version. Figure 2.2 lists a number of standards that might be used to evaluate the nutritional content of your menus.

Modified or Restricted Diet Menus

Often in healthcare settings, menus need to be adjusted to meet the dietary restrictions ordered by medical staff. While many menu items will not need to be altered to meet the dietary restrictions, some items may require ingredient changes or elimination from the menu as planned.

Some managers have gone to a "one pot cooking" method for dealing with dietary restrictions. In essence, whatever the identified ingredient is that requires restriction is eliminated from all or most recipes making the recipe work across all diets. Many dining services have adopted a salt-free, fat-free, and even sugar-free menu to allow for a single gravy, vegetable, and entrée to be served to all clients. While this is a quick and simple answer to the problem, it effectively penalizes all clients to the most restrictive of diets.

Most clients do not need to follow all of these restrictions and find the limited palate of meal options unsatisfactory. Keep in mind that client satisfaction may be related to reimbursements and client retention. Often the access to liberalized diets in senior living facilitates allows for the use of a more acceptable variety of foods on the menu.

When the nutrient analysis of a menu dictates an alternate is required for some clients, the use of a modified recipe or totally different item is in order. Planning a menu with alternate items that mix well with the primary base menu (sides or entrées as appropriate) helps control the number of different items that need to be prepared.

> Specific information on nutrition therapy and food restrictions are covered in the *Nutrition Fundamentals and Medical Nutrition Therapy* textbook which accompanies this textbook in many nutrition and foodservice professional training programs.

GLOSSARY

Dietary Guidelines for Americans
Dietary guidelines that encourage Americans to focus on eating a healthful diet that focuses on foods and beverages that contribute to achieving and maintaining a healthy weight, promote health, and prevent disease

Cultural, Regional, and Religious Considerations

Cultural heritage should be a consideration when planning menus as the U.S. encompasses enormous cultural diversity. People's food preferences stem from their own cultural experiences. It is important to look at the population we serve to determine what menu items should be added to meet cultural diversity. While turkey with mashed potatoes and gravy may be widely accepted as a menu choice, other groups may prefer a rice-based dish with chicken due to cultural preference. Holidays, festivals, and important events each have foods associated with them. On Easter Sunday, lamb is served throughout Italy while a roasted pig is a cultural symbol at a Chinese wedding. The significance of these foods is much deeper than their sheer nutritional values.

Traditional Japanese cuisine, for example, is likely to include sushi, tempura and white rice. Indian food would include curries, which are gravy-like sauce or stew-like dishes with meat, vegetables, or cheese. Swedish cuisine may include the traditional meatballs and brown cream sauce while Mexican meals include staples such as tortillas, rice, and refried beans. Creole cooking, popular in Louisiana, blends French, Spanish, and Caribbean influences. Some examples of classic Creole dishes are jambalaya and gumbo. Our menu choices are as rich and complex as our population itself. The following are commonly seen ethnic groups that have migrated into the United States. Please note that this list is not extensive but a sampling.

Figure 2.2
Nutritional Guides or Standards for Menu Planning

NAME OF GUIDE	SOURCE
Centers for Medicare & Medicaid Services	CMS
Corrections Food Guidelines	Association of Correctional Food Service Affiliates
Dietary Guidelines for Americans	Department of Health and Human Services and U.S. Department of Agriculture:
Exchange Lists for Diabetes or Renal Disease	Diabetes Association. National Kidney Foundation
Facility Diet Manual	Check with facility dietitian or state regulations for a current diet manual or complete an online search for "healthcare diet manual" for additional resources
International Dysphagia Diet Standardisation Initiative	
MyPlate	U.S. Department of Agriculture
National Dysphagia Diet	American Speech-Language-Hearing Association. Nutrition411.com
National School Lunch	USDA Food and Nutrition Service. School Nutrition Association
Recommended Dietary Allowances	Nutrition.gov

View the Supplemental Materials for links.

Hispanics/Latinos. Latinos trace their ancestry to Cuba, Mexico, Puerto Rico, or Central and South America. The largest of these is the Mexican-American population, which represents at least two-thirds of all Hispanics/Latinos. Beans and corn in combination are common sources of protein and are frequent ingredients in Hispanic ethnic meals. Some items typical of Latin American cuisine include tortillas, tamales, tacos, pupusas, and arepas. Various salsas and condiments are used with the food such as guacamole, pico de gallo, mole, chimichurri, chilli, and aji. These spices are generally what give the foods their distinct flavor. Desserts in Latin American cuisine are generally very sweet in taste and include dulce de leche, tres leche cake, and flan.

East Indians. Staples of the Indian cuisine include rice, vegetables, lentils, and bread. Diets are varied depending on regions within India. The basic menu in North India is comprised of Indian breads (roti, a round flatbread made of whole wheat flour; and naan, a bread that uses yeast), a chicken or lamb main dish, vegetables and yogurt. South Indian cuisine is more rice and coconut-based. Dosas are savory stuffed pancakes eaten regularly in South India. India's religious beliefs have also influenced the diet of Indians (e.g., Hindus believe that cows are sacred so they do not eat beef). Curry powder, a mixture of spices, is often used to flavor Indian foods. The heart of Indian cooking is the combination of spices that gives each dish its unique flavor.

Chinese. Noodles are a basic staple in China. Chinese noodles are generally made from wheat flour, rice flour, or mung bean starch. Noodles are often served in soup, or stir-fried with meat, eggs, or vegetables. Plain rice is served at all meals. Sometimes fried rice is served. Pork, poultry, and fish are popular and used in small amounts to flavor the rice. Sticky rice is used in specialty Chinese dishes. Foods are often seasoned with soy sauce. Corn oil, sesame oil, and peanut oil are used for cooking. Within Chinese cuisine, different regions have a varied taste such as sweet Cantonese food, spicy Sichuan cuisine, or hot and sour Hunan cuisine. Cow's milk and dairy products are not used often as lactose intolerance is comparatively common in the Asian population.

Japanese. Japanese food is very different from Chinese food. Although the traditional cuisine of Japan is based on rice, it's served with miso soup and other seasonal dishes. While Chinese food is often stir-fried, Japanese food is often simmered, boiled, steamed, or broiled. Seafood is common, often grilled, but also served raw as sashimi or sushi (assorted seafood wrapped in seaweed and rice). Tempura is food deep-fried in vegetable oil after being coated with a batter. Soba, made from buckwheat flour and udon, from wheat flour are two kinds of Japanese noodles. They are served either in a broth or dipped in sauce and are made in many delicious variations.

Mediterranean and Middle Eastern. Whole grains (including barley, bulgur, faro, rice, polenta, couscous, and pastas), fruits, vegetables, legumes, nuts, and seeds make the foundation of the meal. Vegetables are normally cooked or drizzled with olive oil. Cheeses and yogurt are regular selections in a meal. A Greek specialty is baklava, a baked dessert made with nuts, honey, and filo dough. Common cooking styles are grilling, frying, and stewing.

See Figure 2.3 for cultural food influences. Here are more examples of cultural and ethnic food influences.

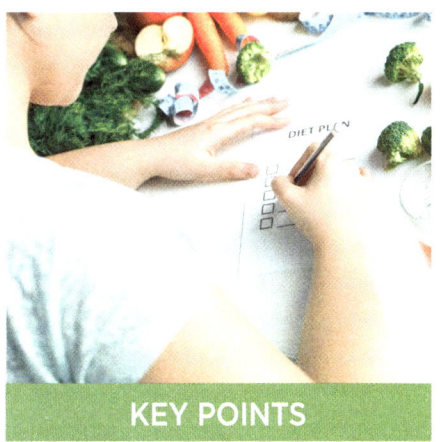

KEY POINTS

Factors Affecting Menu Planning
- Customer Satisfaction
- Cultural, Regional, and Religious Considerations
- Government Regulations
- Aesthetic Appeal
- Management Considerations
- Sustainability Practices

Figure 2.3
Cultural Influences on Food Intake in the U.S.

FOOD GROUP	HISPANIC/LATINO	ASIAN (China, Japan, Korea, Southwest Asia)	MIDDLE EASTERN	EAST INDIAN
Grains	Tortillas (some made with lard) and rice	Rice noodles	Couscous, tahini, pita bread, and filo dough	Rice and whole wheat flatbread (naan)
Vegetables	Cactus, cassava, chayote, jicama, peppers, pinto beans, and tomatoes (salsa)	Garlic, ginger, mung beans, sprouts, bamboo shoots, bok choy, cabbage, and carrots	Tomatoes, olives, lentils, hummus, grape leaves, and eggplant	Red lentils, pigeon peas, legumes, and curries
Fruits	Avocado, bananas, guava, mango, papaya, plantain, and citrus fruits	Mango, banana, citrus fruit, coconut, and pineapple	Dates, figs, and citrus fruits	Coconut, watermelon, and mango
Meats	Chorizo (sausage and other processed meat), goat meat, tongue, and pork	Small amounts of meat, especially fish, eggs, and tofu	Small amounts of lamb, fish, and chicken	Mostly vegetarian—some mutton, chicken, and fish
Dairy	Goat cheese, goat milk, and whole milk	Soy milk	Yogurt and feta cheese	Milk, butter, and yogurt

Note: This is not a complete list of foods. All of these cultures have diets that vary from one region/country to another.

Regional Trends

Part of the cultural heritage unique to the U.S. is the development of regional culinary trends. Often, these trends reflect a mix of native cultures, foods that are grown and harvested in the area, and ethnic traditions contributed by settlers and immigrants over time. For example, New England is known for maple syrup, Boston beans, brown bread, and cranberry muffins. Maine is recognized for lobster. Blueberries are important in New Jersey and in the Midwest, where many are grown. In Pennsylvania and parts of Ohio, the Pennsylvania Dutch heritage gives rise to scrapple (a loaf made from meat scraps, broth, and flour), homemade noodles, and shoofly (molasses) pie.

Vidalia onions are a hallmark of Georgia's cuisine and are the official state vegetable. Peanuts and peaches are also key crops in Georgia. Florida is known for key limes and key lime pie, coquina soup, and other specialties. Kuchen is the official state dessert in South Dakota. Most people associate Idaho with potatoes and New Orleans with Creole cuisine, such as jambalaya, dirty rice, and gumbo. Barbecued meats and pickled okra have special significance in Texas. In the Southwest (Arizona, New Mexico, Oklahoma, Texas), Mexican-style foods such as burritos and tacos are popular. Garlic is so important in California that the town of Gilroy celebrates an annual garlic festival. In fact, food celebrations, such as strawberry harvest festivals, maple syrup festivals, and many others, are key events in all parts of the country.

Religious Practices

Religious beliefs, along with religious customs and rituals, can exert a strong influence on menu planning. Fasting is one practice that many religions observe. The length of time one fasts varies with his/her religion and can range from one day to a month. Some Muslims observe Ramadan, which lasts for one month and fasting occurs from sun up to sun down.

Religious laws will also affect menu planning. For example, the Jewish faith has their own religious beliefs including building kosher kitchens which separate the meat from dairy when cooking. The Islamic faith has guidelines for the sourcing and cooking of halal foods.

Some religious beliefs are specific to the time of child birth and the 6-8 weeks following birth. Many religions and cultures have specific food requirements for their dying loved ones.

Developing a menu has now become more complicated for the Certified Dietary Manager, Certified Food Protection Professional (CDM, CFPP) as they must think about how to include these practices into the process for the facility. Identification of the presence and cultures of various ethnic and religious groups in your local population may require additional research into the food preferences and dietary restrictions of those groups. Ethnic populations may influence large areas of the country, state, or local community.

For example, one-third of all Somalis living in the United States live in Minneapolis, Minnesota. Just 10 miles away in St Paul, you will find the largest single community of Hmong residents in the United States. Both of these cities also share a unique blend of Norwegian, Swedish and Danish heritage along with the significant presence of Native American tribal history. The CDM, CFPP is well-advised to verify the multiple cultures and religions present in their local community and to incorporate the dietary restrictions and food preferences into their menu planning.

Government Regulations

Government regulation is another type of resource that plays a major part in menu planning. These regulations govern the type and quantity of food served at a meal. The Centers for Medicare & Medicaid Services (CMS) is a branch of the U.S. Department of Health and Human Services. CMS is the federal agency that administers the Medicare system and monitors the Medicaid programs offered by each state.

All healthcare facilities have mandatory state licensing requirements. The facility is held to the strictest regulatory requirements, either state or federal. It is important to know and follow local and state regulations. These guidelines are dynamic, meaning they change constantly. Work with your facility administrator to make sure you have the most recent CMS guidelines that impact menu planning.

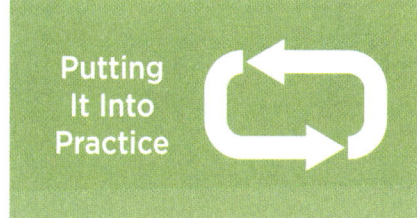

1. As a new CDM, CFPP, you want your menu to address the cultural differences of your customers. What is the first step to implementing cultural changes in your facility?

If you work in a federal or state-funded school system, you will be expected to follow the USDA National School Lunch Program. Critical upgrades were made through the Healthy, Hunger-Free Kids Act of 2010, which provides additional guidelines for school meals. More details on the Nutrition Standards for the National School Lunch Program can be found on the USDA website.

Also work with your school administrator to make sure you have the latest guidelines.

Aesthetic Considerations

Think about this menu: unbreaded baked cod, cauliflower, scalloped potatoes, and vanilla pudding. Everything is white, round, and the meal has strong competing flavors in the fish and cauliflower. This meal is often seen on menus and not widely accepted by clients. While there are times when the flavors and traditions, such as Thanksgiving dinner, warrant a meal of competing flavors, it should not be seen on a regular basis.

Well-written menus not only look at the nutritional balance but also look at the color, texture, mix of strong and mild flavors, and the shape of food on the plate. When the meal looks and tastes good, clients will be more apt to enjoy their food.

One tip would be to prepare the planned menu and take a photo of the plate. This will tell the story around the appearance of the plate and what adjustments may need to be made. Look for all of these characteristics:

- **Color**—Is there a variety and balance?
- **Shape**—Is everything round, linear, wedged?
- **Texture**—Is it diced, chopped, formed, or mushy?
- **Plate Coverage**—Is there a good balance across the plate (too crowded or empty)?
- **Seasoning**—Is there a mix of mild and spicy?
- **Flavor**—Is there bland or mild foods to complement the stronger meats or vegetables?
- **Food Group Balance**—Is there a mix of protein, vegetables, and starches?
- **Consistency**—Is everything in a sauce or gravy?
- **Overall**—Look at the whole meal as served, not just the main plate.
  > The grilled chicken breast with herbed rice and mixed vegetables may look fine until you see the rest of the meal with coleslaw and fruited (fruit cocktail) lemon gelatin, and sugar cookie.
  > Suddenly the whole meal is one color of mostly chopped-up food items.

Sanitation regulations can also play a part in menu planning as they dictate the temperature to which foods must be cooked or reheated prior to service. A beautifully prepared roast beef may have perfect plate presentation when cooked for the time of service. However, the same roast in a cook-chill operation needs to be reheated to a rather well done 160°F prior to service. How quickly food needs to be cooled, the

Photos of the plates and meals assist you in identifying some simple menu standards. It also helps the staff to maintain a consistent plate presentation for the client.

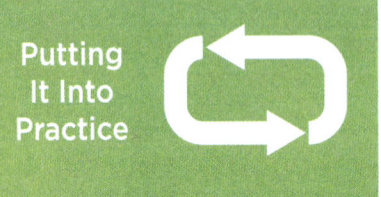

Putting It Into Practice

2. The original menu has baked cod, cauliflower, mashed potatoes, and vanilla pudding. How would you evaluate this aesthetically, and what changes would you make to the menu?

appropriate storage time of cooked and raw foods, and reheating guidelines all affect the safety and often the serving quality of foods.

More will be discussed related to sanitation in Chapter 19. More details on the regulations can be obtained from federal, state, and local agencies.

Management Considerations

Since the menu drives what you do in food production, it also drives your labor and food costs. A number of management-related factors must be considered when menu planning such as the budget, production methods, time and labor available, and finally the equipment and food availability.

- **Budget and Cost:** Next to labor, food cost is the second largest expense for your department and maybe even for the facility. This means managing food cost is a very important part of your job. Many facilities determine their food cost per client, per day and your budget is allocated accordingly. Whether your menu uses foods from raw ingredients or pre-prepared food items, both will impact your budget and your menu planning process. Further discussion of this and other budget controls is in Chapter 26.

- **Production, Service, and Delivery Methods:** Your menu needs to coordinate with your type of service. For instance, if you are doing display cooking, a stir-fry would be a great menu item. However, for cafeteria service where food may be held on a steam table, stir-fried items may lose quality and prove a poor choice. If trays are being plated in the kitchen and delivered to individual patients, menus should include items that sit well during the delivery.

- **Timing and Labor:** How long it takes to prepare each menu item is an important consideration. Some menu items are more time-intensive than others. If you include a product that requires intensive preparation, you may need to pair it with a convenience or low-prep item to balance resources. The production schedule dictated by the menu must be realistic.

In addition, you must match your menu to the skills of employees responsible for producing the menu items. Culinary challenges presented to minimally-trained employees can lead to increased costs through the loss of food or time. On the other hand, a facility that has a trained chef can use this resource to incorporate sophisticated techniques and preparation while holding food costs down. Through focused training, a CDM, CFPP can broaden the skills of food production employees so as to incorporate specific menu items that require specialized techniques.

Your foodservice department management team can help with menu planning by using their respective skills. For instance, the CDM, CFPP may provide input into the menu from the perspective of managing production. An Executive Chef can provide expertise on food items and preparation techniques. The Registered Dietitian Nutritionist can provide specific nutrition and therapeutic diet guidelines. The Diet Office Clerk or Serving Line Checker can identify the items that have frequent call backs for a second choice. The Dishroom Attendant can tell you what is returning on the plates uneaten. Each area of the department can contribute to the development of a better menu for the clients.

- **Equipment:** Menu items may require a broad variety of equipment. Consider each proposed menu item in terms of physical layout and equipment. You also have to consider what equipment will be in use at each time throughout the day. You may not have enough oven space if every menu item for a given meal requires the use of the oven. Storage equipment and transport/delivery requirements can be related concerns.

- **Availability of Food:** What ingredients are available for your menu may be impacted by where your facility is located. Consider a rural facility that is 100 miles from a metropolitan center. You won't be able to get an immediate delivery of a special menu item. With the current emphasis on purchasing locally, your menu may reflect the ingredients that are available in your geographic region, such as Idaho potatoes, Washington apples, or Wisconsin cranberries. Weather may also impact what menu items are available. If there is a freeze in Florida, oranges or orange juice might be available but at a price too high for your department budget. The availability of many of your produce items may be affected by weather and you may have to adjust your menu accordingly.

Sustainability

Sustainability concepts are having an increased influence on menu planning considerations. Customers are interested in the food production process and the story behind what they're eating. There are many lenses through which one can look at food options including: local, organic, seasonal, and water-wise. Often these lenses overlap, but sometimes choices need to be made between various options. Sustainable menu planning typically focuses on one or more of the following:

- Use of locally-grown items
- Limited use of processed food
- Use of "in season" foods
- Replacement of meat entrees with vegetarian entrees

The increased use of local produce often means planning menus based on when local produce is "in season." The term "farm to table" broadly refers to food made from locally-sourced ingredients, often natural or organic. The limited use of processed food would mean an increase in preparing products from "scratch." For example, perhaps you pickle your own vegetables, or make your own salad dressings from fresh ingredients. Finally, a focus on vegetarian rather than meat-based entrees also is deemed sustainable because growing vegetables is less harmful to the environment than livestock production. "Meatless Monday" and increased vegetarian options are factored into menus at restaurants and onsite foodservice operations.

Types of Menus

Now that we have looked at all the factors affecting menu planning, let us discuss a few more types of menus. Beyond the regular **cycle menu** that was discussed in Chapter 1, food service operations may also use a **static menu** or a **single-use menu.**

A static menu is one in which the same menu items are offered daily. The static menu has been a characteristic of many restaurants, but onsite foodservices may use them as well. The single-use menu is a, separate menus are often prepared to use for special events, theme meals or holidays. Many times, these meals are designed to help break the monotony of a cycle menu. These menus may evolve out of a client food committee designed to incorporate their input into the meal planning process.

GLOSSARY

Cycle Menu
Different menu items each day of the cycle and then repeats the entire menu

Static Menu
Offers the same items daily

Single-Use Menu
Used only for one event

3. The menu for the dinner at a group home is Baked Lasagna, Garlic Bread, Oven Roasted Brussels Sprouts, and Apple Pie. How would you adjust this menu so it doesn't overload the same equipment? How would you make this menu more sustainable?

Figure 2.4
Sample Special Menu 1 (St. Patrick's Day) for a Hospital Cafe

Appetizers
- Baked Spinach Artichoke Dip with Pita Chips
- Bruschetta with Edamame Pesto

Entrées
- Corned Beef
- Irish Stew

Accompaniments
- Baked Cabbage with Bacon
- Boiled Potatoes and Carrots

Bread
- Irish Soda Bread with Raisins

Desserts
- Crème de Menthe Pie
- Chocolate Zucchini Cake

A la Carte and Table d'Hote Pricing of Menus

An a la carte menu allows clients to select each item they desire for a meal. In a retail setting, each menu item is priced individually. This may be used in campus dining or in schools. It is also common in many employee and visitor dining cafeterias. With the **Table d'hote** menu, a complete meal is provided at a fixed price. A complete meal may include an appetizer, a salad, an entrée, a starch, a vegetable or fruit, a beverage and possibly a dessert.

Standard Weights and Measures

An essential part of menu planning is using standard food weights, measures, and recipes correctly. Within the menu planning process, consideration has to be given to the food being served in terms of quantity on the plate, nutritional value of the foods, and cost controls. Serving sizes are specified in the menu design itself. If a cup of soup is planned as an appetizer, the quantity is significantly less than a bowl of the same soup served as the entrée of the meal.

The Purchasing Supervisor needs to know the serving sizes and number of servings so they order the appropriate amount of raw ingredients. The production team needs to know the serving sizes of items so they prepare the correct amount of food. The serving staff need to know the serving size of each menu item so they can plate the meal correctly. Registered Dietitian Nutritionist, Dietetic Technician, The Registered/ Nutrition and Dietetic Technician, Registered, and/or Certified Dietary Manager, Certified Food Protection Professional need to know the serving sizes to evaluate the client meal intake for dietary intake tracking.

To plan a menu, you and your staff need to know how many servings in a full-size steam table pan, how many servings from a quart when using a disher/portion scoop,

GLOSSARY

À la Carte
Pricing each menu item separately

Table d'hôte
One price for the entire meal

how many tablespoons in a cup, how many servings you can expect from a case of fresh broccoli, etc. One very helpful book that provides these charts for standard weights and measures is *Food for Fifty* by Mary Molt. This reference also contains many quantity recipes that may help you in revising menus to meet your facility/client needs. The need for accurate weights and measures in the recipe and production process are addressed in Chapters 3 and 4 of this textbook.

Menu Substitutions and Alternates/Standard Write-in Menu

Even with liberalization, another issue often arises—the need for substitutions on the menu. A substitution is a product that replaces a planned menu item when requested by a client or family member because he/she does not like or refuses to eat the food being served. Centers for Medicare & Medicaid Services (CMS) regulations specify that requests for substitutions should be permitted and honored, as long as they are reasonable and achievable. A substitution must be of similar nutritive value. On a selective menu, some CDM, CFPPs use the term menu write-in to describe the same idea. A client may write an item on the menu that was not part of the planned cycle.

Providing substitutions upon request is part of the concept of giving clients control over their care; meal choice is considered a client right. Adjusting offerings to a client's requests helps to ensure optimal nutritional intake. In all, honoring substitution requests contributes to quality of life, especially for nursing facility clients.

What should a CDM, CFPP do with a substitution request? The answer is, honor it or provide an alternate choice. While some choices are not feasible, many options may exist. For a long-term client, a CDM, CFPP may be able to accommodate a special request. Sound management and practical realities dictate that the substitution process be planned and organized as part of the menu.

One way to provide substitutions is simply to offer alternate choices on a menu or in the service setting itself. This eliminates many of the challenges of providing substitutions at the last minute. It is one reason that some long-term care facilities have changed to selective menus. On a selective menu, clients can choose their substitutions or alternates in advance of service, and dining services staff can tally requirements in time for production.

With the goal of honoring client requests, a CDM, CFPP may also develop a list of "Always Available" write-in requests that can be accommodated in the kitchen. The manager can plan production of these items in conjunction with routine meal service or is at least prepared to honor these requests efficiently. Some write-in list offerings may cross over with items prepared daily for another service area, such as a cafeteria. Essentially, this write-in list becomes its own supplementary menu. Designated staff may refer to this menu to guide clients towards practical substitutions.

Special Diets in Long-Term Care

Nursing homes are beginning to use the **International Dysphagia Diet Standardisation Initiative (IDDSI)** as the foundation for texture modified foods and thickened drinks provided to residents. The use of global, standardized terminology and definitions for texture modified foods and thickened drinks help improve the safety and care of residents with dysphagia by helping staff communicate individual resident needs to interdisciplinary teams. Figure 2.5 shows the IDDSI Framework which consists of a continuum of 8 levels (0-7), where drinks are measured from Levels

GLOSSARY

IDDSI
The International Dysphagia Diet Standardisation Initiative is a standardized framework for labeling texture-modified foods and thickened liquids.

Figure 2.5
IDDSI Framework

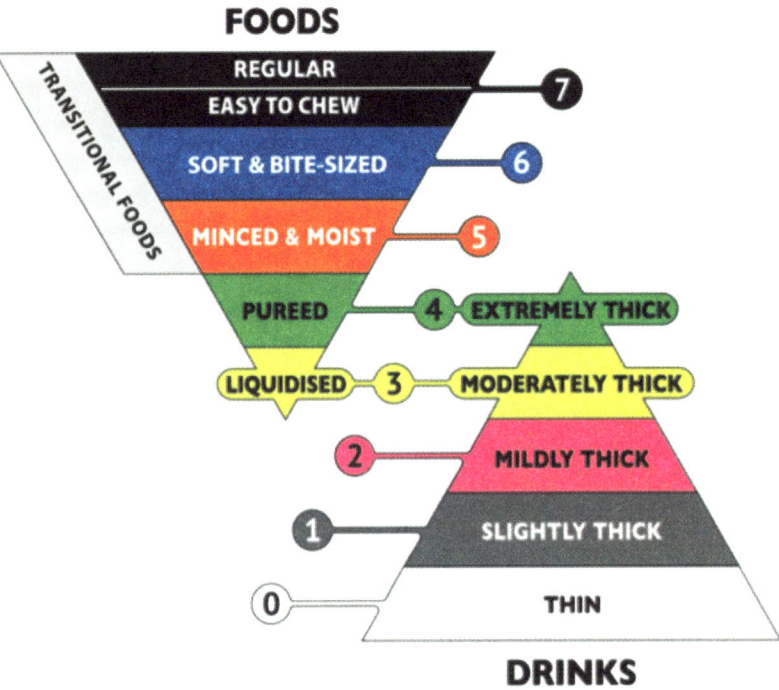

Copyright: The International Dysphagia Diet Standardisation Initiative 2016
@ https://iddsi.org/framework/

View the Supplemental Material for this chapter for more information and resources on IDDSI.

0 – 4, while foods are measured from Levels 3 – 7. The IDDSI Framework provides a common terminology to describe food textures and drink thickness. See Supplemental Material for more IDDSI resources.

Monitoring the Menu and Meal Service

The best meal service starts with a well-planned menu and finishes with a well-trained staff. No matter how well-designed the menu is, staff competencies and performance determine the final presentation of the meal to the client. During the meal service there are several steps that require monitoring.

- Testing of the recipes for product performance and palatability is only the beginning.
- Training of the production team on the techniques required to make the menu items and the use of standardized recipes (discussed in detail in Chapter 3) starts the meal service.
- In addition to the standardized recipes, the use of ingredient pull lists and production sheets with appropriate panning charts ensures the right items come to the serving line in the correct serving pans.
- Specification of portion sizes and serving utensils helps standardize the portion control.
- Pre-line meetings to taste the food and sample plate demonstrated the correct plating of the meal for consistency and presentation, and allows for any corrections to be made prior to the time of service.

- Documented pre-line temperature logs ensure that food is reaching the serving line at the appropriate temperature. It allows for any corrections to be made prior to the time of service; this is for both HOT and COLD food (milk sitting at room temperature during a one hour serving line will be close to room temp by the end of the line).
- Monitor the start and stop times of the meal service, and the time needed to deliver the meals (longer delays cause greater temperature loss).
  > If the serving line is stopping for re-supply of items, either:
    - your production numbers were not correct—or they didn't make the amount specified;
    - the serving size on the line is over-portioned and they are running out;
    - the production team is not keeping up with the batch cooking; or
    - the production team is not focused on their primary task—serving the clients.
- Check random trays for accuracy to the items specified on the menu and compliance with all diet restrictions and allergies.
- Assess the trays for plate presentation, attractiveness, and placement of the items on the tray or table setting.
- Check the mid-line temperature of the food being served—are appropriate temperatures being maintained?
- Monitor the number and frequency of call-backs for a second meal selection.
- Record the over production and run-out/shorts for the line.
  > Why were the production numbers wrong (over or short)?
  > What did you substitute for the products you were short?
- Observe the dishroom after the meal for what is coming back on the plate.
- Conduct meal rounds in the dining rooms talking with the clients or in the patient/resident rooms during the meal service times.
- Conduct test trays/meals.
  > Sample the food as a complete meal at the point of service in the dining room or in a patient/resident room.
    - Take temperatures.
    - Taste the food.
    - Ask nursing and support staff to participate in the test trays.

Information is your friend. Know what you expect and verify the level of service you are providing.

4. You are monitoring the trayline service of your hospital food service. What are some steps you would take to ensure accuracy of the meal service?

Menu Revision

In the foodservice industry, most experts agree that a menu should not become static. For both ongoing and occasional clients, periodic revisions are a necessity. Here are some events that might signal a need for menu revision:

- **Client Feedback.** Client suggestions, along with information gathered through surveys, often begin to show patterns. A suggestion that arises repeatedly—or a complaint about a particular menu—can be triggers for revision.
- **Seasonal Change.** People choose different foods at different times of the year. Summer foods may include salads, chilled entrées, and produce in peak season. Winter foods (where winters are cold) may include more soups, stews, and seasonally available produce.
- **Trends and Fashions.** Ever-changing, the world of food experiences culinary innovations as well as trends. Keeping pace with these helps a facility compete in the industry. For instance: edamame was not well known 20 years ago; today it is a common restaurant menu option.
- **Special Requests.** A CDM, CFPP may monitor items that clients request or add to their own menus. If a request appears repeatedly, it may be time to add the item to the menu or increase its frequency.
- **Sales Records.** If you are monitoring sales records or selection data for the menu, you may discover that certain items are proving unpopular. One of the jobs of a CDM, CFPP is to identify menu "duds" and replace them with products clients prefer.
- **Quality Issues.** Similarly, a CDM, CFPP conducting routine quality checks may determine that a certain item is not holding up well on the menu. There may be a solution. Changing the procedure or the recipe, using different techniques or equipment, or training staff may make a difference. If not, the item may need to be replaced.
- **Changes in the Physical Facility.** Remodeling, renovations, or reallocation of space in a facility may impose changes on the foodservice department. Perhaps the opportunity exists to build an expanded cafeteria. A CDM, CFPP may explore a food court concept and its related menu implications. Or a facility may have an opportunity to build a group dining area, where buffet service is an option. The menu needs to change accordingly.
- **Service Revisions.** Sometimes a CDM, CFPP faces the need to develop new services or serve new clients. In addition, mergers and acquisitions may present new requirements to serve remote facilities. Integrating service changes with existing schemes may provide cause for re-evaluation of the menu as a whole and all related coordination issues.

A proposed menu revision should undergo evaluation for any nutrient standards that apply, as well as for costs. In addition, any menu revision creates ripple effects through the operational flow. To implement a change, systematically examine and plan related revisions required in staffing, service, delivery, inventory, purchasing, and food production.

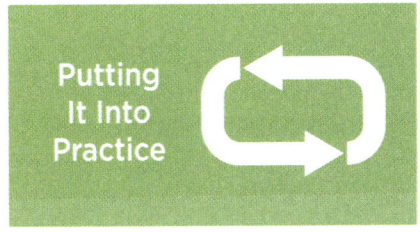

5. As a Certified Dietary Manager, Certified Food Protection Professional you have been asked to evaluate and make necessary changes to the existing menu. What tools would you use for evaluation and revision?

In all, you can see that a menu has great impact on every aspect of the foodservice operation. Designing a menu that meets your clients' needs and expectations and uses your resources effectively is an enormous amount of work. However, the rewards are well worth the effort.

Tailoring Individual Menus—Honoring Legal and Ethical Responsibilities

Every healthcare menu system must have a method for ensuring that every client receives a meal, even if selections have not been made. Clients who do not complete a selective menu receive a house diet or default selection. For a client whose preferences are known, a member of the clinical staff may complete a menu based on care plan or client preference record. This information may be tracked in a diet office software system.

Furthermore, every menu communications system must include control steps to ensure that foods planned for the individual menu meet the current diet order prescribed by the physician. Whether menus are selective or non-selective, spoken or paper-based, or implemented through trayline or buffet service, trained foodservice staff must assist with individual menu review before a client consumes the meal. Figure 2.6 lists some of the criteria for menu review.

Reviewing menus can be time consuming. CDM, CFPPs can structure menu systems to minimize this. For example, there are computer programs to review menu choices in order to check for compliance, calculate totals for restricted nutrients (such as sodium, protein, or fluid), eliminate allergenic foods, or automate routine food additions. This process requires that staff maintain a computerized set of care plans or client preference records.

Figure 2.6
Criteria for Individual Menu Review (Health Care)

Before a client receives a tray and consumes a meal, trained foodservice staff must review individual menus and answer the following questions:

1. Do the selections provide a well-balanced meal, or has the client selected choices from nearly all categories (e.g., entrée, vegetable, starch, beverage, etc.)?
2. If the client's diet order specifies combined modifications, such as sodium-restricted and carbohydrate-controlled, are selections compliant with these restrictions?
3. If the client has a meal pattern or a carbohydrate count, how do the totals compare to the plan?
4. If the client has a fluid restriction, how do the figures add up?
5. If the diet order or kardex lists specific foods to avoid (e.g., allergies or food intolerances), have these items been removed from the menu?
6. Are appropriate condiments included (e.g., margarine for bread, dressing for salad, etc.)?
7. If texture modifications (e.g., mechanical soft diet or National Dysphagia Diet levels) are part of the diet order, does each menu selection comply with the order?
8. Are portion sizes indicated on the menu appropriate for this particular diet order?
9. If the client has requested a substitution, is the request honored?
10. If the diet order or kardex lists specific additions for meals (e.g., nutrition supplements), are these items included?

When a foodservice staff member makes adjustments to a menu, communicating this with the client is important:

- If the client does not know the menu has been adjusted intentionally, the revisions may be perceived as an error.
- Menu review provides an opportunity for a dining services staff member to explain a meal pattern or other adjustment.
- Discussing adjustments opens a dialogue with the client about diet-related needs and preferences.

It is the responsibility of the department director, dining services staff, and CDM, CFPP to provide nutritionally adequate meals to clients. Sometimes there are specific requirements for patients, residents, and school food service or one of customer choice. Planning a menu that meets the needs of both groups in a cost-effective and efficient manner is the goal of every manager.

Chapter References

RESOURCES	
Centers for Medicare & Medicaid Services (CMS)	cms.gov
Dietary Guidelines for Americans 2015-2020	https://health.gov/dietaryguidelines/2015/guidelines/
Food for Fifty	Molt, Mary, Pearson Education, Inc.
Gregoire, Mary (2013). Foodservice Organizations, A managerial and systems approach, 8th ed. Upper Saddle River, NJ: Pearson Prentice Hall	
IDDSI Framework	https://iddsi.org/
Kotschevar, L..H (2008). Management by menu, 4th ed. Hoboken, NJ: John Wiley & Sons	
MyPlate	Choosemyplate.gov
Nutrition Standards for School Meals	https://www.fns.usda.gov/school-meals/nutrition-standards-school-meals
USDA Food and Nutrition Information	https://www.nal.usda.gov/fnic

Prepare Standardized Recipes for Food Production

Overview and Objectives

Even if you work in a corporate-owned facility where menus and recipes are pre-determined, it's important to be able to create and use standardized recipes. A standardized recipe is an essential tool in controlling costs in food service. It is a recipe for managing and controlling many aspects of the foodservice operation. After completing this chapter, you should be able to:

- Identify the different elements of a standardized recipe
- Explain the importance of a standardized recipe as a management tool
- Compute proper portions and measurements using appropriate food charts/references
- List the steps in developing a standardized recipe
- Understand product yields to effectively cost recipes and meals
- Elaborate on the use of standardized recipes in requisitions, portion control, and food allergies
- Evaluate client acceptance of new recipes

A menu serves as a master plan for the food you serve. From the menu, a Certified Dietary Manager®, Certified Food Protection Professional® (CDM®, CFPP®) uses and develops recipes. A standardized recipe is the ultimate formula for the control of food. Each recipe has an effect on quality, cost control, and client satisfaction. A standardized recipe ensures consistency in quality, yield, nutritional value, the time required to prepare it, and staffing requirements. It is a fundamental and essential tool in the foodservice department.

A Standardized Recipe: The Ultimate Formula

A recipe is a formula for preparing a menu item. As such, it plays a strong role in control of your operation. It tells what ingredients to include and in what amounts. It tells how to prepare, portion, and present the food. It specifies what equipment and techniques to use. It controls what nutrients you will be serving clients.

If you are making something as simple as gelatin, the amount of water added to the flavored powder makes all the difference in final quality. For a homemade minestrone soup, think about the seasonings included. Too much or too little can make the product unacceptable. Preparation procedures affect quality, too. For example, a prime fillet of fish will not turn out well if your procedure calls for baking it too long. Or, a stir-fry recipe will not turn out well if your procedure has you simmer the crisp vegetables in sauce for an extended period. In fact, the accuracy of a recipe, the procedures it defines, and even the ingredients it requires all affect final food quality. If you make changes to the recipe, you have to evaluate the quality of the final product, and exercise good judgment.

A **standardized recipe** is a set of written instructions used to consistently prepare a known quantity and quality of food for a specific location. A standardized recipe will produce a product that is close to identical in taste and yield every time it is made, no matter who follows the directions. A standardized recipe tells exactly how much of each ingredient to use, how to add ingredients and in what sequence, and what procedures to use in producing the item. The use of standardized recipes helps all staff to maintain a consistent quality product regardless of who is cooking. This can be a great advantage, particularly in situations where a minimally trained employee may need to produce food or numerous employees may rotate through an assignment.

Quality. The result of using a standardized recipe is that you can produce a product that is consistent in quality, appearance, and tastes the same. Clients notice this consistency, particularly if you have long-term clients, you can count on certain expectations. A client who enjoyed the banana bread last week expects to enjoy the same product again this week, and may be disappointed if it turns out differently.

Yield. A standardized recipe is consistent in **yield** and number of servings at a given portion size. A recipe for 100 servings always yields 100 servings. This is critical in ensuring you have enough food ready for service at any given time. You need to be able to tell a cook how much food to make—and how much of each ingredient to include to ensure this happens.

Nutritional Value. A standardized recipe is also consistent in nutritional value. A serving that contains 8 grams of protein this week will contain 8 grams of protein again next week. In most non-commercial foodservice situations, you are responsible for assuring nutritional consistency. If you are complying with specific nutritional guidelines, standardized recipes become the formula for reliable nutrition. If you are

---

GLOSSARY

Standardized Recipe
A recipe that contains detailed specifications, and has been adapted and tested in your own operation

Yield
The number of servings a recipe will produce at a given portion size

not, you may still be marketing nutritional aspects of your products to clients. For example, the low-fat fare in a business dining setting needs to be reliably low in fat.

Time. In addition, a standardized recipe is consistent in time required for preparation. If it takes 75 minutes to prepare, you can generally count on that time and schedule the product to be ready for service. It is consistent in its labor requirements as well. This time-and-labor aspect of standardization is critical for devising effective employee schedules, and for assuring timeliness of service.

Cost. A standardized recipe is developed with specific amounts of ingredients and a given yield of servings. Because of this factor, you can use a standardized recipe to cost out your menus. What if employees choose not to follow a standardized recipe by increasing ingredient amounts or serving larger portion sizes and the cost has been figured into your department budget? You will be over budget, so making a standardized recipe work requires attention to the human factor as well.

It is important to note that a recipe out of a cookbook does not qualify as a standardized recipe. Why? Because the equipment may vary, cook's interpretation of "cook until done" or "add seasonings to taste" may vary, and the portion utensils and ingredients availability may vary. Each recipe needs to be standardized to your food preparation kitchen and staff.

The bottom line is that standardization allows you to manage the operation effectively. You want to be able to predict the inventory needed for food preparation, quantify purchasing needs, and have ingredients on hand in time for production. You can predict and control expenses in your operation through standardized recipes. You can also predict staffing needs, and prepare an employee schedule far in advance. You need to plan exactly how much food to produce for each meal in order to feed all clients. For each of these tasks, standardization provides a useful planning tool. From the recipes, you know what you will need and can exercise strong management of the entire process.

Components of a Standardized Recipe

Now that you understand the concept of a standardized recipe, let's examine the details that define its consistency. An example of a standardized recipe appears in Figure 3.1. As you can see, the standardized recipe contains some key elements. These are described below.

Title. Each recipe must have its own unique title or name. The title in Figure 3.1 is *Turkey Burrito Bowl*. While the need for recipe names may seem obvious, in operational practice, confusion actually can occur without attention to this detail. Let's say that you have two types of beef stew. One uses traditional carrots and potatoes, while another uses leeks and peas. You will need to distinguish these clearly from each other to avoid production errors. For clients, too, unique names make it easier to distinguish one menu item from another.

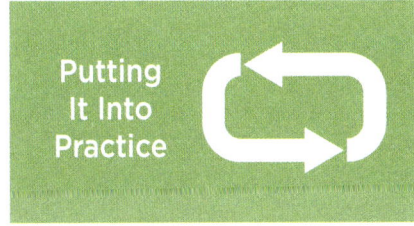

1. As a Certified Dietary Manager, Certified Food Protection Professional (CDM, CFPP) you see the need to standardize all the recipes in your foodservice operation, but the rest of the team thinks it's unnecessary. What advantages would you cite to justify the need for standardization?

Figure 3.1
Standardized Recipe Example

Recipe Title: Turkey Burrito Bowl | **Recipe Category:** Entrée | **Portion Size:** 1 Bowl

RECIPE YIELD
100 SERVINGS

INGREDIENTS	Weight	Measure	DIRECTIONS/HACCP
• Rice, brown, whole grain • Turkey pot roast (CN labeled) • Cheddar cheese, shredded • Beans, black • Romaine lettuce, fresh, untrimmed • Chili powder • Cumin, ground • Garlic, granulated • Oregano, ground	25 cups 15 lbs. + 10 oz. 3 lbs. 4 #10 Cans 1 lb.	 2 cups 1/2 cup 1/4 cup 1/4 cup	**Critical Control Point (CCP):** Before handling ready-to-eat foods, such as fresh fruits and vegetables, hands must be washed and clean gloves must be worn. 1. Prepare rice according to instructions. 2. Remove thawed turkey from the bag and divide it equally in 2" pans. Break apart with a fork. 3. Add the chili powder, cumin, garlic, and oregano. Mix to combine. 4. Cook the turkey at 350°F for 30 minutes or until it reaches an internal temperature of 135°F as measured by a meat thermometer. **CCP:** Heat to 135°F or higher. 5. Remove beans from cans, drain, and rinse. Heat or steam the beans until they reach 135°F as measured by a thermometer. **CCP:** Hold for hot service at 135°F or higher. 6. Assemble for service. Scoop 1 cup cooked rice into the bowl. Add 1/4 cup beans (#16 scoop), 1/2 cup turkey, and 1/8 cup of cheese.

MEAL PATTERN CONTRIBUTION

Meat/Meat Alternate	Grains	Vegetable/Vegetable Subgroup	Fruit
2 oz.	2 oz.	1/4 cup beans/peas (legumes)	0

NUTRIENT ANALYSIS

Calories: 405	Saturated Fat: 1.5 g	Sodium: 900 mg

STANDARDIZED RECIPE COMPONENTS

Recipe Title: Name that describes the recipe

Recipe Category: File location or classification such as an entree, side, or grain

Recipe Number: Optional

Ingredients: Products used in the recipe, be specific

Ingredient Amounts: The quantity of each ingredient listed in weight and/or measure

Directions: Detailed information needed to prepare the recipe and equipment needed. Cooking temperatures, HACCP process, HACCP procedures, cooking, cooling, and holding temperatures should be addressed in the directions

Portion Size: The amount of a single portion in volume and/or weight

Recipe Yield: The total amount of portions the recipe yields

Meal Pattern Contribution: (Optional) Identify the component and the amount the recipe contributes toward the meal pattern

Nutrients per Serving: (Optional) Amount of calories, saturated fat, and sodium per serving

Source: Adapted from Colorado Department of Education

Category. Most facilities use a category designation to help keep recipes organized. Figure 3.2 provides some examples of category designations for recipes. Using categories helps you assign recipe production to the intended staff members. It also helps you group recipes for production on any given day. It helps you locate recipes for special menus as needed. If you use a computerized recipe system, categories help you use search features to find recipes. There is no right or wrong way to develop categories for your own operation. Categorization is simply a logical grouping that is useful to you.

Recipe Number. As you adopt recipes into your own facility, you will probably assign a recipe number to each as an additional way of identifying and controlling your bank of recipes. A computerized system typically requires a recipe number as a way of ensuring a unique identity for each recipe in the database. Some operations use numbering systems that relate to the categories. For example, a series of recipes beginning with 5000 may represent quick breads and muffins. A cinnamon muffin recipe may be number 5001. An apple walnut quick bread recipe may be number 5026 and so forth.

Total Yield. A yield is the number of servings or portions a recipe will produce. Yield is closely related to portion size. Sometimes yield is shown as the total volume of the batch, such as 4 gallons or 7.5 pounds.

Portion Size. This specifies what size each portion will be. It is expressed as a measurement. In the example shown in Figure 3.1, the recipe yields 100 servings of 3/4 cups each. Note that the same recipe would alternately yield 50 servings of 1-1/2 cups each. Thus, it's important to specify portion size in every recipe. Otherwise, the yield becomes meaningless.

Portion sizes occasionally vary for use in different menus. For example, if a soup is an appetizer on a dinner menu, it may be used as a 3/4 cup portion. However, when it is featured as a main lunch entrée, the larger portion may be more appropriate. Traditionally, a "cup" of soup is 3/4 cup and a "bowl" of soup is 1 cup.

Ingredient List. A standardized recipe specifies each ingredient. As with recipe naming, ingredient naming is a task that must always be tackled with precision. For instance, if you use flour in your operation, you need to be sure the names of various types are clearly distinguished. You may have all-purpose flour, self-rising flour, pre-sifted flour, whole wheat flour, cake flour, bread flour, and/or others. The success of a recipe for baked goods will depend on your cook selecting the proper ingredient. Very simply, a clear and precise name for the ingredient, used consistently, helps to make

KEY POINTS

Key elements in a Standardized Recipe include:
- Title
- Category
- Yield
- Batch Quantity
- Portion Size
- Ingredients
- Weights or Measures
- Food Safety Information
- HACCP
- Directions or Procedure
- Nutrition Information
- Recipe Sources

Figure 3.2
Sample Categories for Recipes

STARTERS	ENTREES	SIDES	HOT VEGETABLES	BREADS	DESSERTS
• Soups • Appetizers	• Beef • Pork • Poultry • Seafood • Vegetarian • Salads • Puréed	• Side Salads • Salad Dressings • Rice and Pasta Sides	• Potatoes • Other	• Quick Breads and Muffins • Yeast Breads and Rolls	• Cakes • Cookies • Pies • Fruit • Other

this happen. Computerized systems use ingredient numbers along with names to track, distinguish, and describe ingredients.

Typically, a recipe for quantity food production shows all ingredients in the order in which they are added. It is essential that every ingredient used in a recipe appear on the ingredient list. The list itself may serve as a tool for cooks in organizing their work. A common procedure is to measure each ingredient and have it ready before beginning production. The ingredient list in each recipe forms a basis for evaluating purchasing needs. An item that misses the list may not be purchased, and may not be available when needed. So, oversights in the ingredient list can lead to unnecessary work and error, and thoroughness is worth the effort.

Weights or Measures. An essential control in food production is measurement of ingredients. For most operations, three basic options present themselves. One is to measure ingredients by volume. Another is to measure by weight. Another, only feasible with certain ingredients, is to measure by count, or by "each." Figure 3.3 gives examples of measurements. It is more accurate to weigh large amounts of dry ingredients and more cost effective.

Some foodservice operations control ingredients by using an ingredient room. An ingredient room is a unique location where an assigned employee measures ingredients for all recipes, packages them, and labels them. Pre-measured ingredients are then distributed to assigned preparation staff. The ingredient room concept imposes several forms of control in the kitchen.

First of all, it ensures that ingredients are carefully measured by someone with specialized focus on measurement. This can support consistent yields and adherence to the measurements required for standardized recipes. Secondly, an ingredient room allows managers to limit access to food storage areas, which may be kept locked. This prevents pilferage or theft in a foodservice operation. Beyond these benefits, an ingredient room allows cooks to work very efficiently during the production process. In an ingredient room model, it is very common for all ingredients to be weighed.

Food Safety Information. To support a food safety system, many CDM, CFPPs also provide sanitation-related information on recipes. In a proactive system for managing food safety called **HACCP (Hazard Analysis Critical Control Point)**, a particular

> **GLOSSARY**
>
> **Hazard Analysis Critical Control Point (HACCP)**
> A proactive system for managing food safety in which a particular step of the recipe may be identified as being critical for ensuring food safety

Figure 3.3
Examples of Weights and Measures for Ingredients

BY WEIGHT	BY VOLUME	BY COUNT
• 3.5 lbs. of all-purpose flour	• 9 qts. of all-purpose flour	• 11 fresh, white onions
• 2 oz. iodized salt	• 3/4 cup baking powder	• 3 lemons
• 2.5 lbs. sugar	• 2 Tbsp. ground sage	• 45 bananas
• 12 lbs. turkey roast	• 1-3/4 cups skim milk	• 7 cloves of garlic
• 6.5 lbs. crushed pineapple	• 3 cups margarine	• 3, #10 cans of tomato sauce
• 1 oz. cinnamon		
• 12 lbs. raw apples		
• 5.5 lbs. chopped, fresh white onions		
• 8 lbs. margarine		

step of the recipe may be identified as being critical for ensuring food safety. This step is called a **critical control point (CCP)**. The CCP may be noted on the recipe for reference and use by food preparation employees. The Hazard Analysis Critical Control Point system is also a component of the standardized recipe. Inclusion of safe food handling steps within the recipe helps ensure staff have appropriate guidelines on how to handle at risk ingredients and final cooking temperatures.

Directions or Procedure. Detail and clarity in the directions for preparing a recipe help make it reproducible from one employee to the next. Steps for preparation must be presented in a logical sequence. Specific directions for the order of operations and types of operations are an important part of a standardized recipe. Understanding when to use the term blend versus fold, mix or sauté is essential. Include cooking temperatures and times in the directions to ensure the dish is cooked properly and safely.

Pan Size. Many types of recipes include specifications for a pan size. A cake, for example, may use a 12" x 20" x 2" pan. Instructions for employees should indicate how to portion a pan (e.g., cut 8 x 10), or cut a pie (e.g., 6 slices). The pan specification may also relate to a layout for a steam table. Then, it is especially important that the cook use the right pan, so it will fit the layout. See Figure 3.4 for pan and portion sizes.

Batch Unit. Sometimes called unit of production, this figure tells what the batch size is for the recipe. Batch unit may not appear on all recipes, but is sometimes critical. Often the quantity produced by a recipe does not match the yield you need. So, the recipe has to be scaled.

Scaling. Adjusting the recipe ingredients upward or downward to generate specific yields is called scaling. Other terms for this are extending or factoring the recipe. When you scale recipes, you often have to recognize batch units. Consider this example:

You are making apple pies. Each apple pie yields 6 servings, with a portion of 1/6 of a pie. You need to serve pie to 221 people. To determine how many pies you will need, divide 211 by 6, which gives you 35.17. Since you cannot make a fraction of a pie, you have to round this up to make 36 pies. In portions, this is a yield of 216, or 5 more servings than what you need.

A batch unit may be important for a meatloaf, cake, quick bread, roast, or other products that are conducive to serving groups. When and how you round yields up depends on the batch unit. If you are preparing chili, stew, or soups, and you need 6.1 batches, consider rounding down. You would over-produce too much if you rounded up.

Seasonings (such as salt and sugar) do not always scale up and down as easily as flour or ground beef. Therefore, it's important to test scaled recipes prior to putting them into everyday production.

For some products, the batch unit is irrelevant, because you can scale the recipe into batches of single servings. Examples include sandwiches, individual cold plates, and most single serving entrée items such as chicken pieces and hamburgers.

Nutrition Information. This has become an expected component of a standardized recipe. Clients are asking for information about protein, calories, sodium, and fat content. Identifying the nutritional benefits of menu items, such as "A good source of Vitamin A," helps clients make better choices in their food selections. Posting of nutritional content is being required for multi-unit chain restaurants, and as part of the "nutrition labeling" of pre-packaged and commercially packed food products.

> **GLOSSARY**
>
> **Critical Control Point (CCP)**
> This step is called a critical control point (CCP) and may be noted on the recipe for reference and use by food preparation employees
>
> **Scaling**
> Adjusting standardized recipes upward or downward to provide specific yields

Figure 3.4
Pan and Portion Chart

PAN SIZE	PAN DEPTH	PAN CAPACITY		SIZE OF PORTION		# OF PORTIONS YIELDED*
		Quarts	Cups	Cup	Scoop #	
Full Size 12" x 20"	2-1/4"	7-1/2	30	1/4	18	120
				1/3	12	90
				3/8	10	80
				1/2	8	60
	4"	13	52	1/4	16	206
				1/3	12	156
				3/8	10	138
				1/2	8	104
	6"	19-1/2	78	1/4	16	312
				1/3	12	234
				3/8	10	208
				1/2	8	156
				1	6 oz. ladle	78
Half Size 12" x 10"	2-1/2"	3-3/4	15	1/4	16	60
				1/3	12	45
				3/8	10	40
				1/2	8	30
	4"	6-1/2	26	1/4	16	104
				1/3	12	78
				3/8	10	69
				1/2	8	52
	6"	9-3/4	39	1/4	16	156
				1/3	12	117
				3/8	10	104
				1/2	8	78
				1	8 oz. ladle	39
Third Size 12" x 6-7/8"	2-1/2"	2-2/5	9-3/5	1/8	2 Tbsp.	76
				1/4	16	38
				1/3	12	28
				3/8	10	25
	4"	3-7/8	15-1/2	1/8	2 Tbsp.	124
				1/4	16	62
				1/3	12	46
				3/8	10	41

Adapted from The Foodservice Tune Up by Wayne Toczek, Innovations Services, and Tim Bauman.
* Rounded down to lower portion

When nutrition labeling is not readily available for a product, you may need to calculate the nutrition content based on the ingredients and scaling the quantity of each ingredient within a recipe. We used to rely on books available with tables of nutritional composition such as Bowes and Church's *Food Values of Portions Commonly Used* or the USDA National Nutrient Database. However, looking up individual ingredients, or even ready-to-eat foods, in a printed book format is cumbersome and time-consuming.

Access to the internet or a computerized database of nutritional analysis can make the process much faster and more accurate. The USDA database is available online with thousands of items and detailed nutrient content.

Several commercially available nutrition analysis software programs are used by clinical Registered Dietitian Nutritionists to calculate the nutrient intake of their clients. Access to one of these nutrient analysis tools would make the calculations easier. Likewise, often food distributors offer recipes online that include the nutritional analysis.

The most effective means of determining the nutrient content of a recipe, or a complete menu, is to access the information via a computerized recipe program. In a full-service recipe module, you can edit the ingredients and add items to the recipe. The program will recalculate the nutritional content for the recipe, the meal, or even the entire day's menu based on your edits.

Recipe Sources. Generally, CDM, CFPPs strive to find recipes specifically developed for quantity production. This is primarily a time-saver. Adapting a home recipe to large-scale production has some pitfalls and requires a fair amount of effort. A practical question to ask as you evaluate new recipes is: Has this been refined for quantity production? Even if you have a corporate office providing your recipes, you will want to address the following questions:

- What does this recipe cost per serving?
- What is the labor cost for producing this recipe?
- Do we have the proper equipment to produce it well?
- Do we have the match of skills required to produce a high-quality product?
- How does this recipe meet the nutritional requirements of our menus and recipes?
- How does this recipe fit the tastes, preferences, and needs of our clients?

Computerized Menus and Recipe Management Systems

Computerized menu systems are designed to accomplish a wide variety of tasks, from managing the patient/resident diet orders to standardizing the recipes used to meet those dietary restrictions. The interplay between the menu and the recipes is a little like which came first, the chicken or the egg.

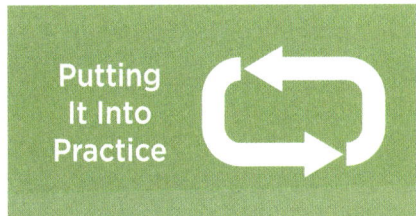

2. Your macaroni and cheese recipe calls for a full size 4" deep pan. Using Figure 3.4, if each person gets a #8 scoop serving, how many portions would you get? What serving size would you need to double the portion yield?

A successful menu uses tested recipes that have high acceptance by the clientele for whom the menu is developed. Often the menu dictates the recipes to be used, but frequently variety is added by reviewing new recipes available. Computerized menu systems often provide a library of quantity foods tested recipes that may meet your needs.

Recipes in a computerized system use a standardized format for the recipes consistent with the points covered above. One of the options available with the computerized recipe is the ability to easily scale the recipes to any number of servings. This can be very handy if a recipe is designed for 50 servings and you need 215 portions.

The scaling of recipes in a computerized system is a simple math function, which may have some unusual side effects. By entering the number of portions needed, the computer automatically divides or multiplies the base recipe to the level needed. However, the computer will not adjust the amount of seasoning in the recipe appropriately. The computer will also scale a recipe with unexpected quantities such as seven cups plus one tablespoon and one teaspoon of water. Remember, computers are very literal and do not round up or down well.

Steps in Adapting and Testing a Recipe

As you find recipes you wish to use in your operation, you are ready to begin adapting and standardizing them. When you obtain a recipe for food service that has already been standardized, you still need to test it in your own facility. Why? The standardization may change a little bit with the specific ingredients and equipment you use. Furthermore, variations occur with altitude. If a recipe for baked goods was tested at sea level, and you are at an altitude of 4,000 feet, you will need to make adjustments to create a similar product. In addition, a standardized recipe that meets one facility's standards may not meet another's. Thus, a safe practice is: *Don't believe it until you prove it in your own facility.* This ensures you know you have standards upon which you can depend.

The steps in adapting and standardizing a recipe are as follows:

Step 1: Verify that directions, techniques, ingredients, and equipment specified all apply to your own facility. Edit them if necessary.

Step 2: Produce the original recipe in your own facility, using the equipment you expect to use for routine production. Portion out servings according to your portion and yield figures, and verify the numbers and acceptability.

Step 3: Name and categorize the recipes in a way that makes sense for your own facility.

Step 4: Specify the portion size you wish to use to comply with your own menu needs.

Step 5: Set the yield for which you wish to standardize the recipe. This should be the yield in which you expect to produce it most often.

3. What steps would you take before introducing a new recipe on the menu?

Step 6: Scale and cost out the recipe accordingly (described under Recipe Math).

Step 7: Assure that measurements are expressed in terms you always use for each ingredient and are easy to understand.

Step 8: Prepare the new recipe. Taste and evaluate the final product for quality. This is often done through a taste panel, a group of individuals who all taste and evaluate the food. A sample evaluation for members of a taste panel appears in Figure 3.5.

Step 9: Document any adjustments needed, and retest if warranted. Some experts advise adjusting only one ingredient at a time, so that you may fully evaluate the impact of each change.

Step 10: Prepare a finalized, clearly documented version of the recipe for reference. At this point, you may be entering it into a computer-based management system, or, you may be filing an original copy in a secure location.

In large facilities, recipe testing occurs in a test kitchen. A test kitchen is a designated location with proper equipment and staffing for trying out, verifying, adjusting, and standardizing recipes. Whether or not you have a test kitchen, the steps are similar.

In this process it is important to be precise and accurate so that you may be certain you have developed a meaningful, standardized recipe.

As you adapt recipes, you may make adjustments that affect both cost and nutrients. Many managers run both cost and nutrient analyses when the standardization is complete, and again verify that all figures are acceptable.

Figure 3.5
Recipe Evaluation for Taste Panel

Date: _____ Menu Item: _Blueberry Muffins_____

Evaluator: _____ Recipe Number: _____

Instructions: Check (✓) your reaction to each of the following factors used to describe the menu item.

Evaluation Factor	Exceptional	Like Very Much	Acceptable	Like Slightly	Unacceptable
Evenly browned.					
Rounded, not peaked top.					
No tunnels.					
Blueberries evenly distributed.					
Cake-like texture.					

Comments:

Recipe Math

Scaling a recipe to produce different yields calls for recipe math. First, you convert the yield from old to new. Then, you adjust all ingredient measurements accordingly. Let's take a closer look at the calculations.

The most common method is to determine a **conversion factor**. A conversion factor is the number by which you will (initially) adjust everything to arrive at a new yield. The steps for scaling a recipe are as follows.

Step 1: Divide the new yield by the original yield. This gives you a conversion factor. Note that when you are reducing a yield, the conversion factor will be less than 1.0. When you are increasing a yield, the conversion factor will be more than 1.0.

Example: Your original recipe yields 100 portions. You want a yield of 225 portions.

New yield ÷ original yield = 225 ÷ 100 = 2.25

2.25 is your conversion factor.

(*Tip:* Remember that n comes before o in the alphabet. To obtain a conversion factor, use *new* yield divided by *old* yield.)

Step 2: Multiply the measurement for each ingredient by the conversion factor.

Example: The original recipe calls for 3 oz. of sugar. The new measurement is:

3 oz. x conversion factor = 3 oz. x 2.25 = 6.75 oz.

Step 3: Consider additional adjustments that may be necessary. Some ingredients do not need to follow the conversion factor precisely. Spices and seasonings, for example, can appear in smaller quantities than you might calculate. Oil used for sautéing vegetables may not need to increase in proportion.

Step 4: Specify and verify the batch unit if applicable. For example, if you are adjusting a recipe for whole pies, be sure the final quantities you have determined will make some number of whole pies. Likewise, if you are working on a recipe that must be prepared in steam table pans, baking pans, or something similar, examine the batch unit.

In Step 2 of this process, many experts suggest you use only weight measurements (e.g., if measuring flour in cups, first change it to pounds and ounces). This is generally the most precise and easiest to convert. To do this, use a reference table of conversions from weights to measures, found in many quantity cookbooks, such as *Food for Fifty*, and built into many computer-based recipe management systems. When you are finished, you can use the same table to convert back to volume measurements if desired. Figure 3.6 shows an example of a set of weight and volume conversions for flour.

Converting a recipe to new yields requires careful attention to the proper calculations. Your final answer may come out as a unit of measure that is not usable in daily operation or, it may come out as a decimal, such as 2.79 teaspoons. In this case, you

GLOSSARY

Conversion Factor
The number by which you adjust each recipe ingredient to arrive at a new yield

View the Supplemental Material for this chapter for videos on recipe math.

Putting It Into Practice

4. The meatloaf recipe has a yield of 25 servings and you need to prepare the menu item for 75 people. What is the conversion factor? Use that conversion factor to determine how much ground beef is needed in the recipe if the old amount was 4 lbs.

need to round the decimal to a usable fraction. Keep in mind how the recipe will be used and strive to make it simple to understand. Finally, after scaling a recipe and converting measurements, be sure to retest the recipe for accuracy.

Figure 3.6
Example of Weight and Volume Conversions for Flour

BACKGROUND

You are scaling a recipe that contains all-purpose flour. Your original recipe calls for 5 cups of flour. You wish to scale this recipe to a higher yield using a conversion factor of 3.3.

1. Convert Cups to a Weight

1. Look up the volume-to-weight equivalent in a cookbook and find that 4 cups of all-purpose flour = 1 lb.
2. Create an equation to show the relationship: 4 cups/1 lb. = 5 cups/? lbs.
   Tip: When you are setting up an equation like this one, always put the volume measurement on the top of each side, and the weight measurement on the bottom of each side (or vice versa). This assures that you have set up the equation correctly.
3. To solve this, you cross multiply the top number (numerator) of one side by the bottom number (denominator) of the other to create a new equation:

   $$\frac{4}{16} \times \frac{5}{x}$$ Cross multiply and then divide

   $4x = (5 \times 16)$
   $4x = 80$ Now divide both sides by 4

   $\frac{4x}{4} = \frac{80}{4}$ $x = 20$ oz.
   $x = \frac{20}{16 \text{ oz. or 1 lb.}}$ $x = 1.25$ lbs.

4. Divide each side by 4
   $5 \div 4 = x$ $x = 1.25$ lbs.

2. Scale the Measurement

Scale the measurement for the new yield. Multiply the original measurement in weight by the conversion factor: 1.25 lbs. x 3.5 = 4.125 lbs.

3. Convert to Volume

This is an optional step. If you measure flour by volume, it is important. If you measure flour by weight, you can stop here. You create an equation to show the relationship.

$$\frac{x}{4.125} \times \frac{4}{1}$$

To solve this, you cross multiply the top number (numerator) of one side by the bottom number (denominator) of the other to create a new equation.

4 x 4.125 = 1 x (x) *or* 4 x 4.125 = 16. 5 cups

To make this measurement easier, convert this final volume measurement to a manageable unit. From a cookbook, you can also learn that 4 cups = 1 quart. So you may change this figure to: 4 pt. + 1/2 cup. Food production references such as *Food for Fifty* by Mary Molt provide direct reading tables so you don't have to calculate.

Using Standardized Recipes to Determine Standard Portion Costs

Additional math used with a standardized recipe is costing. A standardized recipe helps you with cost control because recipe amounts and portions are predetermined. Costing a recipe without using a computer program can be time consuming. As the CDM, CFPP, you should decide whether to include ingredient costs on the standardized recipe. Perhaps you could begin with the recipes that are most expensive, such as your meat items and your supplements.

Regardless of whether you use ingredient costs on your standardized recipes, you need to know how to calculate the cost of a recipe. Here's how to calculate the cost of a recipe.

Step 1: Create a standard recipe costing form such as the one in Figure 3.7 and fill in the ingredient and amount columns.

Step 2: Calculate unit cost and determine the total cost of the ingredient.

Total cost of the ingredient item = unit cost x the quantity/amount of the ingredient.

Unit Cost = Total cost ÷ by number of servings per package

Example of calculating unit cost: You have a 2 lb. package of bacon @ $7.78/pkg. A salad recipe calls for 12 pieces of bacon. Bacon is about 1 oz./piece. Two lbs. = 32 pieces. Determine unit price by dividing the total cost of the package by 32: $7.78 ÷ 32 = $.243 per piece/unit. This becomes the unit price on the recipe. The total cost of that ingredient is then $.243 x 12 pieces called for on the recipe or $2.92.

Step 3: Determine if any recipe ingredients have a different yield from the amount purchased. (See section on Understanding Product Yields.) Calculate the Edible Portion cost.

Step 4: Total all ingredient costs.

Step 5: Divide by the total number of portions for the recipe to determine cost per portion.

Understanding Product Yields

When you purchase fresh produce, you will clean it, peel it, core it, etc. before you use it. This preprocessing reduces the final amount available for a recipe. You might also remove skin from chicken pieces, trim fat from pork chops, or remove bone from a ham steak. You are changing the amount purchased (aka **As Purchased [AP]** to an **Edible Portion [EP]** amount). For costing purposes, you must calculate the cost of the Edible Portion of an ingredient. Thus, the ingredient information in recipes must be adjusted or converted to reflect the cost of what is actually consumed. Use the Yield Factor to determine the As Purchased amount of product needed.

Cooking may also change the amount purchased to an Edible Portion amount. You know when cooking a roast, turkey, or ground beef that the amount you end up with is less than the amount you started with.

How do you know what the Edible Portion (EP) is for any produce you use? You can weigh the product in its As Purchased (AP) form, and then weigh it again after you have completed the preparation or cooking. There are many reliable resources available that provide you with tables showing the yield percentage of an As Purchased amount

---

GLOSSARY

As Purchased (AP)
The raw weight, without any pre-production

Edible Portion (EP)
The final quantity produced after all preparation is done

to an Edible Portion. One such reference is Food For Fifty by Mary Molt. This book includes many food production tables and quantity recipes and would be a valuable resource for any foodservice department.

Calculating Edible Portions from As Purchased Amounts. Most facilities use a yield percentage to determine the ingredient amount from the raw purchased or AP amount. The **yield percentage** is the percentage available after preproduction, portioning, or cooking has been completed.

> Edible portion (EP) cost = AP cost ÷ yield percentage
>
> Example of determining the Edible Portion cost of a recipe ingredient: The yield percentage table (from a reference book) indicates that each pound of 85% lean ground beef yields 0.80 lbs. of cooked, drained ground beef. 10 lbs. x 0.80= 8 lbs. of cooked ground beef. The AP price of 85% lean ground beef is $13.90 for 10 lbs. The EP cost = $13.90 ÷ .80 or $17.38 for 10 lbs. To determine the price per pound, divide the total EP cost of $17.38 by 10 = $1.74 (round up) per EP pound.
>
> Example of determining ingredient cost using yield percentage: Recipe calls for 15 lbs. of fresh green beans. The unit cost of the green beans is $.69 per pound. The yield percentage on fresh green beans is 88% or .88. The EP cost of one pound of green beans then is $.69 ÷ .88 = $.78/pound.

Figure 3.7 shows ingredient costing where the AP and the EP are the same (with the Kaiser Rolls and Au Jus) and an example of calculating an ingredient cost where the AP and EP are different (with the Roast Beef).

Recipe Costing Versus Meal Costing

Recipe costing assumes that you have perfect preparation and portioning of the recipe with no leftovers or waste. With single serve items such as a grilled chicken breast, the number produced and the number consumed can be tracked and the waste factor calculated. With menu items that are not single serve, the number of portions and the actual portioning become a consideration in the cost of the meal.

If you are serving baked fish for lunch, the case of product may cost you $48.75 for 40 – 4 oz. portions.

> The recipe costing would be $48.75 ÷ 40 = $1.22 per portion
>
> You plan to serve 60 portions of fish so your cost would be 60 x $1.22 = $73.20 However, you only served 47 portions and had 13 pieces of fish leftover. Your true Meal Cost for the fish is the total cost divided by the actual number of servings used or $73.20 ÷ 47 = $1.56. (There is no "popular" use for leftover baked fish so the remaining portions will be thrown out.)

> **GLOSSARY**
>
> **Yield Percentage**
> The Edible Portion (EP) weight divided by the As Purchased (AP) weight

5. Your operation has purchased 50 lbs. of potatoes. Upon cleaning and peeling, there are 42.5 lbs. remaining. Using the yield percentage, calculate the ingredient cost of 10 lbs. of peeled potatoes if the AP price is $1.69 per lb.

Figure 3.7
Standardized Recipe Cost Sheet Sample

Menu Item: French Dip Sandwich

Total Yield: 50 Sandwiches | Portion Sizes: 3 oz. meat, 1/4 cup au jus

50 servings x 3 oz. = 150 oz.

150 oz. ÷ 16 oz./lbs. = 9.4 lbs. (round up to 10 lbs., which is the EP Amt required)

10 ÷ 0.66 = 15.1 lbs. (AP Amt. needed for recipe), 15.1 x 2.39 = 36.09 (total cost of Roast Beef)

	INGREDIENTS			INGREDIENT COST	
Item	AP Amt.	Yield %	EP Amt.	AP $	Total Cost
Roast Beef*	15.1 lbs.	66% or 0.66	10 lbs.	$2.39/lbs.	$36.09
Au Jus, Canned Item	12.5 cups or 2, 51 oz. cans			$5.38/can	$10.76
Kaiser Roll	50 each			$0.17 ea.	$8.50

Total Recipe Cost: $55.35

* Roast Beef purchased raw and then cooked.

\# of Portions: 50

Cost per Portion: $1.11

Let's use the meat as the first item to cost for the French Dip Sandwich. To calculate the EP of meat for a total Yield of 50 Sandwiches, we know from the recipe that each sandwich has 3 oz of meat and 1/4 cup au jus. Therefore for 50 sandwiches x 3 oz . = 150 oz of meat will be required. Converted to pounds, 150 oz . ÷ 16 oz = 9 .4 lbs. (round up to 10 lbs which is the EP Amt required).

Now to calculate the AP, we divide this EP by the yield which has been given by the recipe as 0.66. 10/0.66 gives us 15.1 of AP. Given that the meat costs 2.39/lb and we will need to buy 15.1 lbs to give us 10 lbs of EP, the cost of meat in the recipe is 15.1*2.39= $36.09.

Similarly, once the AP for Au jus and the buns have been calculated, they are multiplied with the cost and the total recipe cost is determined.

Recipe costing is a valuable step in the recipe standardization process. It provides you with the beginning calculations for your food cost by meal or patient/resident day. Just keep in mind that the recipe cost is not the same as your food cost. Calculating recipe costs using computer software speeds up calculating food costs. If the software is linked to your electronic inventory program, your recipe costs can be updated as prices change, thereby providing more current information. The more current your recipe costs are, the more accurately you can stay within budget.

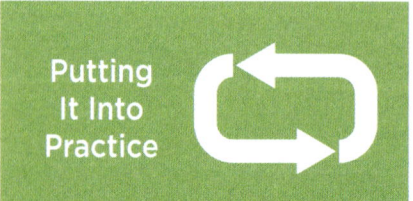

6. Your chef does not think standardized recipes are important. How would you convince him otherwise, and what steps would you take to improve compliance?

Encouraging the Use of Standardized Recipes

Making standardized recipes work requires communication. Remind staff of the importance of standardized recipes by holding short in-services annually to review how and why to use them. Make sure that your department standards (such as standardized recipes) are part of new employee orientation. If you notice over or under production problems, follow up on them immediately with the cooking staff.

Conducting pre-line taste testing panels daily will establish a pattern of evaluating the food items being prepared. This allows you and the entire team to assess the quality of the food being served and ensure a consistent use of the recipes. In addition, there are several ways to make a standardized recipe user-friendly and improve compliance:

Sequence of Ingredients: As you list ingredients on a recipe, verify the sequence of ingredients matches the sequence in which they are used. This helps to prevent oversights and errors.

Consistent Units of Measure: Recognize that there are many ways to measure any given ingredient, and standardize your units of measure for each one you use in your operation. For example, if you decide that flour will be measured by volume, then be sure it is always done this way on every recipe. There may be a few exceptions, where ingredients are used differently in one recipe than another. In a computer-based system, a user may actually specify two different ingredients that can appear on recipes, such as: margarine, measured in 1-lb. blocks; and margarine, measured by volume. Make sure that for whatever measurements you specify, measuring utensils are available. For example, if you use quart measurements, have a quart measure on hand.

Consistent Abbreviations: There are variations in abbreviations used to describe common measurements. For example, teaspoons may be: tsp or t. Tablespoons may be: Tbsp. TB or T. Pounds may be: lbs. or #. There is no right or wrong to any of these designations. However, the use of abbreviations must be standardized and consistent on all recipes to minimize confusion.

Figure 3.8
Common Equivalents

VOLUME MEASUREMENTS	FLUID MEASUREMENTS	WEIGHT MEASUREMENTS
• 1 bushel = 4 pecks	• 1 gallon = 4 quarts	• 1 lb. = 16 oz.
• 1 peck = 8 quarts	• 1 quart = 4 cups	• 1 oz. = 30 grams
• 1 gallon = 4 quarts	• 4 cups = 2 pints	
• 1 quart = 2 pints	• 1 cup = 8 fluid oz.	
• 1 pint = 2 cups	• 1 fluid oz. = 2 Tbsp.	
• 1 cup = 16 Tbsp.		
• 1/2 cup = 8 Tbsp.		
• 1/3 cup = 5-1/3 Tbsp.		
• 1/4 cup = 4 Tbsp.		
• 1 Tbsp. = 3 tsp.		

Consolidated Measures: When scaling a recipe, you may arrive at measurements such as: 18 cups or 24 teaspoons. If you ask staff to make these kinds of measurements, you lengthen the time required for production and increase the opportunity for error. When possible, consolidate smaller measurements to larger units, using a chart of equivalents. For example, 18 cups becomes 4.5 quarts, and 24 teaspoons becomes 1/2 cup. See Figure 3.8 for common equivalents.

Consistent Temperature Standards: It is also helpful to standardize all temperature measurements to one system, such as degrees F (Fahrenheit) or degrees C (Celsius). Generally, this has to match available readings on actual equipment, and many operations use Fahrenheit.

Proofread Recipes: As you finalize tested recipes, take the time to proofread them carefully. Small errors can magnify in the food production kitchen. Imagine the results that could occur if you omitted baking powder from the cornbread recipe, or accidentally noted teaspoons instead of tablespoons, or specified a baking temperature as 425°F instead of 325°F. Check final amounts carefully. In addition, ensure that every ingredient in the ingredient list is used in the text of the procedure—and that every ingredient called for in the procedure appears on the ingredient list. Finally, make sure the procedure is clear and cannot be misunderstood. Attention to detail helps ensure the recipe will be carried out as it is intended to be.

To ensure the ongoing success of standardized recipes, it's also important to encourage feedback from production employees. Tell employees that if they encounter suspected errors in recipes or believe that a standardized recipe is producing unacceptable results, you would like to hear about it. Encouraging communication allows you to pinpoint areas for correction and involve production staff in tweaking recipes that are then updated with the new information.

Employees who feel they cannot talk to the CDM, CFPP about recipe problems are much more likely to make their own adjustments to "fix" a recipe. As a result, a flawed recipe can slip through the system for a long time. When a new employee comes in and prepares the same recipe, it can flop. It's always better to edit the recipe and create a document that can generate reproducible results.

Other Benefits of Using Standardized Recipes

Standardized recipes are useful for more than just production needs. Use them to determine your requisition needs and to improve portion control.

Standardized Recipes and Requisitions

In large facilities, there may be one staff member whose job is to retrieve items from the storeroom for production needs. That person will work from a requisition that lists all of the items needed for the day's production. If your standardized recipes are computerized, your computer software can generate the requisition from those recipes.

If your recipes are not computerized, you can still generate a requisition from the standardized recipes. When starting a new menu cycle write down, or better yet, open a software such as Excel, and enter each ingredient used and the quantity needed in all of the recipes used during the day. If you have the same ingredient used in multiple recipes in the same production area, you could pull it all at one time. For example, if you are making Turkey a la King you might need:

15 lbs.   of turkey breast for the regular entrée
+
1 lb.   for the chopped and ground turkey
+
2 lbs.   for the carb-controlled recipe
+
15 lbs.   for the cafeteria
= 33 lbs. TOTAL

The requisition list would show a total of 33 lbs. needed.

A requisition sheet helps with inventory control, purchasing, and storeroom management. This will improve the storeroom process and staff efficiency by reducing trips to the storeroom for forgotten items.

Standardized Recipes and Portion Control

Ensuring that food served matches portions specified in standardized recipes and on menus is critical because portion control is intertwined with recipe yields. **Portion control** is essential for managing the value of a standardized recipe, such as predictable costs, predictable nutrient content of menu items, and predictable number of servings for each product. Portion control also builds client satisfaction, as the portion sizes of foods are predictable and consistent.

Responsibility for portion control may be shared among various employees, from production staff to trayline employees to servers. For example, portion control for applesauce pre-portioned into dishes in the cold food production area becomes the responsibility of a cold food production employee. Meanwhile, portion control for hot mashed potatoes served on a buffet becomes the responsibility of the server. As the CDM, CFPP, you need to explain and reinforce the importance of portion control to all involved employees, provide training, and allow employees to practice the techniques. For example, have them practice using a common big spoon, a **spoodle**, and a **disher** to portion a set number of portions of mashed potatoes. Usually, these portion sizes will vary and will demonstrate the need for a standard portion utensil.

Carrying through portion control often requires some tools for measurement. For example, when you specify 1/2 cup as a portion size, how do you know it will be served that way? Common measurement tools used in foodservice facilities include portion/dishers, scoops, and ladles. Portion scoops/dishers, and ladles designed for non-commercial food service have standardized sizes and are an aid in portion control. Portion scoops/dishers have designated numbers. For example, a #8 disher equals 1/2 cup, and a #16 equals 1/4 cup. This number is equivalent to the number of servings in a quart or 32 oz. So a #8 disher means 8 servings in a quart. (Note: A disher is frequently called a scoop or an ice cream scoop. The proper term is disher or portion scoop so it is not confused with another utensil called a scoop and used for dry ingredients such as flour.)

For some foods, portioning is achieved by weighing on a scale. For example, the 2-ounce serving of beef for a renal diet may be weighed to ensure compliance with the diet order. However, it is not always practical or cost-effective to weigh every portion of a food. In portioning the roast beef for a trayline service, a cook may weigh several portions in order to establish the thickness and dimensions of a 4-ounce serving and use this as a visual guide for the remaining portions. Finally, managers have many pre-

> **GLOSSARY**
>
> **Portion Control**
> Control of the serving sizes so they are standardized
>
> **Disher/Portion Scoop/Spoodle**
> A portion control serving utensil used for dishing vegetables, fruits, desserts, or starchy items like rice and potatoes

portioned foods available to them today. These eliminate many of the challenges related to portion control. For example, you may purchase pre-portioned chicken breasts or fish fillets for service. Figure 3.9 provides examples of how portions may be measured.

As you have seen, one advantage of standardized recipes is that you can specify standard portion sizes. But how do you know what the portion size should be? There are many references that describe standard portion sizes such as the Academy of Nutrition and Dietetics Exchange Lists.

Standardized Recipes and Food Allergies

The use of standardized recipes is of particular importance to people with food allergies. Food allergies and sensitivities are a potentially life-threatening concern for millions of people. Allergic reactions to the presence of an allergen can vary from an itchy or tingling feeling of the skin, nose, or mouth to anaphylaxis (ana-fil-lax-is).

Anaphylaxis can cause difficulty in breathing, reduced blood pressure, and gastrointestinal symptoms such as vomiting and diarrhea. If untreated, a severe anaphylactic reaction can lead to death. According to the U.S. Food & Drug Administration website:

> Each year in the U.S., it is estimated that anaphylaxis from food results in:
> - 30,000 emergency room visits
> - 2,000 hospitalizations
> - 150 deaths
>
> *https://www.fda.gov/Food/ResourcesForYou/Consumers/ucm079311.htm*

The most common "Big Eight" food allergens are:

1. Peanuts
2. Eggs
3. Milk
4. Fish
5. Shellfish
6. Wheat
7. Soy
8. Tree Nuts

Your clients rely on you to follow your recipes. At home, they can manage the ingredients of the meal items they prepare. However, when they are in your dining room, or when they are living in your care center, residence hall, or detention center, they cannot control the ingredients in their foods.

When asked what is in the apple crisp, standardized recipes provide the staff with the list of ingredients that can be reviewed with clients. The consistent use of standardized recipes ensures that the baker did not add some chopped walnuts (a tree nut) to the apple crisp topping today.

For more information on food allergies and anaphylaxis, refer to websites such as FDA.gov, WebMD, or FoodAllergy.org.

Figure 3.9
How Portions are Measured

PRODUCT	PORTION	METHOD
Diced peaches	1/2 cup	Use a #8 disher/portion scoop to portion individual servings into bowls.
Individual chicken fillets	5 oz. cooked weight	Portion each as one serving.
Vanilla cake	1/24 of pan	Slice cake as a 6x4 equal portions.
Apple pie	1/8 pie	Slice pie into eight equal pieces/portions.
Hearty chicken stew	1 cup	Use 8 oz. ladle to portion into bowls at the time of service.
Mashed potatoes	1/2 cup	Use #8 disher/portion scoop to portion individual servings onto plates.
Whole banana	1 each	Offer one banana each.

Recipe Acceptance

Recipes are planned and edited to provide our clients with meals and menus they will enjoy and that meet their dietary restrictions, if any. Developing a standardized recipe also has to include how well the dining clientele accept the item. Talking with diners during the meal, circulating menu surveys or scorecards, and observing plate waste are all part of the feedback loop as you trial or present new recipes. Sometimes new items are not well accepted just because they are different. Oftentimes though, you may have a great item but the clientele prefers more oregano and less onion. You will not know unless you ask. A good evaluation of client preference is key to recipe acceptance and menu planning.

Chapter References

RESOURCES	
A Brief History of Health Care Quality Assessment	http://www.ncbi.nih.gov/pmc/articles/PMC1022402/pdf/westjmed00067-0065.pdf
Academy of Nutrition and Dietetics	eatright.org
Alaska Seafood Marketing Institute	alaskaseafood.org
Food Allergy Research & Education	foodallergy.org
Food for Fifty	Molt, Mary, Pearson Education, Inc.
Food Resources for Consumers	www.fda.gov/Food/ResourcesForYou/Consumers/ucm079311.htm
Food Values of Portions Commonly Used	Bowes and Church
Gregoire, Mary (2013). Foodservice Organizations: A managerial and systems approach, 8th ed. Upper Saddle River; NJ: Pearson Prentice Hall	
Kotschevar, L.H (2008). Management by menu, 4th ed. Hoboken, NJ: John Wiley & Sons	
The Foodservice Tune Up	Toczek, Wayne & Bauman, Tim
U.S. Food & Drug Administration	FDA.gov
USDA National Nutrient Database	nal.usda.gov/fnic/pubs/foodcomp.pdf
USDA Standard Portion Sizes	https://www.fns.usda,gov/cnpp
USDA Standardized Recipes	https://www.fns.usda.gov/tn/main-dishes
WebMD	www.WebMD.com

Standards and Procedures for Purchasing and Preparing Food

Overview and Objectives

Specifying standards and procedures for purchasing and preparing food is an important consideration in managing production. The Certified Dietary Manager®, Certified Food Protection Professional® (CDM®, CFPP®) needs to understand and establish the standards for food and production as part of the quality management initiatives. This chapter helps us understand food standards and what is involved in the preparation of food. As with all standards, follow-up and continuous coaching of employees will ensure that standards are met. After completing this chapter, you should be able to:

- Write specifications for purchasing food
- Understand food grades and quality standards when buying food products
- List food preparation standards for different foods
- Provide appropriate menu substitutions
- Develop procedures for monitoring food waste control

> **GLOSSARY**
>
> **United States Department of Agriculture (USDA)**
> The United States Department of Agriculture is the primary governing body setting regulations on food supplies in the United States
>
> **Specification**
> Statement that describes the condition or status of a product to safeguard foodservice quality

While menu is the most important control in your foodservice operation, food standards for food purchased and prepared play an important role in ensuring menu integrity. Knowing the quality and quantity of food needed for a particular recipe as well as the manner it needs to be prepared is important for the CDM, CFPP. Most items purchased today in any foodservice organization are prepared, packaged, and processed under some level of government monitoring. Grading of meats, canned goods, and dairy products is provided by the **USDA** (United States Department of Agriculture) and stamped on the labels of the products or cases. Federal guidelines also dictate what labeling is required from the manufacturers: the list of ingredients, nutrition labeling, expiration or use-by date, contact information and pack or lot numbers for tracking purposes. The pack or lot numbers become critically important information in the event of a product recall. Before you purchase foods or write your specifications, you want to identify general information and guidelines about the food you procure. That information can be used to document standards for your facility.

Specifications for Purchasing Food

A **specification** is essentially a statement, readily understood by both buyers and suppliers, of the required quality of products, including the allowable limits of tolerance. It is a list of detailed characteristics desired in a product for a specific use. Written specifications are essential for an efficient foodservice operation. When specifications are written, suppliers, the receiving clerk, and the foodservice manager can all determine if the products received are what was ordered. When writing specifications, one should include the following information:

- Name of product (trade or brand) or standard
- Federal grade, brand, or other quality designation
- Capacity of container (e.g., weight or can size)
- Count per container or approximate number per pound
- Unit on which price will be based
- Product use (e.g., for salads, soups)
- Product test procedures to determine quality compliance (e.g., degree of ripeness, flavor characteristics)

Buyers can write specifications by using the following purchasing standards. These standards constitute a common technical language for buyers and suppliers and are very helpful when determining the types of products to purchase for a specific recipe and/or menu.

Purchasing Standards

Eggs and Dairy Products

Eggs have many uses in most foodservice facilities. You and the chef/cook need to consider what type of eggs best fit the production needs. The type of eggs used will depend upon the number of clients served and the menu. (i.e., Do you have an on-site bakery?) There are three different egg products you might use: fresh, processed (frozen and liquid eggs), or dried eggs.

Fresh Eggs: The USDA provides the following information about shell eggs. There are three consumer grades: U.S. Grade AA, A, and B. The grade is determined by the interior quality of the egg and the appearance and condition of the shell. Eggs of any quality grade may differ in weight (size).

U.S. Grade AA eggs have whites that are thick and firm; yolks that are high, round, and practically free from defects; and clean, unbroken shells. Grade AA and Grade A eggs are best for frying and poaching where appearance is important. U.S. Grade A eggs have characteristics of Grade AA except that the whites are "reasonably" firm. This is the quality most often sold in stores. U.S. Grade B eggs have whites that may be thinner and yolks that may be wider and flatter than eggs of higher grades. The shells must be unbroken, but may show slight stains. This quality is seldom found in retail stores because they are usually used to make liquid, frozen, and dried egg products.

For more than 10 years the FDA and USDA guideline for the use of shell eggs has been to use pasteurized eggs. **Pasteurization of eggs** is a process, using a combination of time and temperature, that heats eggs in the shell, destroying bacteria and eliminating salmonella contamination. After pasteurization, a food-grade wax is added to the shell to prevent recontamination and maintain freshness. Pasteurized eggs are approved for whole egg products such as "sunny-side up," poached, or the making of egg-based sauces such as fresh Hollandaise. Non-pasteurized eggs are intended for use in baking, quiches, or other products where the egg will be *fully* cooked, which eliminates any *Salmonella* contamination. Pasteurized liquid eggs are recommended for most baking, egg bakes, and scrambled products. Healthcare and school surveyors have cited some facilities for having both pasteurized and unpasteurized shell eggs in the same cooler. It may be wise to have only pasteurized eggs in the facility. Refer to the Food Code, CMS, USDA, and state regulations for information pertinent to the specific operation.

Frozen, Liquid, and Dried Eggs: Processed eggs save time when used for baking or cooking omelets and scrambled eggs in large quantities. Processed eggs help meet the food safety regulation that prohibits pooling eggs (breaking raw shell eggs into a container and storing them for later). All processed products are processed under sanitary conditions and must display the USDA inspection mark. Processed eggs are broken and separated into yolks and whites and then pasteurized before processing into dried, frozen, or refrigerated liquid products. There are several different processed liquid and dried egg products. Figure 4.1 shows both liquid and dried egg products, how they are packaged for purchase, their uses, and storage and handling guidelines. Pasteurized dried egg white powder should be used for meringues or desserts that are not cooked. Note: "Egg Substitutes" are comprised of egg whites, food coloring, and some seasoning. They should be handled like liquid egg products.

Cheese

Cheese is important because it can add calcium and protein to menu items. With the wide variety of cheeses available, it can also add unique flavors. There are processed cheeses and natural cheeses.

Processed Cheeses: When you are selecting cheese for use in hot items, such as heated sandwiches, casseroles, or sauces, select a cheese with a suitable flavor and texture that will melt consistently and easily. Processed cheeses are a combination of natural cheeses that have undergone a heat process. They melt more easily and smoothly but

> **GLOSSARY**
>
> **Pasteurization of Eggs**
> A process that uses a combination of time and temperature that heats eggs in the shell, destroying bacteria and eliminating salmonella contamination

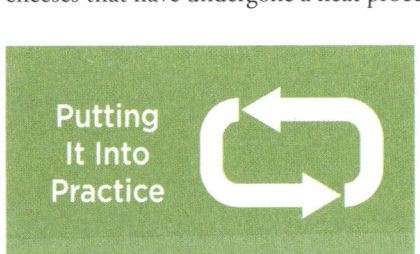

1. Your menu calls for Quiche Florentine. What are the different ways you can write specifications for the eggs required?

Figure 4.1
Egg Products

REFRIGERATED LIQUID EGG PRODUCTS	
<ul><li>Whole eggs, whites, or yolks</li><li>Sugared egg yolks</li><li>Salted whole eggs or yolks</li></ul> <ul><li>Scrambled egg mix</li><li>Extended shelf life whole eggs, whites, yolks, or scrambled egg mix</li></ul>	
Usage	Food service and the commercial food processing industry.
Availability	Bulk tank trucks, totes, metal or plastic containers, polyethylene coated fiber or laminated foil and paper cartons and hermetically sealed polyethylene bags. Container size from small bags to cartons (8 oz. to -lbs.), intermediate size bag in boxes and pails (20 lbs. to 40 lbs.) and larger drums and totes (200 lbs. to 3,500 lbs.).
Advantages	Pasteurized, quick and easy to use.
Storage/ Handling	Refrigerated egg products should be kept at 40°F (4°C) or below, but do not freeze. Use well within expiration dates.
DRIED EGG PRODUCTS	
<ul><li>Whole eggs, white or yolk solids</li><li>Dried egg or scrambled egg mix</li><li>Egg whites</li></ul> <ul><li>Free-flowing whole eggs or yolk solids</li><li>Blends of whole eggs and/or yolk carbohydrates</li></ul>	
Usage	Ingredient especially for the commercial food processing industry.
Availability	Food service: 6 oz. pouches, 3 lbs. and 25 lbs. poly packs Commercial: 25 lbs. and 50 lbs. boxes, 150 lbs., 175 lbs., and 200 lbs. drums
Advantages	Pasteurized, long shelf life, stable, and mixable.
Storage/ Handling	Keep cool at less than 50°F (10°C) to maintain quality. Once containers have been opened, reseal tightly to prevent contamination and absorption of moisture. Dried egg products should flow freely and not be clumped or hardened. Use well within expiration dates.

Source: American Egg Board. Used with permission.

provide less of the variety of unique flavors because they are a combination of cheeses. They work well in casseroles and sauces. If you have a signature hot sandwich, you might have a higher client satisfaction with a natural cheese slice because of the more pronounced cheese flavor. Processed cheeses come in a variety of forms such as sliced, block, or spreads.

Natural Cheeses: The flavor of the natural cheese depends upon the type of milk (cow, goat, or sheep) and the length of time the cheese is aged.

There are several varieties of natural cheeses:
- Fresh cheese such as ricotta, mozzarella, or feta
- Soft cheese such as Brie
- Semisoft such as blue or Monterey Jack
- Firm cheese such as Cheddar, provolone
- Hard grating cheese such as Parmesan

Aging does decrease the lactose content so if you have lactose intolerant clients who prefer cheese, they might be able to tolerate an aged natural cheese. Natural cheeses come in a variety of forms such as grated, sliced, and cubed.

There are hundreds of varieties of cheeses and you can determine which type and form to purchase by reviewing your recipes and consulting the chef/cook. There are many websites that can help you determine the characteristics and purchasing information of cheeses or use a food production book such as *Food for Fifty* by Mary Molt.

Milk

Milk is another staple in the foodservice department and is commonly used in recipes as well as for a beverage.

Fluid Milk: Generally, there are four different types of fluid milk used for beverages:

- Whole milk—contains 8 g of fat per 8 oz. cup and the federal standard requires that whole milk be at least 3.25% fat
- Reduced fat milk—2% fat and contains 4.7 g total fat per cup
- Low-fat milk—1% fat and contains 2.6 g total fat per cup
- Nonfat or skim milk—0.5% fat and contains 0.5 g total fat per cup

The availability of goat milk is increasing and for CDM, CFPPs who work in hospitals, you may need to establish a source for it. Goat milk has a higher concentration of medium chain fatty acids (MCFA) and research has shown that clients with various medical conditions, such as malabsorption syndrome are more tolerant of goat milk. For infants who are allergic to cow's milk, goat milk may be an acceptable alternative.

Sensitivity or intolerance to fluid cow's milk has led to the development of lactose-free dairy products. Alternative "milk" products such as soy, almond, and rice have become easily accessible in grocery stores for customers with intolerance or wanting to decrease their intake of animal-based foods.

Fluid milk products must be **pasteurized** to be served in commercial facilities. Pasteurization means heating fluid milk or cream to a specific temperature for a specified amount of time. Both fluid milk and cream products may also be **ultra-pasteurized**. Ultra-pasteurization takes the pasteurization process to higher temperatures for a shorter period of time. Finally, these products can also be **ultra-high-temperature processed**. The products are heated at a high enough temperature to kill all of the bacteria. Ultra-high-temperature products can be held without refrigeration for up to three months. Once they are opened, they must be treated like all fluid milk or cream products, refrigerated and used within a few days.

Yogurt: Yogurt is a product cultured with lactic acid-producing bacteria. It is available with whole milk, low-fat, or skim milk. Some Greek yogurts have much higher protein content (i.e., 11-14 gm as compared to 7 gm for the traditional yogurt). For cancer clients or those needing increased protein and calories, consider purchasing a whole milk, Greek yogurt. There are many flavorings, sweeteners, and fruits added to increase client acceptance.

Butter

Butter is considered a dairy product because it is made with pasteurized cream and has 80% milkfat content. Butter is usually graded according to federal standards with Grades A or AA. Grade B butter is made from sour cream. When butter is churned, salt or a salty brine is added. Unsalted butter is available as well as whipped butter.

Unsalted butter is called for in some baking recipes because the butter flavor is more pronounced. Whipped butter doesn't convert well in baking recipes; it is used more as a spread.

GLOSSARY

Pasteurization of Milk
Milk or cream is heated to a specific temperature for a specified amount of time

Ultra-Pasteurized
Heated to a higher temperature for a shorter period of time

Ultra-High Temperature Processed Products
Products that are heated to a higher temperature and are shelf stable for up to 3 months

Grains

Grains are the seeds or kernel of cereal grasses. Grains come in many different forms depending upon the amount of milling:

- Whole grains—contain the bran (outer shell providing fiber, B vitamins, trace minerals), the endosperm (provides energy—carbohydrate and protein), and the germ (provides antioxidants, Vitamin E, B-vitamins). Whole grains that are cracked, crushed, or flaked during milling but still retain the same proportion of bran, germ, and endosperm as the original grain are also considered whole grains.
- Pearled grains—bran and germ layers are removed resulting in less fiber but faster cooking times; also known as polished grain.
- Grits—corn or oat kernels cut into smaller pieces so they cook more quickly; they are still considered whole grains. Steel-cut oats is one example.
- Flakes—whole grains that are rolled into a flattened kernel.
- Meal—whole grains that are finely ground; corn meal and graham flour are examples.
- Bran—the outer part of the grain kernel that can be flakes or fibers. Oat bran, wheat bran, and rice bran are examples.
- Germ—the bottom of the grain kernel that contains the fat and fat soluble vitamins; because of the fat content, it has a shorter shelf life.
- Flour—kernels that are ground and sifted; not considered a whole grain if the bran and germ are removed.

Cooking with whole grains and serving whole grains should be encouraged in your facility because of the added nutrient content. There are some new grains on the market that will enhance the nutrient content of your menus if used: Amaranth seeds are higher in protein content and can be used with flour in breads or pancakes. Quinoa (pronounced KEEN-wah) is higher in protein, calcium, and iron than any of the other grains. It is a small seed from South America and is used like rice.

The interest in gluten-free products has skyrocketed in the past several years. Gluten is a type of protein found in many grains. As the CDM, CFPP, you need to know which products are gluten-free to meet the increased demand from your clients. See Figure 4.2 for a table of grains that are considered whole grains, not whole grains, and gluten-free grains.

Flours

Flours can be made from almost any grain. Besides fiber, one of the characteristics that differentiates flour is the amount of gluten it contains. All-purpose flour is blended wheat flour with a lower protein content than bread flour. It serves dual purpose for baking, breading, and general cooking needs. Bread flour, being higher in protein, is also higher in gluten. Gluten helps give yeast breads a higher volume. For pastries such as biscuits and cookies where high gluten content is less desirable, large commercial bakeries use pastry flour that is low-protein flour made from soft wheat. Self-rising flour contains leavening agents and added salt and should be avoided with low-sodium diets.

Corn starch is similar to flour in that it is finely ground endosperm, the starchy part of the kernel. It is used as a thickener in place of flour because the final cooked product is translucent rather than opaque. A substitute for corn starch as a thickener is arrowroot or tapioca.

Figure 4.2
Whole Grains Guide

WHOLE GRAINS	NOT WHOLE GRAINS	GLUTEN-FREE GRAINS
Look for these terms on the label:	Not whole grain if the label reads:	
• Cracked wheat • Crushed wheat • Whole wheat flour • Graham flour • Bromated whole wheat flour • Whole (wheat or corn) • Wheat berries • Oat groats • Rolled oats • Brown rice • Brown rice flour • Wild rice • Amaranth • Whole barley • Quinoa • Kasha/buckwheat groats • Whole millet • Wild rice • Whole rye flour and flakes	• Flour, white flour, wheat flour • All-purpose flour • Unbleached flour • Bromated flour • Instantized flour • Self-rising flour • Any grain product labeled "enriched" • Bread flour • Cake flour • Durum flour • Corn or hominy grits • Farina • Semolina • White rice • Couscous • Pearled barley	• Quinoa • Rice • Sorghum • Teff • Amaranth • Buckwheat • Corn • Hominy • Millet

Pasta

Pasta is made from high-protein wheat flour or durum semolina flour. Pasta comes in a large variety of shapes, most of which can be used with sauces or in casseroles. Your menu, your recipes, and the chef/cook can help decide which pasta shapes to purchase. Ask your foodservice vendor for a poster with the various pasta shapes or do a quick Web search for a guide to pasta shapes and sauces. Another consideration besides the shape is whether the pasta will be made with an egg product, such as egg noodles, and whether you will purchase fresh or dry pasta. Fresh pasta is highly perishable. Some pasta is available frozen.

Some Asian recipes call for other types of noodles such as rice noodles, made from rice, or chow mein noodles, made from wheat. Bean starch noodles or cellophane noodles are made from mung bean starch. Both rice noodles and cellophane noodles can be fried very quickly and added to dishes as a garnish. Asian noodles are usually stir-fried or used as a base or garnish rather than served with a sauce.

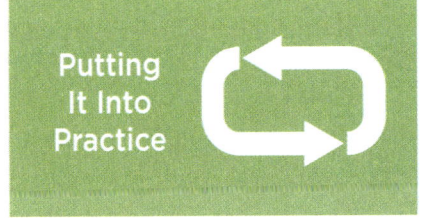

Putting It Into Practice

2. You oversee purchasing milk for a school foodservice operation. What would your specifications include for the milk vendors?

Meats

Beef, Pork, Lamb, and Veal: Meat will obviously be the high dollar item in your food budget. Therefore, knowing about meat quality, how it is handled after delivery, and cooking methods are extremely important. Fortunately, there is help from the **National Association of Meat Purveyors (NAMP)**. They publish a *Meat Buyer's Guide* based on the USDA's **Institutional Meat Purchase Specifications (IMPS)**. The guide is available for purchase at this URL: www.namp.com/namp/Default.asp

Most of the meat today is purchased portioned or a retail, ready-to-use cut rather than in wholesale large cuts such as a hind-quarter. All meat that crosses state lines is required to be inspected by the federal government; if it is processed and sold within a given state, the inspection must be equivalent to the federal standards. Grading of meat, such as prime and choice for beef, is not mandatory. However, the grading process helps to identify for consumers the relative eating quality of the product. If you are responsible for procuring meat in your facility or department, use the *Meat Buyer's Guide* to help you understand the purchasing language and process.

Poultry: The past 10 years has seen an explosion in the selection of cooked and processed poultry products available to CDM, CFPPs. As with the other products, examine your menu and recipes. Together with the chef/cook, decide which poultry products would be the best buy for your facility and clientele. If the chef is skilled at making homemade soups, purchasing whole poultry or cut-up pieces that will yield bones for stock might be a good investment. Would portioned cuts be the best for the skills of the staff? Pulled chicken, rather than uniform diced pieces of chicken, might be needed for salads or casseroles. Before finalizing the purchase order, know what your needs are in terms of the types of poultry cuts.

Poultry has a mandatory inspection for wholesomeness and optional grading. Grade A poultry is most commonly sold to commercial facilities. The grading relates to the fat covering, discolorations, feathers, thickness of flesh, and other overall quality criteria.

Irradiated Stamp

Grade Stamp

Inspection Stamp

Today, both raw meat and raw poultry products may be irradiated to increase product safety and extend the shelf life. The **FDA** requires that irradiated meat and poultry be labeled as such.

Fish and Shellfish: When it comes to purchasing fish and shellfish, fresh is not always the best choice. As soon as fish is caught, it loses its ability to fight off bacteria. Most fish today is quickly frozen within hours of being caught and this fresh-frozen choice may be the best option depending upon your geographic location. If fish are intended for raw or undercooked consumption (such as sushi or cold-smoked salmon), it must be properly frozen before being served to kill worms deeply imbedded inside fish muscle.

GLOSSARY

National Association of Meat Purveyors (NAMP)
They publish the industry standard Meat Buyer's Guide based on the USDA's Institutional Meat Purchase Specifications (IMPS)

The U.S. Food and Drug Administration (FDA)
A federal agency responsible for monitoring trading and safety standards in the food and drug industries

Look for labeling or other information to assure that the fish was properly frozen.

The U.S. Department of Commerce does voluntary inspection of fish and shellfish. Look for the **Packed Under Federal Inspection (PUFI)** mark on packages to assure that the fish is safe, wholesome, and properly labeled. There is also grading for fish similar to other meats. The Grade A stamp assures that the product is free from blemishes and defects, and is of high quality with good flavor and aroma. The **FDA Food Code** recommends that fish be purchased from a state-approved vendor and that it be commercially or legally harvested.

Fish can be purchased in many sizes and shapes. The following are common examples of what you might purchase:

- Fish fillet—product is cut the length of the fish parallel to the backbone; it can be an irregular shape and size
- Portioned cuts—square or rectangular cuts from a block of frozen fish; fish sticks are one example
- Steaks—product is cut across the fish into slices

See Figure 4.3 for a Seafood Buying Guide. The buying guide only addresses commonly served fish and shellfish. If your facility serves high-cost shellfish, be sure you investigate the proper storage and purchasing information for products such as fresh lobster, oysters, clams, and mussels. Make sure that you are purchasing from an approved seafood vendor and that the seafood is "commercially or legally harvested" per the FDA Food Code guidelines.

Fresh and Canned Produce

Fresh or canned produce is most likely part of every meal served so having purchasing standards will be critical to serving quality meals.

> **GLOSSARY**
>
> **Packed Under Federal Inspection (PUFI)**
> Packed Under Federal Inspection mark on packages assures that fish is safe, wholesome, and properly labeled
>
> **FDA Food Code**
> The FDA's best advice for a system of provisions that address the safety and protection of food offered at retail and foodservice outlets

Figure 4.3
Seafood Buying Guide

FISH OR SEAFOOD TYPE	CHARACTERISTICS TO LOOK FOR
Fresh or Thawed Fillets and Steaks	Mild odor; firm, elastic flesh; no bruising, blood spots, or browning
Fresh or Thawed Shrimp—sold by the count per pound (e.g., extra large shrimp are 26-30 shrimp per pound)	Flesh completely fills the shell; no strong odors; no black edges or spots; moist but not slimy feel
Surimi	Firm and moist; possess an off-white color; no strong odors; flesh should have a light pink tint
Frozen Seafood	No signs of frost on seafood or package interior; no signs of drying as in white patches; no strong odors; should be solidly frozen
Smoked Fish	Clean, smoky odor; firm texture; no signs of mold or salt crystals

Fresh Produce

There are changes occurring in the fresh produce industry: 1) purchasing fresh produce at farmer's markets is gaining in popularity; 2) pre-cleaned and cut produce is widely available today and in some cases may be less expensive than the whole product.

Farmers' Markets: Fresh produce is best at peak harvest and you will have the highest quality and nutritional value if you purchase from local farmers. Farmers' markets rarely sell graded products as the USDA grading program is voluntary. They may sell their products under a different name for a grade such as firsts and seconds. Check your menu and recipe needs to determine what level of quality is needed. If exterior appearance is important (i.e., when you are serving whole or pieces of fresh fruit or vegetables), then pay for the top-quality product. If the product is going to be mashed, chopped, or pureed, then choosing the lower quality grade will be your best buy. Check state and local regulations regarding the use of local suppliers and compliance with the "approved vendor" status. Get to know your vendors and how they keep the product fresh between harvesting and market. They might also be willing to deliver products to your facility.

Pre-Cleaned and Cut Produce: Again, you have to know your menu and recipes and what staff time and skill level is available to determine the best produce to purchase. If the pre-cleaned or cut produce is cheaper and meets the needs of the facility, go one step further and make sure vendors have HACCP (Hazard Analysis Critical Control Point) plans in place. Pre-cleaned and cut produce should be processed in clean, cold facilities and delivered in refrigerated trucks.

Canned and Frozen Fruits and Vegetables

Processing slightly reduces nutritional content of canned and frozen products but not enough to abandon the use of them. Frozen products have a higher quality appearance because freezing doesn't cause color and texture changes as much as canning. This is especially true for the **IQF (Individually Quick Frozen)** products. Frozen products can contain more nutrients than fresh because they are processed soon after harvesting. Many fresh products sit in store rooms or produce counters for a long time after harvesting, thus losing nutritional value.

The USDA has voluntary grading of quality for many canned and frozen vegetables and fruits. The most common are U.S. Grade A (Fancy), U.S. Grade B (Extra-select or Choice), and U.S. Grade C (Standard). Grading is paid for by the packer and packers may use different terminology. Grades are based on appearance criteria: color, uniformity of size, shape, lack of blemishes, or lack of stems/leaves. Like fresh produce, purchase only the grade that you need. If you are using canned tomatoes for pasta sauce, you don't need to purchase Grade A or Fancy.

Preparation and Quality Standards

Preparation tips indicated below are not meant to be cooking or production instructions. They offer guidelines and parameters for the foodservice operation in

> **GLOSSARY**
>
> **Individually Quick Frozen (IQF)**
> A process of rapid freezing that yields smaller ice crystals and maintains the individual units of fruits, berries, vegetables, and meat items

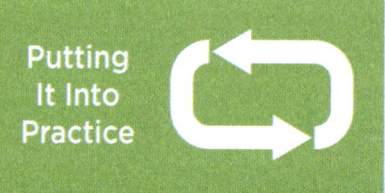

3. Your menu has pasta, wheat tortillas, and bread. What are some substitutes you can offer to your clients with gluten sensitivities? Plan a 5-day menu for lunch and dinner using wheat alternates.

menu planning and maintaining consistency in meal preparation. These standards also serve as a tool in employee training. Consider purchasing a book like *Food for Fifty* by Mary Molt to find recipes and full cooking instructions. Some organizations maintain a notebook of photographs of the final plate presentation for their different menu items. That way, production and serving staff will be reminded what the product should look like, down to the garnishing, when it is completed. You will find more detailed quality standards in *Food for Fifty*.

Eggs, Cheese, and Milk

Eggs

Preparation: The two most important principles for preparing egg products are to use low temperatures and minimize cooking time. It is also helpful to review grades and sizes of shell egg products discussed earlier in this chapter. Pasteurized Grade A or AA is a good choice for eggs that will be prepared whole, such as poached or fried, because the yolks are firm and high. For other uses, Grade B is fine. Eggs are also sized. You will want to match shell egg sizes to sizes specified in any of your standardized recipes.

Menu items featuring eggs can range from scrambled eggs to omelets to frittatas to soufflés. With modified diets, you can use egg whites or egg substitute products that have been modified to reduce cholesterol and saturated fat. Figure 4.4 lists some common egg preparation problems and solutions.

Quality Standards: Quality standards for egg products should include the following:
- Fresh egg products, such as scrambled, omelets and custards, should have a soft, semisolid structure with no water separating from the cooked eggs.
- The color should be a soft yellow with no greening.

Cheese

Preparation: Cheese can add calcium, protein, and unique flavor to menu items. When you are selecting cheese for use in hot items, such as heated sandwiches, casseroles, or sauces, select a cheese with a suitable flavor and texture. Generally, it should be sliced (for sandwiches), shredded, or cubed. Low temperatures, generally no higher than 350°F, help prevent curdling, toughness, and stringiness. For food safety, a foodservice operation should select only pasteurized cheeses.

Quality Standards: A quality product containing cheese will have the cheese evenly distributed and melted with little or no browning on the top. The cheese flavor will blend with the other flavors and not be overpowering.

Milk

Preparation. Your menu and recipes will drive what milk products to purchase for cooking. See Figure 4.5 for descriptions of milk products used in cooking.

When cooking or reheating products containing milk or cream, use a low heat setting. Like cheese, milk is high in protein. When heated too rapidly, protein **coagulates** causing the milk product to potentially curdle. The film on the top of cooked milk or custards is another example of coagulated protein.

Quality Standards: Products containing milk or cream such as cream soups, sauces, and desserts will appear smooth with a uniform texture and no film. The color will be light and opaque. Products containing cream will also have a rich mouth feel and texture.

GLOSSARY

Coagulate
To cause transformation of a liquid into a soft, semisolid, or solid mass

Figure 4.4
Egg Preparation Problems and Solutions

GREENING

PROBLEM: Cooked eggs may turn green (a natural chemical reaction) if held over heat for an extended period of time.

SOLUTION:

Omelets and Scrambled Eggs
- Use fresh eggs (Grade AA or A). Greening is more likely in older eggs.
- Cook eggs in small batches, no larger than three quarts.
- Substitute a medium white sauce for the liquid in the egg mixture. (One part white sauce to five parts egg.)
- Use temperatures of 135°F and above for steam table holding.
- Do not hold hot foods on buffet line for longer than 1 hour.
- Use only stainless steel equipment and utensils.
- Try a liquid egg product if greening is frequent. (Many of these contain citric acid which slows greening.)
- Beat in 1/4 teaspoon lemon juice for every 18 large eggs, or 1/4 teaspoon citric acid crystals for every dozen large eggs.

Hard-Cooked Eggs
- Simmer eggs (185-190°F) in water. Don't boil.
- Cool immediately in cold water. Peel when cool.

WEEPING

PROBLEM: Water separating from cooked eggs is caused by overcooking or by cooking and holding at high heat or from the addition of watery ingredients.

SOLUTION:

Scrambled Eggs
- Prepare eggs in small batches, no larger than three quarts.
- Substitute a medium white sauce for the liquid in the egg mixture. (One part white sauce to five parts egg.)
- Use temperatures 135°F and above for steam table holding.
- Use egg products with stabilizers (i.e., gums) added.
- Limit the amount of added ingredients and make sure they are well-drained.

Meringues
- Lack of volume of the foam during beating or cooking:
  - Beat whites until frothy before adding sugar.
  - Add sugar slowly.
  - Stop frequently and lift whites from bottom of bowl to ensure thorough and even beating.
  - Use a clean metal or glass (not plastic) bowl.
  - Beat until sugar is dissolved, the peaks barely fold over, and whites do not slip from sides when bowl is tilted.
- If the meringue is to be used on a pie, place it on a hot (160°F or above) filling, and brown immediately at 350°F for approximately 15 minutes.
- For pie meringues containing a larger number of egg whites, reduce baking temperature and increase baking time to achieve temperature of 160°F and mixture tests done (knife inserted near center removes cleanly).

RUBBERY AND DRY EGGS

PROBLEM: The problem is the result of overcooking and high heat. It generally follows weeping.

SOLUTION:

Omelets and Scrambled Eggs
- Cook at medium heat until no visible liquid egg remains.
- Cook in small batches, no larger than three quarts.
- Use a medium white sauce as liquid in egg mixture. (One part white sauce to five parts egg.)
- Use temperatures 135°F and above for steam table holding.

Fried Eggs
- Cook over medium heat on preheated grill or pan.
- Use the right amount of fat to avoid toughening, about one teaspoon per egg.
- Baste with fat or steam-baste by adding small amounts of water and covering.

Figure 4.5
Milk Products Used in Cooking

PRODUCT	CHARACTERISTICS
Evaporated Milk	Comes as whole milk, low-fat, or fat free. Fluid milk with about 60% of the water removed.
Sweetened Condensed Milk	Comes as whole or fat free. It is evaporated milk with added sugar and processed to one-third its original volume.
Dry Milk	Comes as whole or low-fat. Dissolves in cold water; whole dry milk has a shorter shelf life because of the fat content.
Buttermilk	Can be purchased as fluid or dry product. The fluid product has a bacteria added to make it thick and tart. Dry buttermilk is dried from the liquid produced when making butter.
Half-and-Half	A mixture of whole milk and cream with 10.5-17% fat. May be used in place of light cream or table cream.
Light Cream, Table Cream	A lower-milkfat cream; cannot be used for whipping.
Light Whipping Cream	Contains a minimum of 30-36% fat and does work for whipping.
Heavy Whipping Cream	Contains a minimum of 36% fat and is preferred for whipped cream because it whips easily and holds its shape.
Sour Cream	A cultured product like yogurt except it's cultured cream. It contains 18-22% fat.

Grains

This section will address products made with grains such as yeast and quick breads, pasta, rice, and dessert products.

Yeast Bread

Preparation: Yeast breads are leavened with yeast and may be a lean dough (using little or no sugar and margarine) or a sweet dough (using sugar, margarine, and/or eggs). Lean dough is appropriate for French bread, sandwich rolls, and similar products; while sweet dough makes good caramel rolls or raisin bread. See Figure 4.6 for preparation problems and solutions.

Quality Standards: Uniform golden brown color, sounds hollow when tapped; crisp, tender crust; uniform grain, moist texture.

Quick Bread

Preparation: Quick breads include biscuits, muffins, and loaves such as banana bread or nut bread. Quick breads can be made from batter (as with muffins) or soft dough (as with biscuits that are rolled and cut).

Figure 4.6
Yeast Bread Preparation Problems and Solutions

PROBLEM	SOLUTION
Coarse, Heavy Texture	Be sure yeast is not killed by water that is too hot in initial stages or excessive equipment-generated heat in processing [use a thermometer; extend kneading time; check proofing time (may be too long or too short)]; check to be sure excessive salt was not used.
Loaf is Cracked	Avoid adding excessive flour when forming the loaf; shape loaf with care, not forcing it.
Loaf is too Big and Light	Check flour ingredient (may be too much gluten); check oven temperature (may be too low); check yeast measurement (may be too much).
Loaf Collapses	Recheck and limit proofing time; make sure oven temperature is not too low.

For any baked product, it is important to measure flour correctly. Be sure to match the product to the recipe, as presifted flour does not have the same volume as unsifted flour.

Some ingredients require packing. An example is brown sugar. Failure to pack the sugar when specified could reduce the sugar in the recipe by as much as 50 percent and affect the final product significantly.

Note that unlike yeast breads, quick breads do not rely on developing the gluten in flour, so mixing should be limited. Too much mixing causes the gluten proteins to develop, resulting in tunnels in the product.

Biscuits contain similar ingredients, but the proportion of flour is higher. A muffin dough has two parts flour to one part liquid, whereas a biscuit dough has three parts flour to one part liquid.

Quality Standards: Muffins and biscuits should be uniform size and shape; have a tender crumb, even cell structure, rounded, not peaked top, pleasing flavor, moist texture, no tunnels and a uniform golden brown color.

Pasta and Rice

Preparation: When preparing rice, macaroni, noodles, spaghetti, or similar products, general cooking principles are:

- Cook quickly in boiling water until tender. Salt the water if specified in the recipe.
    > It is not recommended to totally eliminate salt in the cooking of pasta, rice, or grains as the lack of salt changes the final product to a flat hollow taste.
- Drain quickly and stir in fat, if specified. Do not rinse.
- Avoid washing rice before cooking or rinsing pasta after cooking, as these procedures wash away valuable nutrients such as B-vitamins.

Quality Standards: Pasta should have some resistance to the bite (called al dente or tender to the tooth); not too soft or mushy. Rice grains should also be tender, not too soft, and separate easily.

Figure 4.7
Quick Bread Preparation Problems and Solutions

PROBLEM	SOLUTION
Coarse Texture with Tunnels	Avoid overmixing; recheck measurements of ingredients.
Dry Product	Avoid overbaking; also check flour measurement (may be too much).
Quick Breads Become Soggy	Remove from pans after about 5 minutes; do not let sit in pans too long.
Muffin or Biscuit Texture is Tough or Rubbery	Limit mixing; only moisten dry ingredients.
Biscuits are Dense and Don't "Rise" Much	Mix and handle the dough less.

Meat, Poultry, and Fish Products

The quality of meat products will depend upon the quality of the ingredients, the equipment in place, and the skill level of the cooking staff. Endpoint cooking standards for meat products are extremely important and are located in Chapter 19.

Beef, Pork, Lamb, and Veal

Preparation: When cooking meats, choose a dry or moist heat method. For example, tender cuts that contain little connective tissue, such as steaks and roasts, do well with dry heat methods. These include roasting, baking, broiling (for individual portions that are 1-2" thick), and frying. Less tender cuts of meat with more connective tissue require moist heat to develop tenderness and flavor.

You can use meat timetables as a general guide for cooking meat. Timetables, available in most cookbooks, are useful in determining production scheduling requirements, i.e., when to start the cooking process so that products will be done in time for service. You can measure doneness with a thermometer placed in the center of the product, not touching bone. The temperature of a roast may continue to rise after it is removed from the oven.

Quality Standards: Meat products should be evenly browned, not burned, tender, and moist. To ensure food safety, meat products are cooked to the appropriate time and internal temperature recommendations. (See Chapter 19 for a more detailed discussion on food safety and internal temperature controls of cooked food items.)

Poultry

Preparation: Poultry is available in various cuts, from whole birds to cut pieces. Generally, poultry should be cooked at a low temperature (325°-350°F) to produce a tender, juicy product. Preparation options include roasting, broiling, grilling, oven frying, and other frying methods; as well as moist-heat methods such as braising, stewing, or steaming.

As with meats, you can use timetables as a general guide for cooking poultry. It is important to verify end-point cooking temperatures with a thermometer.

Figure 4.8
Cooking Time and Temperature Guide (Suggested Minimums)

FOOD ITEM	TEMP.	TIME	COMMENTS
All whole cuts of meat such as pork, steaks, roasts, and chops	145°F	15 sec.	Allow the meat to rest for 3 minutes before consuming.
Poultry, game, stuffed fish, stuffed meat, stuffed pasta	165°F	<1 second, instantaneous	
Ground meats (beef, pork, lamb), comminuted (minced or ground) fish, and raw eggs (not prepared for immediate service)	155°F	17 sec.	
Fish, seafood, meats not listed above, raw eggs prepared for immediate service	145°F	15 sec.	
Fruits and vegetables	135°F	N/A	
Food cooked in microwave	165°F	2 min.	Hold time after cooking
Reheating leftovers	165°F	15 sec.	

Source: 2017 Food Code pg. 750

Note: These are standards recommended in the FDA Food Code. Please consult your local standards, which may be different. Also review manufacturers' instructions for processed foods.

Quality Standards: Poultry products should be lightly browned, tender, and moist. To ensure food safety, poultry products are cooked to the appropriate time and internal temperature recommendations.

Fish

Preparation: Fish should generally be cooked at a moderately high temperature, rapidly enough to retain juices and moisture, but slowly enough to ensure thorough cooking. You can match preparation techniques to the product. For example, fatty fish such as salmon lend themselves to baking and broiling. In general, consider 10 minutes cooking time per one inch thickness at 400-425°F.

Quality Standards: Fish products should be juicy, flavorful, and tender. Breaded products should be a uniform golden brown color. To ensure food safety, fish products are cooked to the appropriate time and internal temperature recommendations.

Putting It Into Practice

4. You are planning seafood options for your foodservice operation. What are some purchasing standards you would list for shrimp and salmon?

Fresh Produce

Fresh produce should be prepared as close to serving time as practical to preserve the fresh appearance and nutritional value.

Fresh Vegetables

Preparation: Careful attention to preparation techniques can help preserve nutrient values in produce, as well as flavor, appearance, and overall quality. It's important to consider the needs of the clients served, ensuring that vegetables are tender enough for any clients with chewing limitations. Sometimes chopping or grating vegetables (as in a coleslaw, for example) is an option for serving fresh vegetables. Cook vegetables in small amounts of water or steam them until they are tender but firm. If possible, schedule prep work as close to final service time as practical to maintain quality and minimize nutrient losses.

In the past, some chefs have used baking soda to brighten the color of cooked vegetables. Not only does this make the vegetable mushy, it also decreases the nutrient quantity of the vegetable. When cooking fresh vegetables, pre-cook only until color brightens and the vegetable is still crisp. Plunge into ice cold water, drain, and store in the refrigerator until ready to complete cooking immediately prior to service. This helps to preserve the color and texture. Do not over-blanch the vegetables as it can increase the nutrient loss, particularly antioxidants.

Quality Standards *(this is also appropriate for canned vegetables)*: Vegetables are cut into bite-sized pieces as appropriate for the clientele. They are cooked to a tender but firm consistency. Color is pleasing and appropriate for the vegetable.

Fruit

Preparation: Fresh fruits may be served whole, halved, or in pieces. Wash fresh fruits thoroughly before serving. Some, such as peaches and bananas, can turn brown after slicing. To prevent this, you can dip slices in ascorbic acid or diluted lemon juice after peeling or cutting. As with vegetables, you should cut or prepare fresh fruits as close to service time as practical.

Dried fruits may be served as stewed fruit or in pies, cobblers, crisps, whips, and salads. Frozen fruit should be served as soon as it has thawed (preferably before all the ice crystals have melted).

Quality Standards *(this is also appropriate for canned fruits)*: Fruits are cut into bite-sized pieces as appropriate for the clientele or the fruit recipe. Color is pleasing and appropriate for the fruit. Frozen fruit is not watery and has some ice crystals. Flavor is mildly sweet and appropriate for the fruit.

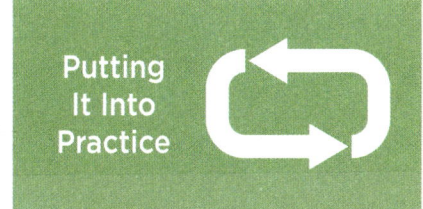

5. Your clients have complained that the breakfast eggs are watery, the bread is hard, and the meat is tough. What are some solutions you would provide to the cook during training?

Sauce

Preparation: There are several basic sauces; not all of them are thickened with a grain or starch based process:

- **Simple sauces:** A simple sauce is the au jus made from the drippings of roasted meat. The caramelized drippings are dissolved in water by stirring over heat with no thickening added. Concentrated canned soups may be used as a sauce (with no or minimal dilution); simply heat and serve hot.
- **Butter sauces:** Butter or margarine adds richness and flavor as a sauce and holds additional seasonings well. To make a butter sauce, stir seasonings into melted butter or margarine.
- **Bread sauces:** To prepare dry bread sauce, stir and brown breadcrumbs in a hot skillet with melted butter. For moist bread sauce, use two ounces of dry breadcrumbs to thicken one quart of stock.
- **Sauces thickened with egg:** These include mayonnaise and cooked sauces such as Hollandaise. The principles involved in the preparation of these sauces include the absorption of fat into the egg yolk and the ability of the egg yolk to act as an emulsifying agent and hold oil in suspension, as is the case in mayonnaise. Select pasteurized egg products for these recipes.
- **Tart or savory sauces:** Examples are barbecue sauce or teriyaki sauce. These sauces are often used on baked, broiled, and grilled meat, poultry, and fish. Marinades can be used to flavor and tenderize meats. Some include acid ingredients to help tenderize meat. If meat is marinated, do it under refrigeration. Discard the excess marinade before cooking.
- **Starch-thickened sauces:** These products use starch ingredients such as flour, cornstarch, tapioca, or others to thicken the product while heating. Cereal starch requires a boiling temperature to complete gelatinization, or the swelling of the starch granules which causes thickening to take place. Boiling must continue for five minutes to ensure complete swelling. Root starch begins to gelatinize when heated to 150°-160°F, and complete swelling is accomplished before boiling. If boiling continues, the starch granules will break down; the sauce will lose its thick appearance and become sticky. When preparing a starch-thickened sauce, it's important to stir continuously to prevent lumps.

A basic method for preparing a starch-based sauce begins by mixing the starch with fat. This is called a **roux**. To make a roux, blend an equal weight of melted fat and flour, and cook together three to five minutes for a white roux, five to seven minutes for a blond roux, and ten minutes for a brown roux. Next, remove roux from the heat and add to the hot liquid, whipping with a wire whip. Return to heat while stirring until it reaches a boil. Cooking thickens the sauce and removes the starchy flavor.

Quality Standards: Quality standards for gravies and sauces should include: smooth texture; not too thick; lightly salted. The appearance and texture depends upon the type of sauce or gravy:

- White sauce (made with milk): White, opaque color
- Cream sauce (made with cream): Light yellow, rich mouth-feel
- Béchamel (made with part milk or cream and chicken or fish stock): Light yellow, rich mouth-feel
- Veloute (made only with chicken or fish stock): Light yellow
- Brown sauce (made with browned roux): Rich brown color, lightly toasted flavor, has a slight sheen

---

GLOSSARY

Roux
Is made from equal parts fat and flour and used to thicken sauces and gravies

Ingredient Substitutions and Monitoring Food Waste

During food production, sometimes things go wrong. An ingredient may be unavailable due to a delayed delivery, a shortage from the supplier, or an error. Or a recipe may fail due to errors in standardization, changes in ingredients, or errors made by a cook. In each of these situations, a CDM, CFPP is likely to be called upon to solve the problem.

Substitutions

When ingredients are not available, the CDM, CFPP needs to make a decision about substituting ingredients. A reasonable policy is to have substitutions routinely approved by a manager, rather than left to the cook's discretion. This policy ensures that the manager will become aware of supply problems. This allows the manager to further investigate the problems and take steps to ensure against repeated shortages.

Work with the staff to develop a standard ingredient substitution list. Some ingredients do not substitute well. However, many common ingredients can be changed. Figure 4.9 lists examples of common ingredient substitutions that may be acceptable in many recipes.

Occasionally, it may also be necessary to substitute entire products in a menu, due to shortages. To make these decisions, look for the most similar product you can identify. For example, a substitution for breaded chicken strips might be breaded chicken breasts. A substitution for meatloaf might be Salisbury steak or a ground beef patty. A substitution for cooked oatmeal might be cream of wheat. In each of these decisions, double check the intended substitution for each special diet served. Key nutritional components, such as calories, protein, fat, and carbohydrates, should remain about the same. Also give special consideration to any client with unique restrictions, such as food allergies or intolerances.

Beyond the substitution issue, sometimes there is an error in production leading to unacceptable products or recipe flops. Figure 4.10 lists ideas for dealing with common production problems.

Monitoring Food Waste

There is an old management adage in food service: "You can't control what you don't measure." When it comes to controlling food costs and food production, you also need controls for what food is wasted. Implement a waste log and ask employees to record what was wasted and why. This waste is then calculated as part of the food cost.

It is also important to occasionally monitor items that are discarded daily. There have been incidents where employees have hidden food in trash bags and then transferred it to their vehicle.

View the Supplemental Material for a Food Leftover Usage Chart.

Another control is using food waste that is edible (such as leftovers) that can't be used for another meal, as donations to hunger relief charities.

As follow-up to any problem that arises during food production, investigate the causes and seek to make improvements. Whether the situation relates to inventory management, reliability of suppliers, errors in standardized recipes, or skills of employees, it is up to the CDM, CFPP to implement improvements.

Figure 4.9
Common Ingredient Substitutions

These substitutions work in some recipes, but not all. Substitution decisions require culinary experience and sound judgment.

INGREDIENT	INGREDIENT SUBSTITUTE
1 lb. butter	1 lb. margarine
1 cup milk	1/4 cup dry milk plus 1 cup water
1 cup buttermilk	1 cup plain yogurt or 7/8 cup milk plus 1 Tbsp. vinegar or lemon juice
1 tsp. baking powder	1/3 tsp. baking soda plus 1/2 tsp. cream of tartar
1 cup cracker crumbs	1 cup bread crumbs
1 Tbsp. cornstarch (for thickening)	2 Tbsp. flour
1 clove garlic, minced	1/8 tsp. garlic powder
1 tsp. lemon juice	1/2 tsp. vinegar or 1 tsp. lime juice
1 lb. dried beans	Approx. 5 cups cooked beans (adjust liquids)
1 cup packed brown sugar	1 cup granulated sugar (may add 1 Tbsp. molasses)

Figure 4.10
Solutions for Common Production Problems

PROBLEM	SOLUTION
Soup or sauce curdles	Add milk and beat rapidly
Chips are stale	Heat in oven at 350°F for 10 minutes
Soup is under yield	Add broth, tomato juice, or other liquid as appropriate
Baked product is overly browned	Cut off dark edges
Product is too salty	Add a small amount of sugar (if not for special diets) or if it is a soup
Product is too dry	Add a small amount of sauce or gravy

Source: Adapted from F&N Training Paks, © 1998, The Grossbauer Group

Nutrient Control and Special Diets

If you are serving special diets, you may have the responsibility to supervise the amounts of certain nutrients during food production. Foods served to clients following sodium (salt) limitations, for example, need to provide consistent and reliable amounts of sodium. The same is true for fats, as well as many other nutrients.

Meanwhile, many clients who have no special diet orders may still follow special nutritional guidelines, through personal choice and attention to healthful practices. For these clients, you also have a responsibility to standardize and control nutrient content of menu items. Furthermore, if you label foods served by nutritional content, you have an obligation to ensure the labeling is truthful on an ongoing basis.

To ensure this control, specify salt, fats, and other ingredients in standardized recipes. Avoid using phrases like, "salt and pepper to taste" or "add butter as desired" or "pour olive oil liberally over all." Instead, test and standardize quantities for these ingredients. It is also important to standardize amounts of salt to add to water for pasta, rice, and vegetables.

Vegetables, stir-fries, hamburgers, and many other foods can be produced on a batch basis throughout service. Often, cooking in small, continuous batches minimizes holding times, preserves nutrients, and boosts final quality of products at the time of service. This is called **batch cooking**.

It is also essential to practice meticulous portion control. Not only does portion control affect the success of standardized recipe yields and food costing plans, it also affects nutrient control. Over-portioning a product by 10 percent increases calories, fat, sodium, protein, and other nutrients by 10 percent. An accumulation of portion control errors through a one-day menu can seriously violate the controls intended by a special diet.

In producing food, also pay special attention to texture and consistency, especially for products served to clients with swallowing disorders. Variations from standards established for product consistency can make mealtime difficult, or even dangerous, for a client with a swallowing disorder.

Making special diets appealing sometimes requires culinary creativity and a flair for presentation. Particularly in a healthcare or a correctional facility, you may be serving clients whose appetites are compromised due to illness, disability, side effects from medications, psychological stress, or even depression. Extra attention to presentation, attractive **garnishing**, and other visual details can play a strong therapeutic role.

Dysphagia/puréed diets in particular require planning. In a skilled nursing facility, a quarter of clients (or more) may be eating from a texture-modified menu containing plain puréed foods. These foods typically offer little visual appeal (such as pale brown for puréed meat).

> **GLOSSARY**
>
> **Batch Cooking**
> Cooking in small continuous batches to preserve nutrients and food quality
>
> **Garnishing**
> Enhancing food appearance by adding edible decorations

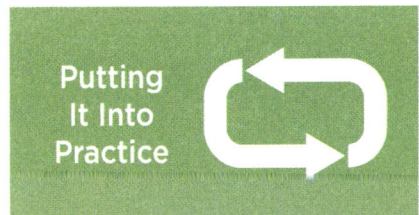

6. What are some different ways you can garnish the Grilled Salmon with Wild Rice before serving it to your clients?

Experienced CDM, CFPPs use food processors to blend casseroles, rather than serving plain foods. They also emphasize using seasonings, thickening ordinary foods, serving slurries, and adding milk or other ingredients to bring entrées up to required protein and calorie needs.

Today, healthcare foodservice managers use specially-developed recipes, color combinations, flavor combinations, and safe garnishes to make puréed menu items interesting, attractive, and appealing. Puréed meat products can also be molded to look more like their source foods.

Garnishing

Garnishing foods is a small touch that goes a long way. A simple garnish provides a polished appearance with professional zest and can entice appetites. Garnishes can be part of many standardized recipes, and foodservice staff can benefit from training in presenting food. An appropriate garnish is always edible and safe to eat. Often, it complements the color and flavor of the food, such as a lemon wedge on fish or minced parsley on soup. Remember to calculate the cost of garnishes. While there are many possibilities for garnishing, here are a few ideas:

- Lemon or orange wedge (on fish, chicken, salads)
- Fruit sliced in a fan shape
- Melon balls (with cold plates)
- Cucumber and/or carrot curls; cherry tomatoes (with sandwiches)
- Croutons (on soups or salads)
- Grated cheese (on soups, salads, or hot vegetables)
- Parsley, dill, or rosemary sprig (with meat, poultry, or fish entrées)
- Minced herbs (on soups or casseroles)
- Whipped cream (on desserts or beverages)
- Maraschino cherry (on desserts)
- Flavored syrup (drizzled on cakes in a zigzag pattern)
- Carved vegetables (with entrées or cold items)
- Paprika and/or minced chives (on potato products)
- Grated summer squash on salads

Chapter References

RESOURCES	
American Egg Board	https://www.aeb.org/food-manufacturers/where-to-buy-egg-products
Dairy Good	https://dairygood.org/health-and-wellness
FDA Food Code	fda.gov
Food for Fifty	Molt, Mary, Pearson Education, Inc.
Goat World	http://goatworld.com/articles/goatmanagement.shtml
Gregoire, Mary (2013). Foodservice Organizations, A managerial and systems approach, 8th ed. Upper Saddle River; NJ: Pearson Prentice Hall	
National Association of Meat Purveyors (NAMP) *Meat Buyer's Guide*	https://www.meatinstitute.org/index.php?ht=d/sp/i/107919/pid/107919
The Diamond Approach to Quality Improvement in Food Service: Eck Mills, Linda S., Dietary Manager, May 2010, pgs. 25-27	
USDA Leftover Food Usage Policy	https://fns-prod.azureedge.net/sites/default/files/sfsp/SMT-LeftoverMeals.pdf
USDA Specifications and U.S. Grade Standards	https://www.fns.usda.gov/fdd/specifications-us-grade-standards

Food Production Systems

Overview and Objectives

Many factors go into the production and distribution of food. The difference between quality food service and poor food service is the Certified Dietary Manager®, Certified Food Protection Professional® (CDM®, CFPP®) who compares the key standards to current practice and takes necessary action to ensure quality production. After completing this chapter, you should be able to:

- Identify the type of food production system used by a foodservice operation
- Use production planning tools effectively and write out a production schedule for a menu
- Provide a forecast for a menu item
- Train staff on food quality control and ingredient control

Food production is the step that links the menu and purchasing to the actual service of a meal to your client. Chapter 2 discussed the menu as an important control in any foodservice operation while Chapters 3 and 4 addressed production controls and standards such as standardized recipes, purchasing, preparation standards, and portioning. This chapter looks at the various food production systems and other controls in the production and distribution process that affect the quality and quantity of food.

Food Production Systems

Food production can vary in complexity depending on the type of kitchen, the menu produced, the skilled labor force available, and the number of people to be served. It will also change as the distance between the kitchen and the service area increases. The simplest type of food production is a **conventional or traditional food service**. Here food is purchased for an individual operation, and production, distribution, and service are completed on the same premises. Following production, foods are held hot or refrigerated per the menu requirements and served as soon as possible. Foods prepared in a conventional food service may be distributed for service directly in an adjacent or nearby serving area such as in many senior care facilities or using tray service as in a hospital foodservice operation. With conventional food service, a big disadvantage is the labor cost as menu items are produced for immediate service. **Ready prepared food service** has evolved as a solution to the erratic labor needs of a traditional foodservice. Here menu items are produced and held chilled or frozen until heated for service.

Cook-chill and cook-freeze are two methods used in ready prepared food service. The food is prepared in advance, often in a production center, and either "blast chilled" or frozen and held for service later. Food items may be distributed for reheating in bulk and served in a satellite dining room such as congregate meals or a remote facility. Individual meals may be pre-plated cold on a trayline system and reheated in specialty equipment prior to service. Meals are shipped to other buildings or transported by carts to nursing units for rethermalizing. Often, cook-chill is a model used by school systems, where food production is centralized, and food is transported to individual school cafeterias for plating at the time of service.

The **commissary foodservice** system (also known as central kitchen, central food production) centralizes food production, and food is transported to satellites (receiving kitchens) where it is served to customers. Food usually is purchased with minimal processing, and food production is done in the central kitchen, which results in lower food costs. Labor costs also are lower because of the centralization of food preparation. This foodservice system takes advantage of economies of scale, so it is most effective when mass food production is required. The airline industry is a good example of where a commissary food production system is used. Many large school districts also use a central kitchen for food production and then food is transported to various satellite kitchens to be reheated and served at individual schools.

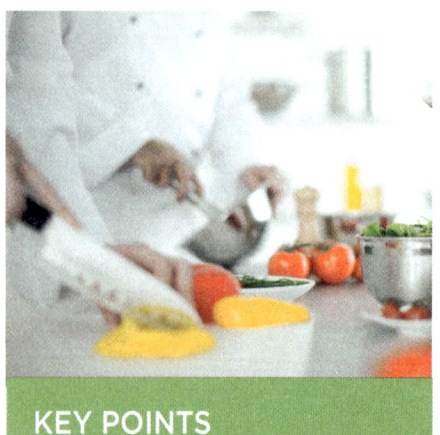

KEY POINTS

The key types of food production are:
- Traditional or Conventional
- Ready Prepared (cook-chill and cook-freeze)
- Commissary
- Assembly-serve

Putting It Into Practice

1. Your facility runs a conventional foodservice operation. However, it's challenging to prepare food right before service for every menu item. What are some changes you would make to the menu to ease the labor schedule?

In today's environment labor is scarce and expensive. Also, there are many choices of foods that can be bought pre-cooked and only require heating and serving prior to service. This bring us to the fourth type of production system, which is **assembly-serve food service**. Here food is purchased partly or fully processed. The purchased food is stored either frozen or chilled for later use. It is then portioned, reheated, and served to customers. The assembly-serve foodservice system traditionally has been the least common, although that is changing due to the current operating environment.

Many foodservice operations will use a combination of these four production systems. A traditional foodservice operation may purchase frozen chicken nuggets which are then reheated and served to customers with minimal preparation. This reduces the pressure on their labor schedule although it raises the food cost of the product since it has not been prepared from scratch.

Time and Temperature Controls in Food Production

One of the greatest influences on the quality and quantity of food served is controlling time and temperature. So far, examples of quality standards for preparation addressed criteria such as purchasing the appropriate quality of product, using low heat when preparing high protein foods, and comparing end products to expectations prior to service. Time and temperature controls should be added to your standardized recipes so that foods are cooked to the proper temperature, within a given amount of time, and then cooled and stored properly. These standards, combined with the sanitation guidelines from the **Food & Drug Administration (FDA Food Code),** help ensure food safety for your clients. They also help to improve the quality of food.

> **GLOSSARY**
>
> **FDA Food Code**
> The FDA's best advice for a system of provisions that address the safety and protection of food offered at retail and foodservice outlets

How do you supervise time and temperature to ensure food quality and quantity? Let's assume that you have procedures in place to take the temperature of foods at the time of delivery and before, during, and after service. As the CDM, CFPP, your job is to make sure that those procedures are in place, they are working, and you take any necessary corrective action. In this instance, you can do that by checking the temperature documentation and taking the temperature yourself occasionally to compare to the documentation.

What if food is being served at an improper temperature? What is the corrective action? The immediate action is to pull the food from service and adjust the food temperature. For instance, if the food is too cold, reheat the food to 165°F for 15 seconds and return it to service, which addresses the temperature issue but may create a food quality problem. The second action is to address the performance problem with the staff member responsible.

Deal with the performance issue as early as possible. If the problem occurred due to lack of training, arrange for one-on-one training right away. If the problem occurred due to lack of equipment (thermometers weren't readily available), fix it. If the person can do the job properly and just didn't do it, review the standard and hold the person accountable.

You should also have a policy that foods are tasted prior to service at each meal. Pre-meal test plates allow you to evaluate the meal to be served for consistency with the recipes as they were standardized. This step can assist in defining the plating of the meal for presentation to the client and taking temperatures of the food as it is coming off the serving line. While pre-meal test plates seem unnecessary for an established menu (after all, everyone should know how to plate and serve this meal) it becomes even more important to ensure a quality product, that you not assume compliance.

Production Planning Tools

Supervising the production and distribution of food requires using production planning tools. These tools include forecasting, food production scheduling, supervision of quality, and training for production staff.

Forecasting

Have you ever wondered how CDM, CFPPs know the amount of food to prepare for any given meal or event? **Forecasting** is the process of estimating future needs for food. It identifies both how much food to produce and how much food to order. Based on your own facility, you will determine how far in advance you need to forecast. About a week ahead is not uncommon. Based on the menu, purchasing systems, and inventory management system, a timetable or schedule for forecasting becomes a routine part of the daily operation. To create a forecast, there are several types of information typically used.

Production History: Many CDM, CFPPs keep records of the quantity of food served in the past. Maintain a production history of your past production numbers and usage. Using a menu cycle, along with past production sheets, allows you to track how much was produced the last time the item was on the menu and how much was used. Knowing if you were over by 50 servings or short by 10 servings helps refine the number of servings to be produced next time. If a computerized menu system is being used, the production history is automatically tracked for future reference.

Census Figures: Depending on the facility, this may be available in one or more forms. In a healthcare environment, the manager may use the overall daily census, or more specifically, the client count of patients/residents receiving each of a variety of menus or diet types on corresponding days of the menu cycle. Keeping track of census can be as simple as writing the count on a wall calendar every day.

Tally Figures: In a computerized menu system, the program may tally each item selected or served on a menu. These tallies become valuable detail for the next forecast. In this system, a CDM, CFPP essentially transfers the tally figures on the computer from a past menu cycle day to the next one, making any manual adjustments desired.

If you are conducting a manual tally of items for production, keep in mind that the only recipes that really need to be tallied are those for items that are made by the each at the time of service. A tally counted at 10:00 for Beef Stew to be served at 11:45 is of no value to the production team. You have already thawed the beef and made the stew in enough quantity to meet the needs based on prior history (forecasting). However, an accurate count of how many of the made-to-order Roasted Turkey on a Croissant cold plates you will need is very important.

Using historical data such as census and tallies, a CDM, CFPP also must evaluate whether the predictions were accurate the last time around. For example, did the service line run out of food before the service ended? Or, did the cook report large quantities of leftovers of any item? These must be considered for the next estimate. A standard procedure is to provide a form for documenting shortages and **leftovers**. Managers may include an over/short column on the Production Sheets that the cooks use, or on the Panning Charts that the serving line uses. See Figure 5.1 in the Supplemental Material.

Keep these records for at least two or three times through the menu cycle and review them frequently. If there are excessive leftovers, this can be a sign that the forecast

---

GLOSSARY

Forecasting
Estimating future product needs for menu items

Production History
Maintain a history of the production levels and usage as the basis for estimating future needs

Census Figures
The count of clients and customers present or available to access your services

Tally Figures
The actual count of individual items needed for a meal service

Leftovers
The number of servings remaining after a meal has been served

View the Supplemental Material for this chapter for Figure 5.1, Sample of a Simple Production Sheet with Over/Short.

needs to be decreased. However, if a particular product consistently runs out before service ends, this is a sign that more should be produced. It is particularly important to encourage employees to complete production records accurately when service ends, and to monitor overproduction and underproduction for continued planning.

Weather plays a big part in how many meals are served for different facilities. Attendance at K-12 schools, a college or university, and a retirement center or senior housing may all be dramatically affected by the weather. Along with your census figures, make a note about the weather. If you have a record of how many were served on a rainy day, you can use this information for future rainy days. Even though forecasting figures might be pre-set in your electronic software, the system can be overridden to adjust the forecast on days when weather or campus events are likely to affect the count.

Catering can significantly impact your forecasted and tallied numbers. Typically, you ask for advance notice of catering events so you can plan appropriately for production and staffing needs. Many meetings and activities are on a regular schedule, such as the third Thursday of the month. Maintaining a calendar of known catering events helps to better forecast the impact of those events on the daily production schedule.

For a catered event, you generally have an advance client count that can be used in forecasting. The last minute notice of catering needs, while not desired but often unavoidable, can be disruptive to production planning.

Point of Sale (POS) Records: Another source for historical figures is a point of sale (POS) system or computer-based cash register system that tabulates menu items sold. This is useful in a cafeteria setting. The data may be available as a printout tape from the POS system, and/or the system may include software for forecasting that electronically accepts sales records.

To determine a forecasting methodology, ask the following questions:
- How can I best capture historical figures about the amount of food served?
- How can I verify whether these figures will carry through to the future?
- How can I capture and incorporate notes about food shortages or leftovers?
- How much variation is typical for my facility, and how much do I need to pad the figures?

A forecast is expressed in the number of servings for each menu item. Products served on multiple menus are totaled for a final count. In order to avoid shortages, a common practice is to **pad** or increase the forecast figure by a small increment, such as three to ten percent. You never want to cut the forecast so closely that you cannot serve a few more clients. The amount of padding needed depends on how much variation is normal for client count.

A forecast is more than number-crunching. It requires a willingness to make judgment calls. It is not an exact science. Effective methods for predicting needs are not universal but vary from one facility to another. Client groups, menus, and service models all affect the forecast. Starting with standard approaches, most CDM, CFPPs learn from experience, and refine their forecasting methods to the individual facility. In addition, foodservice facilities with very stable client counts on a cycle menu often devise a standard forecast that is used routinely, with only minor adjustments from cycle to cycle.

GLOSSARY

Point of Sale (POS)
Refers to the computer-based cash register systems menu item counts

Pad
The amount added to a forecasted menu item to ensure adequate quantities are available

The results of effective forecasting include:
- Smooth operations, as products are available when they are needed
- Satisfaction, as clients receive the foods they expect
- Cost control, as accuracy minimizes food waste

Food Production Scheduling

With quantities of food to deliver at single points in time, a CDM, CFPP needs to give special attention to **advance preparation** practices. Advance preparation is a general term that describes any tasks that can or must be completed before main production takes place. To determine what steps of advanced production should be completed, ask questions such as these about each recipe:

- What ingredients need to be thawed before a cook will be able to use them in this recipe (and how long will it take to thaw them following safe techniques)?
- What sub-recipes have to be produced in order to make the main recipe?

A sub-recipe is a distinct recipe routine that must be completed before production of a main recipe is possible. An example of a sub-recipe is the tomato sauce that will be used in lasagna, the pie crust that will be used in chicken pot pie, or the cooked shrimp that will be used in shrimp salad.

- What pre-preparation processing is required to bring an inventory product into the form required by the recipe?

Examples of advance processing include washing lettuce, peeling and slicing apples or potatoes, trimming fat from meat, dicing meat, crushing garlic, chopping onions, soaking dry beans, and many others.

- What products need to be pre-portioned before production can begin?

It is not always necessary to perform all possible advance preparation as a separate group of tasks. However, doing work in advance when possible often eases the workload in the few hours before service and makes it easier to meet service requirements.

Once the tasks are identified that can be performed in advance, it is helpful to establish timetables. For example, thawing frozen meat in the refrigerator may take several days. So, the **production schedule** or **daily production sheets** should indicate the need to transfer it in time. This may be referred to as the **pull list** and included at the bottom of the daily production sheets. Figure 5.2 lists tips for thawing foods.

Production Schedule Resource Management. As you build your production schedule around standardized recipes with controlled inventory and trained staff, the equipment that is available must also be considered. A production schedule that requires oven space for 10 hotel pans may not work in a kitchen with only one oven. While fryer

GLOSSARY

Advance Preparation
Any tasks that can be completed prior to the time of recipe production such as thawing meats, chopping vegetables, or making sauces

Production Schedule/Daily Production Sheet
A document that outlines what to produce, how much to make, and who is responsible

Pull List
Typically included on the Daily Production Sheet for items to be pulled from the freezer for future use

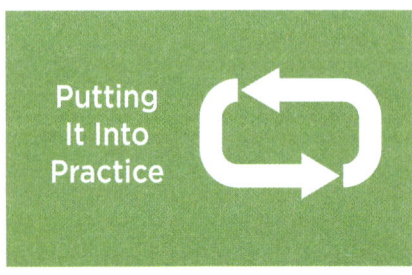

Putting It Into Practice

2. Your hospital menu has BBQ chicken on Fridays. About 65% of the cafeteria clients purchase chicken on Fridays and there are about 470 average customers. The chicken is also on the trayline menu. You serve 280 patients but currently 210 eat solid food and 40% choose BBQ chicken as their main entrée choice. How many servings of chicken will you ask to be produced for the day based on forecasting and historical records? Will you pad the forecast?

space may be no problem to meet the production needs, you may not have the staff to assign to each of the fryers.

Designing a production schedule requires you to think backwards. Not everything can come out of the oven at the same time. Scheduling when items are made is like a big jigsaw puzzle based on their equipment needs, cooking time, finishing time, and if the item can be prepped and then held in a hot box until the time of service.

- Start with the defined meal service time.
- To meet that schedule how much time do you need for final handwork on the menu item, such as slicing of the meat or panning up of the soups?
- What is the cooking time needed to get to the finishing handwork?
- Add how much prep time is needed prior to the cooking time.
- This is the recipe production time.
- Can you cook and hold it (even a day in advance) or is this a cook and serve item?

During the menu planning process, discussed in Chapter 2, consideration must be made for the needed recipe production time, equipment available, and staffing coverage. A fabulous menu that exceeds your production resources, equipment, labor, or time will frustrate the staff and fail to meet client expectations.

Production Schedule Communication: As you forecast production, plan staffing, and schedule activities, it becomes clear there is another critical piece in the flow of food production. This is communication. Scheduling production is an excellent example of a task that requires clear and precise communications for assigned staff. The main production activities require direction, too. A cook needs to know what to make, how many servings to make, when to have items ready, and where to deliver the finished products.

How this is communicated varies by facility. In some small facilities, actual food tallies or counts reach the cooks before preparation. For example, in a healthcare environment, automated menu counts may be handed to the cooks on a daily production sheet with an instruction to add a pad of several servings per item. A sample production sheet appears in Figure 5.3 (see Supplemental Material for this chapter).

View the Supplemental Material for this chapter for Figure 5.3, Sample Production Sheet.

Figure 5.2
Thawing Tips and Times

THAWING TIPS	THAWING TIMES
• Schedule thawing so that meat will be cooked soon after thawing is complete. • Do not thaw at room temperature. Use one of the approved thawing methods. • Withdraw from freezer only the amount of meat/poultry needed for one-day use. • Remove from carton and thaw in original wrappings in the refrigerator. • Space packages on refrigerator shelves so that air can circulate around them.	• Timing for large meat roasts: 4-7 hrs. per pound of meat • Timing for small meat roasts: 3-5 hrs. per pound of meat • Timing for chops, steaks: 12-14 hrs. • Timing for chicken, whole: 1 day • Timing for chicken pieces: 12-14 hrs. • Timing for whole turkey—18 lbs. or larger: 4-5 days • Timing for whole turkey—under 18 lbs.: 2-3 days • Timing for seafood in blocks: 1-2 days

> **GLOSSARY**
>
> **Pre-Preparation Recipes**
> Items that are scheduled to be produced prior to the day of service and used as part of a different recipe

The daily production sheet identifies meal, product, number of servings, and distribution instructions. Details like the number of servings needed for patient/resident meals, with a separate count for a cafeteria and yet another count for the doctor's dining room or the administrator's board meeting, are all included on the production sheets. As explained above, daily production sheets can also include the items to be pulled from the freezer (pull list) and **pre-preparation recipes** of products that will be used tomorrow or the next day.

After production, it is also important to document leftovers and shortages of each product. This information helps with future forecasting, and careful attention to this process can both improve service (supply) and reduce food waste.

Supervision of Quality

Another aspect of ongoing food production management is the supervision of quality. A CDM, CFPP should look at foods during both production and service. In addition, some facilities set up small taste panels of foods produced, either daily or at periodic intervals. Production and management personnel join together to taste samples of all products, evaluate for quality of appearance, flavor and texture (especially for texture-modified products), and make suggestions for improvement.

Another point to monitor is plate waste. Spend some time in the room where plates are being returned or in the dining room. What is on the plate? Are you seeing servings of the same food item uneaten? What is the appropriate corrective action? The initial response is to test the food still on the serving line and assess the item for current problems, over-salting or even salting, when it should have been sugar, are mistakes that happens.

Determine if the problem is an issue with the recipe itself, the ingredients used, the cook who did or did not follow the recipe, the visual presentation of the item, or does the product not meet local food preferences. When you understand what caused the issue, you can take the right steps to fix it.

Throughout the food production process, a manager should be highly visible and accessible to cooks, trayline or plating staff, and the servers. A manager needs to monitor activities and observe practices related to culinary technique, food, and employee safety. A manager should be a coach to employees who are learning new skills. In addition, a manager should be ready to intervene when it appears that production is behind schedule and make decisions when problems or substitution needs arise.

Finally, a manager needs to listen to the concerns and suggestions raised by preparation staff, servers, and the clients. For example, a staff member may suggest an improvement to a standardized recipe, an alternate production method, or an idea for presenting food more attractively. An effective manager continually seeks feedback and input from their team members in order to improve quality.

3. You are planning Thanksgiving dinner for the senior home. The menu is comprised of turkey with mashed potato and gravy, stuffing, sweet potatoes, a green salad, and premade frozen pumpkin pies. Put together a production schedule for that day indicating the items that need advance preparation.

Staff Training for Production Employees

As production employees perform their work, technique becomes critical. Many aspects of final quality rest with the cooks, including measuring, preparation techniques, presentation, and garnishing. Not every cook enters a facility with special training. However, someone in the facility should have a high level of culinary expertise.

This may be the CDM, CFPP, an executive chef, or an experienced production manager. In turn, this person should coach other members of the staff to develop skills and talents. Some facilities have a short production meeting each day to make sure production questions are answered.

Each cook needs some special training about food production. For example, a cook needs to know:

- The purpose of standardized recipes
- Standard terms used on each recipe, such as yield, portion size, etc.
- Ingredient descriptions and the distinctions among products (e.g., the difference between kosher salt and iodized salt; all-purpose flour and self-rising flour, sifted or unsifted flour, etc.)
- Utensils and methods for measuring ingredients
- Abbreviation system for measurements
- Food safety and/or HACCP standards in place for each recipe
- Procedures for requisitioning ingredients
- Cooking terms used throughout the recipe, such as sauté, simmer, bake, broil, roux, etc. A list of common cooking terms appears in Figure 5.4 (see Supplemental Material for this chapter)
- Employee safety and ergonomic practices that protect the cook and others from injury
- Proper methods for using all required equipment
- Methods for portioning and/or panning food
- Methods for holding food and/or transporting it to service
- Established timetables for production
- Procedures for addressing questions and problems

As a basic work process, a cook can follow several steps to ensure an efficient work flow:

- Read through the production sheet and be sure all assignments are clear
   > Question anything that is unclear
- Read through each recipe, and be sure all instructions are clear
- Assemble all needed ingredients
- Verify that all needed equipment, bowls, knives, and utensils are available and ready for use

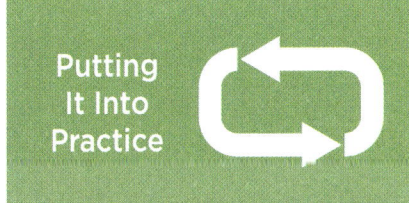

4. Plate waste at your foodservice operation is high. What steps would you take to ensure quality of food meets client acceptance?

View the Supplemental Material for this chapter for Figure 5.4, Common Cooking Terms.

- Follow the recipe procedure exactly, taking each step in sequence
- Clean up between tasks and keep the work area orderly
- Follow established sanitation guidelines
- Group errands (such as trips to the storeroom, dishroom, or trash area) and work as efficiently as possible
- Review upcoming needs for thawed products and generate advance thawing schedules that tell a storage clerk when to transfer products to refrigeration.

Use of an automated system makes it more practical to consolidate and manage production schedules without risking oversights and emergencies.

Beyond basic orientation, many foodservice employees enjoy further culinary training. You may ask your most skilled culinary employee to present cooking classes featuring basic techniques, garnishing tips, and more. When a culinary expert is not available on staff, consider inviting a local talent to present a special in-service session or series of classes.

Another option for training is to use culinary instructional videos, which are readily available from many sources. Culinary reference information, slide shows, and even video clips illustrating culinary techniques are available free on several websites. When feasible, schedule production employees to attend food and trade shows. Finally, if your facility offers a continuing education program, you may encourage employees to attend seminars or classes in preparation and culinary techniques.

It is important to encourage, acknowledge, and reward advances in knowledge and skill. Follow up to ensure the training is implemented. Often, the simple availability of training is enough to motivate employees to challenge themselves and tap into their own talents. Skillful food production brings on the immediate rewards of seeing a product that looks good, tastes good, and generates positive satisfaction ratings.

5. What would you monitor to assure production staff training has been effective? What should you do if you find the training was not effective?

Chapter References

RESOURCES	
FDA Food Code	fda.gov
Gregoire, Mary (2013). Foodservice Organizations: A managerial and systems approach, 8th ed. Upper Saddle River, NJ: Pearson Prentice Hall	
Menu Production Records Forms	https://www.cde.ca.gov/ls/nu/he/mnprodfrm.asp
Nutrition411.com Performance Improvement Worksheet	Nutrition411.com/content/performance-improvement-worksheet
Sergio, Bryan Dave. Foodservice Systems A Guide to Centralized Foodservice Systems, Introduction to Foodservice Systems, Academia.edu	

Preparation and Delivery of Between-Meal Snacks and Supplements

Overview and Objectives

A large percentage of clients receive some type of between-meal supplements. Certified Dietary Manager®, Certified Food Protection Professionals® (CDM®, CFPPs®) have to be prepared to manage the preparation and service of these supplements as well as manage the burgeoning cost of supplements. After completing this chapter, you should be able to:

- Understand types of nutrition support and their role in patient care
- Identify protocol in the implementation of special nourishments and supplemental feedings
- Monitor the cost of supplements and the audit to ensure quality compliance
- Understand F-tags and legal implications

> **GLOSSARY**
>
> **Nutrition Support**
> General term for providing foods and liquids to improve nutrition status
>
> **Nutritional Supplements**
> A food or commercial product intended to enhance nutritional intake
>
> **Enteral Nutrition**
> Supplemental feeding, by mouth or by tube, of liquid formulas that contain essential nutrients

The dual role of meeting nutritional needs and satisfying the personal menu requests of your clients is a challenge. Protein and calorie malnutrition is fairly prevalent today, and you will have clients who need specialized nutrition support. The diet order will be the primary tool used to identify clients who need nourishments or supplemental feedings. You may also gather information for the Registered Dietitian Nutritionist (RDN) on clients in poor nutritional status or with high nutrient needs. These clients are often in need of concentrated sources of nutrition. **Nutrition support** is a general term for providing foods and liquids to improve nutrition status and support good medicine.

Nutritional supplements refers to products that are used to complement a client's dietary needs (e.g., total parenteral products, enteral products, and meal replacement products). The decision to provide nutrition support of any kind beyond what the normal diet provides has clinical and financial impacts that must be considered.

Not all clients benefit from more food in general, and often require less food overall, but more calories or specific nutrients. Nutrition support can start with the addition of "regular foods" to the existing menu. This can be highly effective, particularly for seniors. For example, adding margarine or sweeteners to menu items or adding half a sandwich as a bedtime snack can boost the daily intake for calories.

To effectively impact the nutritional status of a client, it is important to start the dietary recommendations with a complete diet history and discuss food tastes, preferences, and tolerances with a client. This helps to identify good candidates for "regular food" menu enhancements or those who will be better served through a commercially-prepared supplement. See Figure 6.1 for menu planning techniques for nutrition support.

Use food first as a supplement. Providing foods at meals that the client likes will encourage them to eat better. In some cases this may not be the menu of the day. If a resident wants a sandwich at every meal and they eat it, that is better than giving the meal of the day and only having a 25 percent meal consumption.

The use of commercially-prepared nutritional supplements and tube feedings often requires medical staff approval. Nutrition formulas are available to supplement what a client is already consuming or may provide 100 percent of a resident/patients' nutritional needs in a liquid form. There are literally hundreds of different products from several different manufacturers, each designed to meet a specific need.

Enteral nutrition refers to the feeding, by mouth or by tube, of liquid formulas that contain essential nutrients. It requires that the gastrointestinal tract be functioning. Specialized commercial products exist for providing nutrition support. A standard enteral formula provides one calorie per milliliter (ml). (About 240 ml equals one cup.) Other enteral formulas may provide 1.2, 1.5, or 2 cal/ml. A complete enteral product contains a nutritional balance of protein, carbohydrates, fat, vitamins, and minerals. Some are flavored so they can be taken orally.

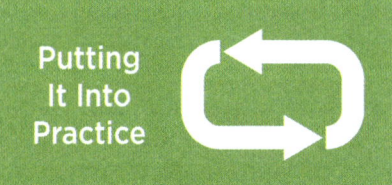

1. You are working with the interdisciplinary team in the nutrition care process for an older client who needs additional calories between meals. What steps would you take to enhance her diet and ensure that the meal supplements meet her needs?

Figure 6.1
Menu Planning Techniques for Nutrition Support

- Use margarine liberally on bread, toast, vegetables, rice, pasta, and in sandwiches.
- Add gravies or sauces to entrées and side dishes.
- Add sour cream to potatoes, casseroles, and fruits.
- Use real whipped cream on top of desserts and fruits.
- Add 2 tablespoons dried milk powder to each cup of whole milk. Use for drinking and when making cream soups, hot cereal, pudding, custard, hot chocolate, mashed potatoes, casseroles, milkshakes, and creamed dishes.
- Add dried milk powder to scrambled eggs, gravies, casseroles, meatloaf, and meatballs.
- Spread peanut butter or other nut butters on toast, English muffins, crackers, cookies, apple slices, and celery sticks.
- Add cheese to sandwiches, scrambled eggs, casseroles, vegetables, and sauces.
- Add chopped eggs and diced or ground meat to salads, sauces, casseroles, and sandwiches.
- Use mayonnaise liberally on sandwiches.
- Choose desserts such as custard, bread pudding, rice pudding, and fruited yogurt. Serve with real whipped cream or ice cream.
- Offer whole milk products or cream in place of skim milk, or offer milkshakes as beverages.
- Cook cream soups or hot cereal with whole milk; add margarine or butter.
- Serve six small meals rather than three large ones.
- Add ice cream to enteral products as a milkshake.
- Use enteral pudding supplements as a topping for cake desserts.
- Add olive oil or flavored oils to potatoes and vegetables.

Incomplete nutritional supplements offer another way to boost nutritional intake. For example, a product of carbohydrate powder with minimal flavor can be stirred into beverages, soups, applesauce, and other foods to add almost invisible calories. Another commercial product is protein powder used to boost protein content when added to mashed potatoes, hot cereal, soup, or other products.

Another type of commercially-prepared products are the formulas for parenteral nutrition. **Parenteral nutrition** is the administration of simple essential nutrients into a vein. Parenteral solutions may contain dextrose, lipids, amino acids, electrolytes, vitamins, and trace elements. They may be used in cases where the client's gastrointestinal tract is no longer able to digest and absorb food properly; to maintain fluid and electrolyte balance both before and after surgery; or when a client is not receiving enough nourishment by other feeding methods.

Implementation of Special Nourishments and Supplemental Feedings

Work with your Registered Dietitian Nutritionist to select special nourishments and supplemental feedings. In selecting an enteral product for oral or tube feeding, a nutrition caregiver should consider the following:

- Taste, texture, and individual client acceptance in an oral supplement
- Tolerance of lactose
- Product concentration of specific nutrients
- The need for nutritionally complete formulation
- Needs for modification in carbohydrate, fat, or protein composition
- Location of the feeding tube if tube fed
- Whether or not to include fiber
- Cost

GLOSSARY

Parenteral Nutrition
The administration of simple essential nutrients into a vein

CLINICAL NOTE

The Registered Dietitian Nutritionist should work with the clinical staff and medical provider in establishing the use of medically-appropriate nutrition support (from basic supplements to parenteral nutrition) to meet the needs of the client. Likewise, the clinical team should regularly assess the effectiveness and impact on the clinical outcomes of the nutrition support and implement changes as needed.

GLOSSARY

Formulary
A list of nutritional products approved for use

Many of the commercial manufacturers have developed a "decision tree" to assist clinicians in the selection of the most appropriate product (See Figure 6.2). Work with dietitians, pharmacists, nursing managers, and purchasing to define a **formulary** of products that will be stocked in your organization and define the criteria for each product's use. Approval and support from the Medical Staff Director is usually required and will help "ease" the transition by all medical staff to a defined number of products.

Advantages and Disadvantages of Commercial Supplements for Your Own Facility

Does the staff have the expertise and/or the time to prepare your own supplements and nourishments? Perhaps you can combine commercial products with conventional foods. For example, a client who does not enjoy a liquid supplement may enjoy a milkshake made from the supplement plus ice cream. Instead of purchasing protein powder, consider adding nonfat dried milk (NFDM) to mashed potatoes, soups, and desserts.

For your clients who prefer it—or for certain dysphagia diets—specialized nutritional pudding products represent another choice. Pudding supplements are nutritionally similar to the liquid supplements that are available. A garnish of real whipped cream, chocolate shavings, or fruits may also make these products more appealing.

Some disadvantages to commercial supplements include acceptance and cost. Client acceptance may vary, as clients may perceive a flavor described as "medicinal" or tasting "like vitamin supplements." On the other hand, these products are available in a variety of flavors and textures that may help to overcome this drawback.

When offering commercial supplements, it is important to allow a client to taste several products and choose what seems most enjoyable. Some facilities have a client taste panel to help determine what supplements the dining services department will purchase.

The cost of nutrition supplements can range from less than the cost of a typical snack to being outrageously expensive. As the CDM, CFPP, you may be expected to manage these expenses as part of your food costs. Some facilities purchase their supplements through the pharmacy and the cost is not allocated to dietary. In some cases tube feedings are paid for by nursing and oral feedings by dining services. Whatever purchasing policy your facility has, it is important to remember cost cannot be the only consideration; it is just one of them.

Keep in mind that the cost of the items used should be directly related to the beneficial clinical outcome. If the client has not consumed the mid-afternoon strawberry flavored supplement because she has been having it daily and is now tired of it, the staff all believe the client is receiving added nutrients when, in reality, the product is being thrown away. This is where a rotation of different snacks can reduce the flavor fatigue and increase supplement intakes.

Nourishment Delivery Systems

Many of the liquid supplements are better accepted when served very cold. If your delivery system isn't efficient, those supplements may arrive too warm and therefore may not be consumed. When managing nutrition supplements it is important to consider when and how they are delivered to clients.

Nearly all healthcare facilities offer snacks to clients. Not all snacks are supplements. A snack may be a simple cookie offered midmorning or birthday cake in the afternoon.

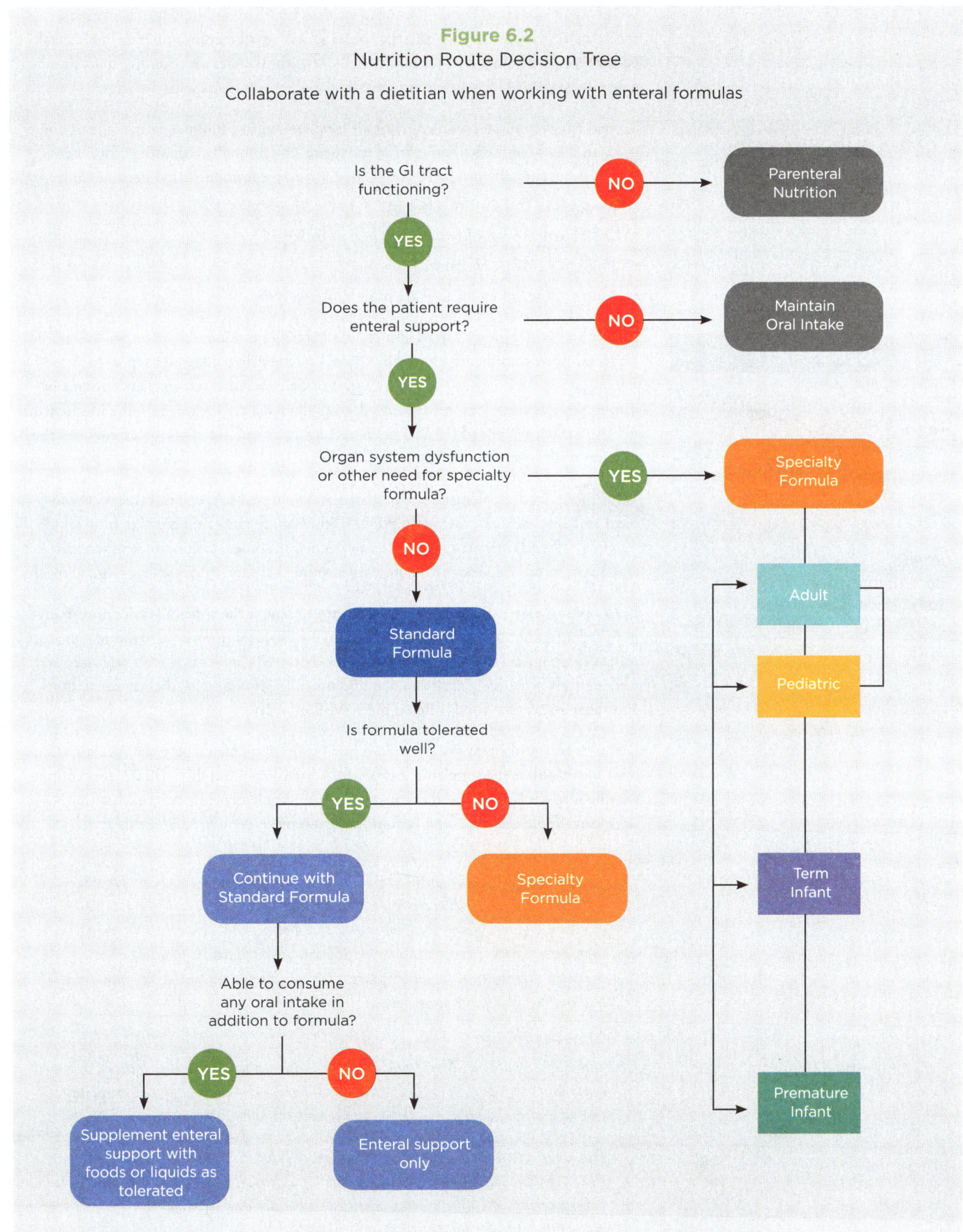

Figure 6.2
Nutrition Route Decision Tree
Collaborate with a dietitian when working with enteral formulas

Source: Excerpt from Enteral Nutrition Formulary Guide

Snacks may be part of the daily routine or may be scheduled only for clients with specified dietary needs, such as a diet order for six small feedings each day or a snack coordinated with insulin injection for a client with diabetes. An evening snack is generally standard for senior living residents and most clients with diabetes.

To make it even more confusing, not all supplements are commercially made or come in a can. Many of the items available today are "nutritionally enhanced" food items, not pharmaceutically produced supplements. Some commonly used items include:

- A packet of Instant Breakfast and 8 ounces of milk
- Individual cartons of frozen enriched milkshakes
- High protein power drinks
- Many of the "sport drinks" are high in electrolytes

Snacks and nourishments must comply with the diet order and may be pre-assembled by an assigned staff member or team. These may be delivered as a group to each nursing station for delivery by nursing staff or delivered directly to clients' rooms by dining services staff. In some settings the supplements are included on the **Medication Administration Record (MAR)** or **eMAR** for electronic versions which requires the nursing staff to verify consumption of the item.

While prescribed supplements are prepared and delivered to specific clients, between-meal and evening snacks are often provided through nursing unit pantries from which nursing staff withdraw items requested by clients. In some locations, dining services employees travel from room to room with a rolling cart and offer diet-appropriate snacks.

Both options allow clients to choose what they want at the time of service and receive personal attention to their requests. In many cases they improve turnaround time for processing requests and may also streamline labor requirements. Dining services and nursing staff providing snacks on demand must be familiar with dietary restrictions and must assure that foods offered meet the diet order.

Part of your supplement system should be to give supplements between meals and not with meals unless the supplement is part of a fortified liquid diet. This is to encourage the client to eat the meal and not just drink the supplement. Be careful that the nutrition supplement does not become a meal replacement. Consider this scenario:

> *It is 11:15 and lunch is served at 11:30. The dining room tables are set for the residents. The assigned location for Mrs. Jones includes the place setting, a glass of water, a glass of juice, a cup of coffee, and a glass with a chocolate flavored supplement. Mrs. Jones chats some with her tablemates and is sipping on the beverages. By the time the lunch plate is served, Mrs. Jones has half a glass of water left and has drunk the other fluids.*
>
> *At the end of lunch, a nurse asks Mrs. Jones why she did not eat the baked chicken and mashed potatoes. Mrs. Jones replies that she just wasn't all that hungry. The nurse notes that Mrs. Jones only ate 25% of her meal—maybe, given her recent weight loss, she needs a between-meal supplement to boost her nutritional intake.*
>
> *Did you see that Mrs. Jones drank the 6 oz. of juice PLUS the 6 oz. of coffee PLUS the 8 oz. of supplement PLUS 3 oz. of water? She had 25 ounces of fluid in her stomach by the time lunch was served at her table and you wonder why she did not eat much of her lunch.*

GLOSSARY

Medication Administration Record (MAR)
Medical Administration Record that is a documentation system for patient and resident med pass

eMAR
Electronic versions of Medical Administration Records

Every facility will have a different variation on their nourishment delivery systems. It will be important to meet with your **interdisciplinary team** to discuss the best process for your facility. Then develop a policy and procedure that outlines what part the dining services department plays in this process. The Supplemental Material for this chapter contains a sample policy and procedure for delivery of between-meal snacks.

Between-Meal Snack and Supplement Cost Implications

While the cost of between-meal snacks and supplements seems minor, it can become a black hole of expenses. The labor to make the items and deliver them to the unit or the client directly can add up. The cost of the products themselves quickly moves from cents to dollars. It is important to track the cost invested in supplements and snacks.

If you are making milkshakes with supplements for calories or protein, look at your labor cost. How much was the ingredient cost? Did the client consume it? The cost is over a dollar for each milkshake. Was it consumed or thrown away because it was melted, wrong flavor, no longer needed, etc…?

Floor stock intended for client snacks between meals costs thousands of dollars a year. What are you supplying those units with? How much is needed on a daily or weekly basis?

Consider the earlier example of Mrs. Jones. Has the use of supplements and between-meal snacks resulted in her being served two different diets a day; a regular food diet which she does not eat because of the liquid supplements diet that she has consumed? What is the cost of the double meal service? What is the nutritional impact on her medical outcome?

Sometimes our best intentions have unintended consequences that come at an unexpected price.

Quality Improvement (QI) Monitoring Between-Meal Snacks and Supplements

Client needs change, their health status changes, taste fatigue sets in, staff availability changes. Lots of events can impact the making, passing, and consumption of the between-meal snacks and supplements.

Since supplements are prescribed with the intent of impacting the client's medical condition it is important to conduct regular audits to verify their use. Tracking of the supplements should include:

- Order is appropriate to client needs and follows the decision tree process
- The item is prepared according to the recipe (ensure the nutritional composition)
- The item is delivered on time to the client
    > Appropriately refrigerated if needed for a delayed service time, i.e., late night or bedtime snack

> **GLOSSARY**
>
> **Interdisciplinary Team**
> A team of healthcare professionals working in support of an individual client

View the Supplemental Material for this chapter for a sample policy and procedure for delivery of between-meal snacks.

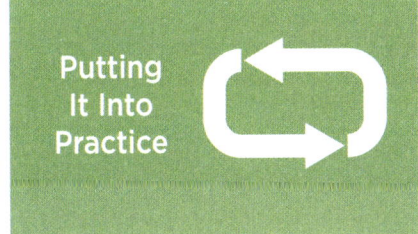

Putting It Into Practice

2. Based on the Decision Tree, enteral nutrition has been recommended for a patient. What steps would you take to ensure effective implementation of enteral feedings?

- All items served to clients, and/or held in the refrigerator, are dated and current
- The item is within reach of the client and ready for consumption
- The amount consumed by the client
- Client comments when appropriate
- The medical record and recommendations for change are entered when appropriate

Conducting the QI audits on a quarterly basis helps keep the focus on the client's needs.

Legal Implications

CMS (Centers for Medicare & Medicaid Services) is a federal agency that administers the Medicare programs and monitors the Medicaid programs offered by each state. CMS provides Investigative Protocols that define guidelines for the surveyors. CMS guidelines use **F-Tag** numbers to identify specific guidance for long-term care. Healthcare facilities also have differing levels of mandatory state licensing requirements. A list of revised F-Tags can be found on www.cms.gov.

A CDM, CFPP is responsible for making sure that clients know what their diet order is and offering a choice of whether to receive the diet (e.g., a choice about whether to receive nourishments or tube feedings). If the client refuses a tube feeding or additional nourishments, the client, facility, medical care provider, and Registered Dietitian Nutritionist collaborate to identify pertinent alternatives.

During a survey, an F-Tag was issued for a tube-fed client who had asked to receive food and drink by mouth. (The facility failed to address F-552: Resident's Right to be Informed/Make Treatment Decisions. With the CMS guidelines (revised 2016), you have to acknowledge the following:

- Promote care in a manner and in an environment that maintains or enhances each resident's dignity and respect. CMS F-550 Interpretive Guidance: Resident Rights/Exercise of Rights promoting resident independence and dignity in dining.
- The resident or representative has the right to make informed choices about accepting or declining care and treatment, Resident Rights/Exercise of Rights.
- Decisions about the appropriateness of tube feeding for a resident are developed with the resident, his/her family, surrogate, or representative as part of determining the plan of care. This requirement is also intended to prevent the use of tube feeding when ordered over the objection of the resident, Tube Feeding Management/Restore Eating Skills CMS F-693.
- Check with your administrator to review the regulations that cover dining services. Make sure you and your staff are aware of all regulations and their implications for meal service, including the service of nourishments and tube feedings.

> **GLOSSARY**
>
> **F-Tag**
> Numbers used by CMS to identify specific guidance for long-term care

3. You have been assigned to audit the meal supplement delivery system of your facility. Prepare an audit checklist and corrective steps to ensure quality compliance.

Chapter References

RESOURCES	
CMS F-Tag List	https://www.cms.gov/Medicare/Provider-Enrollment-and-Certification/GuidanceforLawsAndRegulations/Downloads/List-of-Revised-FTags.pdf
Enteral Nutrition Formulary Guide	https://kr.ihc.com/ext/Dcmnt?ncid=520448890
F-Tags in Review	https://www.lw-consult.com/resources/f-tags-in-review-f800-food-and-nutrition
Nutrition Support Therapy	https://www.nutritioncare.org/About_Clinical_Nutrition/What_is_Nutrition_Support_Therapy/

Evaluate Food Acceptance and Satisfaction

Overview and Objectives

Providing high quality meals that are responsive to the client's needs is the aim of every foodservice operation. Use the information in this chapter to examine how clients' needs influence the foodservice operation, and identify techniques for gathering meaningful data about client satisfaction. A successful foodservice department knows who their clients are and routinely surveys each group. Survey results lead to recommendations and changes to improve the level of service. After completing this chapter, you should be able to:

- Know your client and their expectations
- Identify factors that influence client dietary needs and satisfaction
- Learn techniques to assess client satisfaction
- Develop and conduct food acceptance surveys

Who are your clients? Everyone you provide meal service to is considered a client. Each of them has different needs and different expectations. Your clients may be called patients, clients, residents, students, inmates, or employees. A successful dining service department regularly identifies their clients and their needs. The client defines the role food plays in a facility and even the role your department plays in meeting their nutritional needs.

If you are in health care and started describing the hospital patients or nursing home clients, you would be partially correct. They are a very important part of the client base. Another segment is the staff that work and eat in your facility. Members of the community, such as those receiving meals on wheels or participating in congregate dining services, are also your clients. Special functions and catering events expand the clientele base to family members and conference/meeting attendees. What other groups that you serve aren't mentioned here?

Most operations have a variety of client groups. Along with primary clients, who may comprise the largest group of people you serve, there are others. In a school, for example, services are usually provided for teachers and employees as well as students. In a hospital you may be serving employees, physicians, visitors, and even the community at large. Figure 7.1 lists examples of client groups you may serve in various foodservice settings.

Figure 7.1
Examples of Client Groups

PUBLIC SCHOOL
- Teachers
- Other employees
- Visitors
- Consultants
- Professional groups (meetings, seminars)

UNIVERSITY
- Faculty members
- Other employees
- Visitors and guests
- Prospective students and families
- Sports teams
- Consultants and inspectors
- Sales representatives
- Professional groups (meetings, seminars)
- Conference attendees

CORRECTIONAL FACILITY
- Guards and other employees
- Consultants and inspectors
- Sales representatives

SKILLED NURSING FACILITY
- Potential residents and families
- Employees
- Physicians
- Community members
- Consultants and inspectors
- Sales representatives
- Professional groups (meetings, seminars)

BUSINESS DINING
- Consultants and inspectors
- Visitors and guests
- Clients and prospective clients
- Professional groups (meetings, seminars)
- Children enrolled in onsite daycare

HOSPITAL
- Visitors
- Employees
- Physicians
- Community members
- Students (in training)
- Consultants and inspectors
- Sales representatives
- Outpatients
- Professional groups (meetings, seminars)

CHILD DAY CARE CENTER
- Teachers
- Other employees

REHABILITATION CENTER
- Potential residents and families
- Employees
- Physicians
- Community members
- Consultants and inspectors
- Sales representatives
- Professional groups (meetings, seminars)

Why Are Clients Important?

In a non-commercial environment (hospitals, senior living, and residential facilities), clients are almost always named in the mission statement. Regardless of the specifics, it is clear that the facility exists to take care of its clients. This alone dictates the need for a clear focus on clients in dining services. When planning for **optimal food service**, several questions need to be addressed regarding the clients and their needs. Ultimately what constitutes a good decision for one group of clients may not be a good decision for another.

The bottom line is that the sum total of your decisions creates a dining services operation that gives the clients exactly what they need, the way they need it, and when they need it. In other words, it's really your clients who define the answers to the questions. They do not tell you how to accomplish the job, but they do tell you what the results need to be.

Often the challenge a Certified Dietary Manager®, Certified Food Protection Professional® (CDM®, CFPP®) faces is how to satisfy clients' needs, while also addressing many additional constraints. Some of these constraints may include budgetary limitations and requirements from external factors such as laws, regulations, and accreditation standards. Non-commercial dining operations perform a continuous balancing act to work within all established limits while using available resources most effectively to meet the needs of clients.

Managers in non-commercial dining services are quickly abandoning the traditional view of their clients as a captive audience. Successful players in the field, including successful foodservice contract companies, have adopted a new outlook. While the presentation and quality of the dining services may not be the deciding factor for most clients, it is a consideration and has become a marketing opportunity for the organization. Recognizing the client as a true customer is changing the provision of services to better meet the client's needs and expectations of their dining experience.

Factors Influencing Client Dietary Needs and Satisfaction

Unique Needs of Clients. What do your clients need? What do they like? Answers vary because many factors affect clients' food-related needs, meal expectations, service needs, and even their ability to enjoy food. Clients' unique needs may relate to likes and dislikes, expectations, variety, choice, appetite, sense of taste, drug therapies, allergies and intolerances, cultural and ethnic influences, lifestyle, routines, timing, religious convictions, emotional overtones, and personal values about food and nutrition. In addition, further needs may be dictated by presentation, environment, disabilities, language, literacy, culinary trends, and health status. Beyond these factors, some clients have very specific foodservice needs and follow special diets (therapeutic diets). See Figure 7.2 for a closer look at these factors.

KEY POINTS

To plan for optimal food service:
- Who are our clients and what are their primary needs?
- What type of service do our clients want?
- What types of foods should we include (or exclude)?
- Where will we serve people?
- What range of meal services will we provide?
- How many meals should we serve?
- What will the presentation and environment look like?
- How will we accommodate unique client needs and preferences?

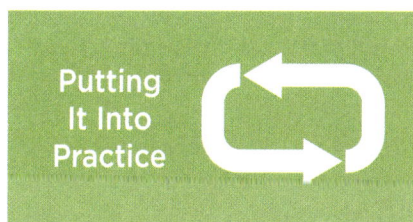

1. You are planning a menu for a skilled nursing facility. Using Figure 7.1 and the questions in the Key Points above, plan an optimal meal service that meets your clients' needs and expectations.

Figure 7.2
Factors that Influence Client Dietary Needs

Likes and Dislikes	The most powerful influence on food choices are personal preferences. Find out what they are for your clients.
Expectations	Your dining room and food service paint a picture that shapes the expectations of your clients. Do you have an elegant dining room? Are your signs scribbled or neatly lettered? Is your staff smiling during service? What picture are you painting?
Variety	You know the old saying, "Variety is the spice of life." Offering variety is especially essential in healthcare, school, and correctional food service.
Choice	Room service, selective menus, restaurant style service, self-service bars, coffee kiosks, and food courts all improve client satisfaction through increased choices.
Appetite	Your clients may be impacted by both physiological and emotional factors that may affect their appetite. Offering a variety of portion sizes will help to meet client needs.
Sense of Taste and Smell	Your client's sense of taste and smell greatly factor into their enjoyment of food. Know your client's condition and work with them to add additional herbs and spices.
Drug Therapies	Medications may impact taste and smell. It is important to note and be aware that clients taking several medications may request additional salt or sugar to achieve the same taste sensations. This may not comply with the diet order. Consulting with the Registered Dietitian Nutritionist may be necessary.
Allergies and Intolerances	Lactose intolerance (the inability to digest milk sugar) and allergies (such as nuts or wheat) mean providing accurate identification of products that may contain allergens. Know the allergies and intolerances of your clients.
Cultural and Ethnic Influences	Cultural and ethnic foods, ingredients, and/or seasoning styles relate to familiarity and comfort. These play a part in clients' expectations and perceptions of meal services.
Lifestyle	People are busier today and often eat on the go. You may meet your client needs by offering take-out food, sack lunches, and even room service.
Religious Convictions	For any clients whose religious beliefs influence eating choices, it is essential to acknowledge those choices and offer suitable options. Chapter One of the *Nutrition Fundamentals and Medical Nutrition Therapy* textbook offers a full discussion of cultural, ethnic, and religious influences on menu options.
Personal Values	Both food choices and service concepts relate to clients' personal value systems. An example of this is vegetarianism or people who feel strongly about healthy eating. You will be expected to identify these needs and develop services and alternatives that accommodate them.
Language and Literacy	Language or literacy barriers may require you to evaluate carefully how best to communicate with clients, to relate menus, to offer services, and to gather requests and choices.
Dietary and Clinical	Medical conditions may dictate food restrictions and/or limitations; for example, significant protein restriction for renal patients or texture modifications for clients with swallowing disorders.

Client Satisfaction. In some situations, the element of choice works a bit differently. In a hospital or a skilled nursing facility, for example, the clients may not have the option of eating somewhere else. However, their satisfaction is still critical to the operation. How will clients choose which hospital to use? Choices may hinge on previous experiences in the hospital, impressions of the hospital, and reputation within the community. The Centers for Medicare & Medicaid Services (CMS) conducts the Hospital Consumer Assessment of Healthcare Providers and Systems Survey (HCAHPS) of discharged hospital patients to measure their perspectives of hospital care. Although there is not a unique section for food & nutrition services (FNS) on the HCAHPS Survey, there are several sections where a positive or negative experience with FNS could affect scores. Ensuring that patient food preferences, intolerances, and allergies, as well as the patient's diet order, are properly recorded can enhance the patient's experience and consequently the survey rating.

For a skilled nursing facility a similar model applies. Among other things, when a potential client and their family are selecting a facility they will evaluate the quality of the environment and care they can expect from each option. Dining Services is a major contributor to the image a facility builds, to community perceptions of quality of care, and ultimately—to the decision-making process of potential clients of a facility.

In health care, physicians are also clients of the dining services department. A physician brings business to the facility and often has the choice of selecting one facility or another. Although insurance coverage may dictate which hospital the patient is admitted to, the physician's perception of patient satisfaction based on patient comments is certainly a consideration.

In prisons, satisfaction takes on yet a different aspect. An inmate most certainly has no choice of one facility over another. Yet satisfaction looms as a critical issue in ensuring smooth operations. A case study of food innovation in a Danish correctional system found that effective management of food systems may improve outcomes for incarcerated people.

School and university clients have a totally different view of what they expect of dining services. The need to balance food preferences with current fads and nutritionally sound dining options in the meal plans is a challenge. The school and university clientele often want more variety in their choices while maintaining easy access to the popular items.

Essentially, know what your client needs are and then work to satisfy them. Once you have identified your clients and their needs, you can continue to improve satisfaction and image by adopting and implementing standards. For instance, the Disney Institute recommends adopting service standards such as, "safety, courtesy, efficiency, and show."

Client satisfaction directly affects **participation rate**. If you are in a hospital and are serving employees, you may be concerned with participation rate for lunch in the hospital cafeteria. If half of employees eat in the cafeteria, you have a participation rate of 50 percent. Participation rate is very important in the school foodservice market, where a key impetus is to encourage more students to use school meal services. Likewise, in universities, the drive is often to encourage students to use the campus dining plan which brings about an improved profitability of the financial bottom line.

GLOSSARY

Participation Rate
The proportion of a potential client group that patronizes non-commercial food service

Client Loyalty. If a foodservice operation does a successful job of appealing to clients' needs, it can gain a following. Just like a favorite restaurant, the operation develops a sense of loyalty from clients. They want to keep coming back and choose this operation over an alternative. Loyalty is very valuable to any business and non-commercial food service is no exception. Loyalty means repeat patronage, and a certain level of security in ongoing revenues to the operation.

Competition. In many cases, non-commercial dining services are competing side-by-side with other forms of commercial and retail operations. For example:

- Employees of a large company can eat in the employee cafeteria or food court. Or they can take advantage of the growing fast-food industry and walk to the chicken franchise around the corner, go to the coffee shop next door, or pack their own lunch (brown bag).
- College students may choose to eat in the dining hall. Or they can: order food for delivery to their residence hall or run to the local convenience store for a take-out submarine sandwich.
- A resident of an assisted living community who wishes to go out to eat may choose the community's onsite restaurant. Or they can drive a mile to a different, privately-owned restaurant.
- A professional group holding a meeting in your facility may have the option of bringing in refreshments from a private catering service, or using yours; likewise with a fundraising group holding a black-tie dinner.

Professional programs can help identify your client base and improve service through knowing the needs of your potential clients. For example, the Disney Institute offers several programs to improve customer satisfaction and coined the terms "Guestology," which is managing the organization from the guest's point of view (GPOV).

As you can see, competing in the marketplace, bolstering satisfaction, boosting participation rates, and developing loyalty all feed into the mission and objectives of many facilities. Success in each of these areas requires a serious commitment to clients and their needs. Furthermore, success requires making the effort to get to know your own client groups, understand their needs, and respond to their preferences. The more effectively you do this, the more readily you can achieve a valid competitive edge in this evolving marketplace.

Techniques to Assess Client Satisfaction

Customer satisfaction is an important part of a successful food service operation. An effective CDM, CFPP continues to monitor clients and obtain feedback and suggestions. Customer satisfaction involves the perceptions of clients related to the food they were served, the service provided to them, and the overall dining experience.

2. As a CDM, CFPP at a hospital cafeteria food service, identify the factors that affect your cafeteria clients' needs and offer solutions to boost satisfaction, participation, and maintain customer loyalty.

There are a variety of techniques to determine the level of client satisfaction. Gathering input from customers as they are finishing dining provides the most accurate information as it is a recent experience and does not rely on memory. Figure 7.3 lists examples of formal and informal ways to assess client satisfaction.

Client Satisfaction Survey. A client satisfaction survey provides an excellent formal means of learning more about your clients. The results of a survey, examined carefully, can assist in refining menu offerings, service mechanisms, and more. What is a satisfaction survey? A satisfaction survey is a series of questions designed to elicit feedback from clients in a systematic fashion. Among the considerations for implementing a survey are: the method you choose for offering the survey, the way you select clients to participate, and the actual questions you ask.

> **GLOSSARY**
>
> **Satisfaction Survey**
> A series of questions designed to elicit feedback from clients in a systematic fashion

Figure 7.3
Methods to Assess Client Satisfaction

INFORMAL METHODS	FORMAL METHODS
• Be present during meal times and observe. • Talk to clients during meal times and ask friendly questions about the meal. • Talk to dining services staff involved in serving and ask about feedback and requests they receive from clients. • Accept any complaint as valuable feedback and use it to evaluate needs. • Talk to related staff, such as wait staff, nurses, or other staff, and ask what they are noticing or hearing. • After a catered function, talk to the person(s) who requested the catering and ask for feedback. • Wear a name tag that identifies your role or title in the facility and make eye contact with people you see. This makes it easy for clients to approach you to give you feedback. • Talk to your peers in similar organizations and share observations about trends that are developing. • Read foodservice trade journals to learn more about trends and issues.	• Create a suggestion box for use by both clients and employees. Review suggestions carefully. • Provide a comment card on tables where clients dine. • Tabulate plate waste. This is the food that is left on a plate returned with soiled dishes. Systematically calculate what is left uneaten, and examine percentages of uneaten food for each menu item. Sometimes, uneaten food gives you a good measure of what clients did not enjoy. • Monitor menu mix and product sales. Sales figures often provide a good indicator of what menu items clients are enjoying. • Use technology to provide an interactive method for clients to provide feedback from tables or bedsides (in a healthcare facility). • In a healthcare setting, ask clinical staff to gather information about the needs of clients, to pass along relevant needs, and to help assure that individual needs are addressed. • Create an advisory committee or focus group comprised of clients and ask them to help provide feedback and suggestions. • Conduct formal satisfaction surveys. • Using a mix of clients, evaluate test trays for temperature and quality. • Use an outside source (e.g., Press Ganey). • Utilize Mystery Shoppers—individuals who act as guests/clients and then write a report on their experience.

There are many methods for offering a survey.
- Print a questionnaire and deliver it with meals.
- Allow clients to "grade" the dining services with a menu scorecard for five items served in the last week.
- Visit clients in person and ask them to answer a series of questions through a brief interview process.
- Telephone clients to ask questions.
- Send a mailing to past clients asking them to answer questions.
- Offer a questionnaire on your dining services website and invite clients to complete it.
- Use other technology, such as a computer-based kiosk (free-standing station), or a handheld computer at tables.

Each method has advantages and disadvantages, and it's important to consider what method will be most effective for your client group. For example: If you are planning to use printed materials, consider whether all your clients will be able to read them and whether you are communicating in a language they know. A printed piece is easy to ignore. It is inconvenient, and may elicit responses only from those clients who have strong positive or negative feelings. In addition, it can leave out anyone who is unable to read and anyone who is not physically strong enough to complete a form.

If you are planning to use technology through interactive online surveys, evaluate clients' comfort level with the devices. In a university environment, for example, technology is frequently used to gather feedback from students. This is a natural fit for a population that uses computers and the Internet on a daily basis. However, among clients in an eldercare community, a smaller percentage of clients may feel comfortable interacting with the technology.

A personal interaction offers its own advantages. Clients are keenly aware of your interest in their satisfaction and may also feel free to tell you more. A disadvantage is that some clients worry about hurting the feelings of the survey taker and will therefore hesitate to express concerns.

Food committees or focus groups have been utilized in many settings. Regular meetings with a team of representative clients can provide information on what the community wants. It can also become a gripe session if issues are not resolved or effectively addressed before the next meeting.

In some situations, a broad-scale client survey mechanism may already be in place. Sometimes the entire survey process is outsourced or administered by an outside firm (such as using Press Ganey). Dining services satisfaction may be one of several topics addressed on a broad-scale survey of satisfaction.

KEY POINTS

Topics for Client Satisfaction Surveys
- Food Related: Appearance, taste, flavor, temperature, price, menu selections, portion size
- Facilities Related: Cleanliness, noise level, lighting, location, décor
- Service Related: Timeliness of order, accuracy of order, friendliness of staff, attentiveness, knowledge of menu items

Putting It Into Practice

3. Client satisfaction is a key component of your university dining service. What techniques would you use to assess your customer satisfaction?

Foodservice Management—By Design

Evaluate Food Acceptance and Satisfaction • C7 | 109

The most effective selection method includes a cross-section of clients and potential clients (if relevant). This means you have a representative sample from all groups. You may select all your clients for a survey, or take a like percentage from each group you identify.

The content of the survey will vary depending on what is the most important issue for the foodservice operation at that time. It can include questions on the food, facilities, and/or service.

In addition, there are several ways to allow a participant to answer a question. An **open-ended question** allows the participant to answer freely, saying whatever comes to mind. It cannot be answered with a "yes" or "no," or with a number. It invites free expression. In Figure 7.4, neutral questions 1, 2, and 4 are all open-ended questions. There are so many possible responses that without an open-ended question, you could miss some feedback you really need to hear! Realistically there is no way to ask enough questions to cover all the bases and elicit each of these answers without an open-ended question.

On the other hand, a **closed-ended question**, or closed question, with a limited number of specific answers also has value in a survey. In Figure 7.4, leading question 3 is an example of a closed question. When you ask, "How often do you use the convenience store?"—you can provide choices for the answers, such as: Every day, 2-5 times per week, less than once a week, or never.

Answer choices can measure frequency, such as these. Alternately, they can be ratings. A common rating technique uses the **Likert Scale**, which is a system for allowing people to rate how they feel about something by choosing a word or a number. For example, a survey question that says, "Rate your satisfaction on a scale of 1 to 5" is using a Likert Scale. Some surveyors avoid numbers in a survey, because users may make errors in interpreting the numeric scale. Words are more clear. Figure 7.5 shows sample questions from a survey that uses the Likert Scale.

From closed questions with answers that rate frequency or a Likert Scale, you can develop specific figures that identify areas for action and measure trends over time. For example, you can calculate participation rates in the use of the convenience store. Or, you can calculate how many clients feel their hot foods are hot enough when they are served. If you ask the same closed questions again in a few months, you can measure the success of any corrective actions and interventions.

GLOSSARY

Open-Ended Question
A question that allows the participant to respond freely with any qualifying comments added

Closed-Ended Question
A question with a limited number of answers such as a simple yes or no

Likert Scale
A common rating technique that uses words or numbers

Figure 7.4
Ways to Ask a Question

LEADING	NEUTRAL
1. You like the food we deliver to you, don't you?	1. How do you feel about the food we deliver to you?
2. The food reaches you on time, doesn't it?	2. How is the timing of your deliveries?
3. You use the convenience store, right?	3. How often do you use the convenience store?
4. You haven't had any problems with the service in the cafe, have you?	4. How do you feel about the service at the cafe?

Figure 7.5
Survey Using a Likert Scale

Another advantage to closed questions is that they are easier to ask than open-ended questions. Closed questions can be delivered on a survey form. Too many open-ended questions on a survey require participants to do a lot of writing, and some simply won't do it. Yet another advantage of closed questions is that they elicit answers that are easy to tabulate and summarize.

To learn about your clients, use both types of questions on a survey. On a survey that offers answers on the Likert Scale, for example, you may wish to include one open-ended question at the end, such as, "What other comments would you like to make about the food services?" A CDM, CFPP who is focused on clients will use a variety of formal and informal techniques, as well as a mix of question types, in order to gather feedback and keep in touch with clients.

As you gather information from formal and informal interactions, how can you summarize and evaluate it?

- As you receive answers to open-ended questions the most important thing to do is listen and think about the responses one by one.
- Follow through on anything that surprises you, and make your own observations.
- Notice similarities among answers.
  > Group answers and tally them.
  > For example, if 11 people say that the convenience store closes too early in the day, you can tally this information and use it in your planning.
- If you are sharing answers with your boss or others in your organization, you may also just make a list of responses so that reviewers can read them one by one.

How about closed questions? Here, you can tally answers to each question and calculate rates of responses. Figure 7.6 shows how to calculate percentage rates for responses to a closed survey question.

4. Develop a client satisfaction survey for your long-term care facility. Determine the topics and type of questions for the survey. How would you best evaluate the survey results?

What do the results of the question in Figure 7.6 tell you? Overall, they indicate that you are doing a great job of offering items the clients want to see in the convenience store. They also tell you that a small proportion of clients are looking for something they are not finding at the store. Hopefully, on this same survey, there are open-ended questions that generate client comments. You may want to look through these to see if anyone has named items they wish you would carry.

What follow-up would be appropriate for these results?

- Work with employees staffing the convenience store and ask them what clients are looking for.
- Provide scripting for them to ask each client, "Are you finding everything you need?"
- Have the staff maintain a list of items that clients ask for but do not find.
- Meet with vendors to select new items for the store to carry.
- Ask clients to participate in an advisory committee to help evaluate product availability.

Figure 7.6
Calculating Percentages for a Survey Response

First ask: How many people responded to the survey?

Next, ask: How many people gave each answer to a question?

Then for each possible response, divide the number of responses by the total number of people who responded to the survey. If you do this on a calculator, you can generally round your answer to two decimal places. If you remove the decimal, now you have a percentage.

Example: A sample survey given to clients of Axl Healthcare included the following question:

How would you rate the offerings in the convenience store? (circle one)

poor   below average   average   good   excellent

Your count says 65 people completed the survey.

On this question, 41 answered "excellent;" 12 answered "good;" 6 answered "average;" 4 answered "below average;" and 2 answered "poor."

Your summary shows:

        Excellent   41 ÷ 65 = 0.6308 or about 63%
            Good   12 ÷ 65 = 0.1846 or about 18%
         Average   6 ÷ 65 = 0.0923 or about 9%
Below Average   4 ÷ 65 = 0.0615 or about 6%
            Poor   2 ÷ 65 = 0.0308 or about 3%

Note: The percentages add up to 99% due to rounding; i.e., 0.0923 was rounded to 9%. Either round the 0.1846 up to 19% (then the total equals 100%) OR accept (and know) that the total is 99% due to rounding.

After a period of time, re-survey clients to measure the effectiveness of actions you have taken.

Thoughtful interpretation of a survey can help you improve products and services, identify client needs, and even develop new concepts. As an ongoing process, use surveys to keep a pulse. Surveys are not only useful in solving problems but are helpful in preventing them too. They also ensure successful competition, quality client participation and customer loyalty.

Chapter References

RESOURCES	
Disney Institute Customer Service	https://www.disneyinstitute.com/blog/customer-service-101-four-ways-to-make-your/
Gregoire, Mary (2013). Foodservice Organizations: A managerial and systems approach, 8th ed. Upper Saddle River, NJ: Pearson Prentice Hall	
HCAHPS: Patients' Perspectives of Care Survey	https://www.cms.gov/Medicare/Quality-Initiatives-Patient-Assessment-Instruments/HospitalQualityInits/HospitalHCAHPS
Sample Online Food Service Questionnaire at Kentucky State University	https://kysu.edu/administration-governance/finance-business/auxiliary-services/campus-dining/cafeteria-satisfaction-survey/
Smoyer A.B; Kjaer Minke L. (2016) Food Systems in Correctional Settings: A Literature Review and Case Study, World Health Organization	

The Quality Process

Overview and Objectives

The quality of products and services is the aim of virtually every organization. Quality is the adherence to standards, processes, and outcomes. In this chapter you will discover why a Certified Dietary Manager®, Certified Food Protection Professional® (CDM®, CFPP®) needs to take a proactive approach towards managing quality and identify techniques for verifying quality. After completing this chapter, you should be able to:

- Define the Quality Management Process
- Identify specific quality indicators for Dining Services
- Develop audits to monitor procedures and effectiveness of quality indicators
- Evaluate the data collected and recommend changes
- Identify the key certification agencies
- Describe the role of the CDM, CFPP in the certification process of the facility

Food quality management is an essential element of any foodservice operation to ensure that the client's needs are continually met. The Quality Management Process uses tools such as HACCP and auditing to describe processes, examine what could go wrong, put procedures in place to prevent things from going wrong, check that systems are working, and identify actions to take if things do go wrong.

The Centers for Medicare & Medicaid Services (CMS) calls the quality management system QAPI, which is the coordinated application of two aspects: Quality Assurance (QA) and Performance Improvement (PI). QAPI takes a systematic, comprehensive, and data-driven approach to maintaining and improving safety and quality in nursing homes while involving all nursing home caregivers in practical and creative problem-solving. Although this may sound complicated, Quality Assurance and Performance Improvement can be found rooted in foodservice operations.

In order to better understand the Quality Management Process, it is important to become familiar with key terms.

- **Quality Assessment** is an evaluation of a process and/or outcomes of a process to determine if a defined standard of quality is being achieved.
- **Quality Assurance** is the organizational structure, processes, and procedures designed to ensure that the care practices are consistently applied and the facility meets or exceeds an expected standard of quality. Quality assurance includes the implementation of principles of Continuous Quality Improvement (CQI). Think about Quality Assurance as it relates to food service—this includes everything from inspecting food deliveries to rotating product in the storeroom.
- **Quality Improvement** (QI), also called Performance Improvement, is the continuous study and improvement of processes with the intent to better services or outcomes, and prevent or decrease the likelihood of problems, by identifying areas of opportunity and testing new approaches to fix underlying causes of persistent/systemic problems or barriers to improvement. QI in nursing homes aims to improve processes involved in healthcare delivery and resident quality of life. Examples of Performance Improvement in foodservice operations would include resident satisfaction surveys, test tray reviews, and development of policies and procedures for various areas of the operation.

While your facility probably has some type of quality initiative, most follow common practices. CMS mandates five elements of QAPI in nursing homes:

- A QAPI program must be ongoing and comprehensive and should address clinical care, quality of life, and resident choice. The food services in a nursing home will have in place a written QAPI plan.
- There is a governing body that assures the QAPI program is adequately resourced, and that staff are adequately trained and held accountable. QAPI should be a team effort. Be sure to communicate the principles of QAPI to your foodservice team. Create a bulletin board in the kitchen to share goals, progress, and achievements.
- The foodservice operation has a feedback mechanism and Performance Indicators to monitor a wide range of care processes and outcomes and review findings against benchmarks and/or targets the facility has established for performance. Some suggested tools to measure and monitor the quality of the Dining Services Department may include meal satisfaction forms, tray accuracy and temperature audit forms, handwashing audit tool, resident satisfaction questionnaire, and food temperature logs.

GLOSSARY

Quality Assessment
The evaluation of processes and/or outcomes

Quality Assurance
The overall structure, processes, and procedures designed to ensure that the facility meets or exceeds an expected standard of quality

Quality Improvement
The ongoing process to improve the delivery of food, services, and client outcomes

- The facility conducts Performance Improvement Projects (PIPs) to examine and improve care or services in areas that are identified as needing attention. QAPI is about pulling together Quality Assurance with Performance Improvement to track changes and progress. A QAPI plan should establish areas for focus along with measurement tools for ongoing assessment and monitoring.
- Finally, the facility is expected to develop policies and procedures and look comprehensively across all involved systems to maintain continuous QI. Consider having a policy in place for quality control in dining services. The policy may also include procedures and tools such as a Dining Room Inspection Form or Kitchen Inspection Form.

Once a process to improve is selected, the next acronym relates to the plan itself. **PDCA** means:

P— Plan: Decide what you will do to improve the process. Decide what information to collect, and how to measure the outcomes.

D—Do: Make the improvements.

C—Check (Study): Collect and review data, and evaluate how the plan is working.

A— Act: Act on what has been learned. If there is a successful improvement, ensure that it becomes part of your policies and procedures. If not, consider an alternate plan.

The Institute for Healthcare Improvement (www.ihi.org) has developed a worksheet that can help you with the Plan-Do-Study-Act (PDSA) process for performance improvement. This tool is shown in Figure 8.1 in the Supplemental Material. The Medicare Quality Improvement Community (MedQIC) website is "a free online resource for quality improvement interventions and associated tools, toolkits, presentations, and links to other resources." The website is funded by CMS to provide a site to share resources based on the CMS scope of work.

Establishing Standards and Quality Processes

Measuring quality really means ensuring that your operation is meeting certain standards. These standards become the backbone of the quality processes. A **quality standard** is your facility's definition of what constitutes quality for a product (such as food) or a service. A single product or service may have a list of criteria to meet. For example, a quality standard for steak tenderloin might stipulate that the steak is tender, the temperature is 145°F or higher, and the food is neatly presented on a plate, with a garnish.

A quality standard for cafeteria checkout might stipulate that the customer will be able to check out within three minutes, the transaction will be accurate, and the customer will receive a receipt. A quality standard for nutritional assessment might specify that an assessment will be completed within three days of admission to the facility. The same standard might also specify what types of information will be included in the assessment.

For food production, some operations use photographs to show how products should look upon completion. Along with photos, specific standards may be listed. These standards may include both qualitative specifications and food safety or Hazard Analysis Critical Control Point (HACCP) specifications.

It is not always necessary, or even worthwhile, to write a quality standard for everything your operation does. However, through ongoing communications with both

> **GLOSSARY**
>
> **PDCA**
> A cycle of process improvement: Plan, Do, Check, Act. Sometimes referred to as PDSA: Plan, Do, Study, Act
>
> **Quality Standard**
> A facility's definition of what constitutes quality for an item or service

View the Supplemental Material for this chapter to see Figure 8.1, PDSA Worksheet for Testing Change.

clients and directors, it is practical to target specific products and/or services for which to specify standards. These standards themselves may need to be revisited and revised periodically.

Once quality standards are defined, you can evaluate and monitor quality. These standards also provide support to the process of training employees. In other words, every time you train an employee on what to do, also train him or her about what the results of the work should be. Incorporate the quality standards into the ongoing in-service education for all staff. This sets up a clear expectation and provides essential direction.

Effective Foodservice Quality Control Processes

Effective control of the quality process requires a proactive approach. Rather than waiting for a complaint or a set of poor survey results to surface, a quality-oriented CDM, CFPP monitors and improves quality continuously.

Quality management stems from clearly defined operating objectives and relates to all other aspects of the operation, including the following:

- Service and delivery systems
- Menu development
- Purchasing specifications
- Standardized recipe development
- Food production
- Scheduling of employees and tasks
- Employee performance standards
- Employee training
- And even the budget

Figure 8.2 illustrates the broad picture of how quality management fits into a manager's responsibilities. These are as follows:

Step 1: The dining services department objectives are established. These should be in harmony with the broad purposes of the organization.

Step 2: Strategies to attain objectives are planned.

Step 3: Specific operating procedures are developed. These may relate to product specifications, standardized recipes, equipment specifications, schedules, delivery procedures, and much more. Developing good initial procedures requires knowledge of the full scope of the dining operations as well as good judgment.

Step 4: Quality standards are developed. It is helpful to clarify these before beginning a new procedure. Objectively, these standards help define how you will know whether a procedure is effective. They provide a way to begin measuring effectiveness immediately.

Step 5: Employees become aware of specific outcomes that you as a team need to achieve. By knowing what these outcomes are, employees can more readily help with adjusting the process down the line. Training is essential to ensure that everyone is working towards the same objectives. Essential to the success of any quality management program is the involvement of employees.

Step 6: After specific operating procedures have been developed, they must be implemented.

Step 7: The CDM, CFPP begins to evaluate the effectiveness of the dining services. The type of questions that will help in this evaluation may include:

- How do quality results compare with the standards established?
- Did a procedure produce any unintentional or unexpected results?
  > If so, which of these is acceptable/not acceptable?
- When results do not meet quality standards, what is the cause (or causes)?
- What interventions will address these causes?
- Is the procedure itself sound, or does it need to be revised?

Following evaluation, a CDM, CFPP needs to assess any revisions or adjustments that may be in order. Any intervention or procedural revision should be evaluated again. Sometimes several rounds of edits or revisions are required to achieve the intended results. In addition, involvement of employees and a team-oriented quality effort are typically the most effective in raising the quality of services or products. When employees are engaged in the process they have greater ownership of the outcomes.

With this big picture in mind, let's examine some of the tools a manager can use to gather information related to quality standards. These include taste panels, test meals, temperature logs, satisfaction surveys, plate waste studies, performance standards, and checklists or self audits. Employee Performance Standards will be addressed in Chapter 12.

Taste Panels

A **taste panel** can help determine whether a product meets the given standards. It can also help achieve an improved outcome of client satisfaction with the food. The people on the panel should be knowledgeable about food standards and they should be able to distinguish flavors. When practical, it may also be appropriate to include a few clients in a taste panel. For example, a dining services committee composed of clients in an assisted living community may be an excellent source of taste panelists.

In a formal taste panel, participants rate each product using a score sheet, such as the one shown in Figure 8.3 in the Supplemental Materials. The score sheet notes taste, odor, flavor, color, texture, and appearance of the sample product.

> **GLOSSARY**
>
> **Taste Panel**
> The evaluation or rating of items by a group of tasters

Figure 8.2
Quality Management Overview

1. Establish objectives for the dining services operation.
2. Plan strategies to attain these objectives including interdisciplinary team (IDT).
3. Develop specific operating procedures and standards.
4. Identify quality outcomes and indicators for measuring effectiveness of these procedures.
5. Communicate standards to employees and provide needed training.
6. Implement operating procedures.
7. Establish a program for monitoring process compliant with standards and evaluate quality outcomes. Revise procedures as needed to improve standards.

View the Supplemental Material for this chapter to see Figure 8.3, Product Score Sheet.

The tastes, such as sweet, salty, bitter, and sour, along with the smell of a food, contribute to how people experience flavor. Taste sensitivity decreases with age, increasing the need for seasoning.

Color is also important. Many foods have characteristic colors closely identified with certain highly acceptable qualities. For example, the desired color of an apple is the color present when the fruit is at its peak of maturity. If the color is darkened or faded, the fruit is not perceived as being high in quality. Color sometimes does not reflect quality, as in the example of oranges. They may be mature in flavor but still be green in color. Thus, color is often a subjective—but very important—evaluation.

Texture is judged by the food item's characteristic texture, which may be stringy, smooth, crisp, mushy, tough, tender, or hard.

Appearance refers to the exterior, interior, and portion size of food in a bowl or on a plate. Factors to consider include a characteristic and/or regular shape, unbroken pieces, correct portion size, proper moistness level, and good color. Questions to consider include: Is the interior appealing in terms of texture and color? Does the portion look attractive? Does it fit the container in which it is to be served?

Figure 8.4 outlines suggested quality standards for common food products. Note that the evaluation of a product is somewhat subjective and will reflect individual tastes and preferences. The information or feedback received through a taste panel, however, is very valuable. A manager can use taste panel feedback to adjust recipes and impact the quality of individual food products.

Several guidelines can help with managing food product quality. Both training programs and the use of standardized recipes help an operation to produce food that is consistently high in quality. It is best to interact with employees during food production, and to involve them in the evaluation process. To achieve a consistent food quality, several things must happen:

- An expectation (standard) must be established and communicated to the employees.
- Employees need to be provided with products or ingredients consistent with the quality standard.
- Employees must receive proper operational support to make the quality of the product possible.
  - > This means you need to furnish the proper tools and equipment for the job, and schedule employees in such a way that necessary procedures and time frames are feasible.
- All recipes need to be tested, scaled, and standardized prior to inclusion on the menu.
- Before being served, the final product must be checked for quality.
  - > Work with employees if the product does not meet the standard to coach them through problems and questions.

1. A student taste panel will be rating bean and cheese burritos for introduction into the menu. Design a product score sheet for the taste panel. What attributes would be important to evaluate for the burrito?

Client reactions to the final product should be shared with employees. When the product receives praise, do not hesitate to pass this recognition on to the staff members who produced the food item. Information about a product that has been overcooked or over-seasoned should also be shared. Discuss whether the equipment is at fault, the recipe is a problem, or human error played a part in the unacceptable product.

Test Meals

Periodically, it is a good practice to prepare a **test meal** as a way of evaluating the service and the quality of foods as handled through a normal meal assembly system. A test meal (tray) is one assembled as part of the usual process, specifically for the purpose of quality evaluation. Some managers create a test meal by inserting a "dummy" tray card or menu ticket into the stack for meal assembly. For a realistic measure, a manager often does not identify this to tray employees as a test.

One strategy in preparing test meals is to make one that will test the outer limits of quality, or the worst case that may be occurring in the process. To evaluate the outer limits of quality, some managers position a test tray as one that will be created late in the tray assembly process, and/or one traveling the greatest distance for delivery.

> **GLOSSARY**
>
> **Test Meal**
> The evaluation of a sample meal as it is served

Figure 8.4
Suggested Quality Standards for Common Food Products

Yeast Bread	Golden brown color, symmetrical, uniform shape, rounded top, good volume, free of tunnels, moist, elastic crumb, nutlike flavor
Muffins	Golden brown color, well shaped with slightly rounded top, moist crumb, light and tender, good flavor, bumpy crust (smooth crust for cake-style muffins), free of tunnels, moist, elastic crumb, nutlike flavor
Cake	Golden brown color (except chocolate cake), smooth surface, slightly rounded top, high volume, fine grain, light but not crumbly, soft/moist texture, tender crumb, delicate sweet and well-blended flavor
Cookies	Uniform shape and color, good flavor, crisp or chewy texture (depending on type of cookie)
Pastry	Golden brown color, blistery surface, uniform and attractive edges, fits pan well, flaky or mealy texture, cuts easily, pleasant/bland flavor
Cream of Vegetable Soup	Thin white sauce base with off-white color; smooth texture that coats a spoon lightly, well blended flavor; vegetables should be finely chopped but have a shape
Scalloped Potatoes	Potato slices uniform in size, potatoes are tender yet firm, has creamy white sauce, finely chopped onions cling to the potatoes, mild potato flavor with delicate flavor of sauce
Pasta	Cooked al dente, uniformly moist and tender to the bite, not sticky, mild starchy flavor
Oatmeal	Grains are tender, consistency is soft and forms a soft mass in the bowl; not gummy or sticky

Adapted in part from Molt, M., Food for Fifty, 13th ed. Pearson Education, Inc., 2011.

Give this tray of food the same treatment as other trays. Deliver it to the service area and evaluate it. You can compare the tray to the established standards by asking questions such as:

- Are hot foods served at or above 140°F?
- Are cold foods served at or below 41°F?
- Are colors bright?
- Are items on the tray in the correct locations?
- Are products served accurately (according to diet order)?
- Is food palatable and enjoyable?
- Is the meal attractively plated?

If "no" was the answer to any one of the questions, you can research the causes and make corrections.

Temperature and Quality

Note that temperature also plays a role in quality, even aside from food safety issues. Temperature often affects the texture of foods and it even affects flavor. Keep in mind that temperature affects the aromatic characteristics of food and smell contributes to taste. A hot food that has cooled may give off less aroma and prove less flavorful. A cold food that has been warmed can also lose something. Think about a warm soda pop with less fizz. This may help explain why seniors rate temperature over flavor in defining food quality.

Temperature and food quality are issues throughout the holding and service process. For example, frozen sweet peas placed in boiling water or steamed to an internal temperature of 200°F for 1-1/2 minutes will be hot and tasty. They will have a bright green color and be slightly crunchy. Frozen sweet peas held on a 212°F steam table for 80 minutes will look pale green and be mushy in texture. This is one reason for batch cooking vegetables and other products that are sensitive to the holding process.

Always monitor the temperature of the food during preparation and service such as:

- Check the temperature when panning up the food for the service line.
  - > Do not transfer hot food to the trayline if the product is below standard.
  - > Plan ahead and preheat the hot wells to avoid temperature loss on the line.
- Check the temperature of food just before serving.
- Take the temperature again midway through the service.
- Recheck the temperatures of backup items in a "hot-box"/oven before restocking the service line.

Another aspect of temperature management is the balance between food safety and food preparation guidelines. In efforts to comply with food safety requirements,

2. You are evaluating a test tray for temperature and quality and find the chicken breast is well below 140°F and the plate is missing the vegetable side. How would you best address this?

employees sometimes overcook foods by bringing them to temperatures that are too high, or cooking for excessive periods of time or both.

An example is a hamburger. To meet the 2017 FDA Food Code recommendations, it must reach a temperature of 155°F for 15 seconds. To be safe, a standard practice is to overshoot the mark, and cook to a higher temperature. However, if the temperature goes much beyond 165°F, the burger may begin to become dry and unappealing. This is a delicate balance that requires careful planning and management. Some operations establish both minimum and maximum temperatures for certain products, especially for meats.

Satisfaction Surveys/Process Improvement

Identifying individual clients' food preferences should be a continual process and a component of clinical nutrition care in a healthcare facility. Beyond the individual care plan, information, or tray cards generated for healthcare clients, a manager should monitor trends in preferences and food acceptance. A manager's role is to be continually alert to the changing expectations of the dining experience. For example, if a high number of clients request a substitution for meatloaf at lunch, this may be a clue that the meatloaf has undergone a quality issue, or that the menu item itself is not a good choice for this group. Chapter 7 provides a more in-depth discussion of food acceptance surveys.

Plate Waste Studies

A **plate waste study** can also provide valuable information about food acceptance. Figure 8.5 illustrates a format for collecting plate waste information. In this process you review soiled trays before breaking them down and tabulate wasted or uneaten food. To make this information meaningful, it is important to randomly select a good proportion of soiled trays at any single meal. The benefit from conducting a plate waste study is the overall information you receive about specific food products. One example was a plate waste study where shrimp was served. Many plates contained wasted shrimp. Further investigation showed that too many shrimps were being served so the serving size was changed. If a product is repeatedly refused, you may reassess its quality, adjust, and recheck its acceptance in another plate waste study. Or maybe remove it from the menu. You can also use this method to document the intake of specific clients being monitored through the nutrition care process. This would help you achieve an outcome for a specific client who needs to gain weight.

Plate waste studies are particularly helpful in identifying items to be replaced when planning a new menu and evaluating the approval of new items on the menu. In addition to the formal plate waste study is an ongoing dialog with, and observation of, the dishroom crew. They can tell you on a daily basis what food items are coming back on the trays as poorly eaten or not even touched.

Another source of plate waste information is the diet office. Frequent requests for second trays or substitute items for particular meals is a clear indication of a problem menu.

> **GLOSSARY**
>
> **Plate Waste Study**
> The evaluation of uneaten food items returned for disposal

GLOSSARY

Self-Audit
A systematic internal "self" review of a process or procedure

Checklists and Self-Audits

To ensure ongoing compliance with standards and regulations a CDM, CFPP can use checklists and **self-audits**. An audit is a systematic, documented method of evaluating an operation in comparison with established standards. When you perform a self-audit, your own operation (rather than surveyors from the outside) is conducting the audit as an internal quality management activity.

A self-audit identifies exceptions or problems that can lead to an immediate plan to correct them. The benefit of performing a self-audit is that you can proactively identify problem areas and correct them without waiting for a surveyor to point them out.

By establishing a scheduled routine for self-audits, you can assure ongoing compliance. In fact, the best preparation for a survey—whether by a health department, **The Joint Commission (TJC)**, or a **Centers for Medicare & Medicaid Services (CMS)** survey team—is simply to comply with standards all the time. One example is by consistently following the set of quality standards for common food products listed in Figure 8.4.

Figure 8.5
Plate Waste Information

In the second column, tally the number of people who refused the product; use the third column to show how many plates came back with half the product, and the fourth column for empty plates.

CYCLE MENU:			
Wk 1, Day 3, Meal 3	Plate Full of Product	Half the Food Consumed	Empty Plate
Soup	III	IIII	IIII IIII II
Juice			
Salad	I	II	IIII IIII IIII II
Entrée	II	IIII I	IIII IIII II
Vegetable	IIII II	IIII IIII	III
Dessert	I	II	IIII IIII IIII II

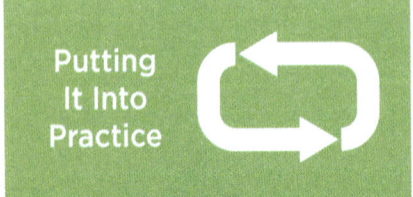

Putting It Into Practice

3. The plate waste study shows that all whole fruits, such as apples and oranges, served in the cafeteria are being thrown into the trash. What suggestions can be made to reduce plate waste?

To create a self-audit tool, you can use the following steps:

1. Review all the standards with which you need to comply, along with your internal quality standards, and list criteria for quality and compliance.
   > When you have multiple standards, such as some from CMS, some from the health department, and some from your own facility, your job as a manager is to consolidate them into one list.
2. Translate each standard into clear, specific, measurable/observable inspection criteria that identify what you need to see to know that the criteria have been met.
   > It is not enough to say: The dining room will be pleasant. Instead list the factors that make the dining room pleasant, such as adequate lighting, cleanliness, minimal noise, attractive table settings, etc. By doing this, you develop a tool that leaves nothing to judgment or imagination. Your criteria can be applied consistently with clear expectations.
3. Group these inspection criteria by logical or functional area to create several different audits.
   > For example, you may develop a meal service audit, a food production audit, a food sanitation audit, a safety audit, a clinical care audit, and perhaps a few others. Ultimately, each tool you create should be clear-cut and easy to use. It should not be so long that no one wants to complete it!

See Figure 8.6 in the Supplemental Material for a sample meal service self-audit tool.

A CDM, CFPP typically delegates some auditing responsibilities to work teams. For example, an audit of the dining room service can include a supervisor and/or a few employees in this service area. Any time you place the audit into the hands of employees, you empower them to manage quality within their own realms of responsibility. You also give them the message that they are expected to work together to make quality a reality. An audit tool can also be a very effective training tool for new employees, and an aid for reviewing required procedures with experienced staff members.

View the Supplemental Material for this chapter to see Figure 8.6, Meal Service Self-Audit Tool.

In conducting a self-audit, the assigned person should review the criteria, use a checkmark or other system to indicate whether the criteria are met, and add a plan for corrective action if warranted. Often, a problem can be corrected on the spot, and this is ideal. The employee who completes an audit should also date and sign the document, acknowledge responsibility and accountability, and return the form to the supervisor or manager.

Even when audits are conducted by others in your department it is important to review every completed audit document. Sometimes an audit will reveal chronic problems with procedures, training, equipment, or other issues that a manager needs to address.

Ultimately, the manager is responsible for compliance with all established standards. Also, the manager should maintain completed audit documents for future reference and for surveyors who may request to see them.

In all, an ongoing self-audit procedure is an essential tool for managing quality. To ensure that audits occur, it is a good idea to create a schedule for audits and assign responsibility on a calendar. Then monitor this to ensure that audits are completed on a timely and thorough basis and problems are addressed.

The Role of Expectations/Outcomes

Outcomes and expectations are related. When determining outcomes as a service in a facility, look at what your clients are expecting. Outcomes should address both their needs and their expectations.

To understand how clients perceive and rank quality, it is critical to understand what is expected. Part of the evaluation of taste and quality boils down to whether a food matches what a client expects. Individually, we each have an idea of what a food should be like, and this can vary among all of us. Being different or putting a new twist on a traditional product is sometimes effective, but only if it is communicated in advance, so that the client will not be unhappily surprised.

Often quality becomes a gauge of whether the food a client receives is the food he or she expected. In any facility, this factor merits special attention. A recent poll of restaurant customers found the number one reason for dissatisfaction was not receiving the food as ordered or expected.

In serving clients who have given up some control of their own meals, it's especially important to evaluate expectations and plate accuracy. Tray assembly service systems require attention to how meal choices are obtained and provided. The move to restaurant service and room service models have improved client satisfaction results simply by offering more choices and allowing the client to select the meal as they want it.

In surveys, sometimes clients will comment that meals are not "accurate." This affects your client satisfaction outcomes. When this occurs, carefully evaluate what this means. Possible sources of a comment such as this may include the following:

- The client did not complete a selective menu.
- The client completed a selective menu, but did not understand which meal it indicated.
- The client selected foods from a menu or by placing a phone call, and clinical staff had to adjust selections to meet a diet order.
- The client has experienced a change in diet order that affected food choices on the tray.
- The client asked the nurse for a specific food, and the request was not passed on to the dining services department.
- The client asked for foods that are not available ("write-ins").
- A clinical staff person has not taken food preferences for the client or has not communicated them to tray assembly employees.
- An error was made in processing orders, tray tickets, or plates.
- An error was made in tray assembly.
- A food shortage occurred, and the manager had to make a substitution.
- A tray was properly assembled according to client's order and food was removed during transit or delivery.

Clearly, many factors contribute to a perception of accuracy. When concerns about tray/plate accuracy arise, a manager should track the meal service process and identify where the breakdown occurred. Feedback in this can also help to pinpoint areas that require stronger communications.

Consider this example: You learn that the clients rated meal accuracy poorly for a certain meal. In tracking the service, you note that a macaroni and cheese was substituted for scalloped potato casserole. Two questions should come to mind:

- How did this occur, and what steps can be taken to prevent this in the future?

    > A solution may be as simple as revising the forecast figures for this product.

- Was the substitution explained to the clients?

    > If it wasn't, then from a client's perspective, the switch was a mistake.

Although substitutions are not desirable in meal service, they are occasionally unavoidable. Some operations keep small substitution cards on hand and place these on trays when a substitution has to occur. This at least lets the clients know that the dining services department knows of the change and that it was not an error. A substitution card may say something like:

> "Sorry! The item you requested was not available today and we had to make a substitution. For further assistance with your meal service, please call extension 404."

Outcome measurements help bring the focus of all you do back to the client's needs and expectations.

External Standards for Quality

Some standards begin with sources external to your operation. In fact, both governmental and private associations may be involved in the evaluation of dining services—and thus, with the establishment of standards. For example, to support a healthcare facility with maintaining accreditation, you will need to assure that the dining services operation meets the standards established by The Joint Commission (TJC). If your facility receives Medicare reimbursement for services, you may also be subject to certain standards enforced by the Centers for Medicare & Medicaid Services (CMS). In addition, you may be responsible for complying with specific standards for state and local agencies, as well as with sanitation standards as enforced by a state and/or local health department.

External standards form a backdrop for quality management in many healthcare organizations.

In a correctional facility, there may be other sets of standards affecting the dining services operation. For example, federal law stipulates religious freedom for inmates. This means that the foodservice operation will honor and provide their food choices as related to their religious convictions. The state departments of corrections may also apply certain standards.

In a public school setting, standards for menu planning and program management come from the USDA for schools participating in the National School Lunch Program and seeking reimbursements and commodity foods.

The Joint Commission (TJC)

There are several for-profit agencies that offer voluntary accreditation according to their established standards of care. They are not to be confused with the requirements of a state license or for the requirement to certify for federal funds. The most known accreditation agency is The Joint Commission (TJC).

Originally, The Joint Commission only accredited hospitals but it has moved into other healthcare facilities such as long-term care. The CMS recognizes The Joint Commission as an "accreditation organization (AO)" approved to provide the routine surveys to determine compliance for Medicare certification. According to The Joint Commission, their mission is:

> *To continuously improve healthcare for the public, in collaboration with other stakeholders, by evaluating healthcare organizations and inspiring them to excel in providing safe and effective care of the highest quality and value.*

The Joint Commission has established standards that each facility is measured against.

To comply with TJC standards, it is essential to review the current standards with others in your own organization. Check those labeled as pertaining to nutritional services, and then review those labeled under other categories too, as many standards are somewhat universal throughout the organization. For example, one standard will explain how to verify staff credentials and assure that they are up-to-date. Another will address disaster planning which is a facility-wide function.

Next, clarify any standards that are unclear. Your own standards, the ones from the in-house experts, a consulting dietitian, and colleagues may be sources of information.

Governmental Agencies and CMS

The Social Security Act mandates that facilities participating in Medicare and Medicaid programs meet minimum health and safety standards. Medicare is a federal entitlement program where those 65 or older or people in other categories receive health insurance. Medicaid is a state administered, federally aided entitlement health and medical care program for certain people with low income or limited resources. The requirements pertain to hospitals, skilled nursing facilities, and a wide range of other providers and suppliers of health services.

The Medicare program is administered by the CMS, an agency of the U.S. Department of Health and Human Services. The states may also establish additional requirements under the Medicaid program. Typically, the federal government sets the minimum standards, while the states may develop more specific standards. When this occurs, those that provide the greatest degree of control will apply.

An agency is designated in each state to carry out the requirements of the Social Security Act. Among other requirements is the need to visit facilities to assure that minimum standards are met and to complete various records.

While state-level officials are generally responsible for conducting on-site surveys for Medicare and Medicaid requirements, the federal government has several responsibilities. These are to:

- Review the survey and certification reports submitted by state agencies.
- Evaluate the fiscal, administrative, and procedural aspects of its agreements with the states.
- Conduct some on-site surveys of Medicare and Medicaid facilities.
- Review and approve state budgets and expense reports dealing with survey/certification activities.

The Survey Process

Both TJC and CMS use surveys as part of their accreditation or enforcement effort. CMS contracts with state agencies for surveys of healthcare facilities. As part of its enforcement effort, CMS and its contracted state agencies conduct on-site surveys of healthcare facilities. Each time a team of surveyors arrives to evaluate the compliance of a healthcare facility with CMS regulations, all managers become involved. A survey is typically unannounced and may occur on any day of the week. A standard long-term care (LTC) survey is designed to review compliance with CMS regulations, including all the detail of the various regulations known as F-Tags. A new survey process for long-term care was beta-tested in six states. It is called the CMS **Quality Indicator Survey (QIS)**. National implementation of the QIS is progressing state-by-state as resources are available to conduct training of state and federal surveyors. The QIS process provides for the review of larger samples of clients based on the **Minimum Data Set (MDS)**, observations, interviews, and clinical record reviews.

A CDM, CFPP is involved in many quality management issues. Interdisciplinary effort is a strong focus of quality management and CMS regulations. Thus neither surveyors nor administrators divide up the CMS regulations and hand a section to a single manager for responses. Nonetheless, the manager is often the most accessible person during a survey. Therefore, you need to understand the regulations, your facility's quality assessment process, and how your data supports your performance improvement program.

Each state agency designated to administer the Medicare and Medicaid programs has several duties, which taken together are referred to as the certification process. Since the standards used change, they are not included in this text.

These basic standards may be combined into an overall facility requirement. The state agency is responsible for the following:

- Identify as many qualified providers and suppliers of health services as possible. There must be eligible facilities on a state-wide basis.
- Conduct investigations and fact-finding surveys to determine how well participating facilities comply with requirements. Often this investigation is done in conjunction with the state's own licensure and other regulatory programs.
- Complete certification, recertification, and periodic follow-up reports dealing with whether facilities are qualified to participate in programs.
- Provide consultative services to providers and suppliers and to those seeking eligibility for the program in order to help them maintain required standards and qualify for participation.

> **GLOSSARY**
>
> **Quality Indicator Survey (QIS)**
> Automated review of client data to help systemize the survey process
>
> **Minimum Data Set (MDS)**
> A standardized record of client screening and assessment required for Medicare clients

As CDM, CFPP, it is your responsibility to be very familiar with the rules and regulations established in the state for the type of facility where you work. It is also your responsibility to work collaboratively and cooperatively with the interdisciplinary team (IDT).

In the most general terms, the manager must provide a nutritionally adequate diet. The diet should supply the nutrients for the age group being served. The modified diets ordered by the doctor or medical care provider should be followed using the guidelines set forth in the diet manual approved at the facility. The authorized clinical nutrition representative (Certified Dietary Manager, Registered Dietitian Nutritionist; or Dietetics Technician, Registered) may make suggesstions for diet changes in the medical record, but the individual who has ultimate responsibility to issue an order should be carefully considered; in some states and/or facilities, this choice may be dictated by licensure laws and/or policies of the facility.

There are food and nutrition-related guidelines incorporated throughout the Medicare and state requirements for certification. F-Tags related to resident dignity and the use of tube feedings were given as examples in Chapter 7. In addition, the minimum time allowed between the last meal in the evening to the first meal in the morning may be specified in requirements (e.g., 14 hours between the evening meal or major evening snack and breakfast).

A facility that participates in Medicare must also meet the conditions established by the federal government. Discuss these conditions with the administrator in order to understand the role that dining services plays in meeting the requirements.

Survey and Certification

There is a close relationship among the certification process, state license requirements, programs for professional accreditation (such as TJC), and medical assistance standards. Typically, the relationships among these standards require close coordination and information exchange. For example, healthcare facilities cannot qualify for Medicare assistance unless they have first been licensed by the state. Standards used by TJC generally meet many of the standards issued by the federal government. Thus, the facility is not faced with sets of conflicting standards which make compliance with any defined standards impossible. The guidelines, recommendations, standards, and interpretations of each regulatory agency and professional association interface to provide guidelines for managing healthcare facilities.

It is important to be up-to-date with a set of current requirements. CMS regulations change continuously. Unlike TJC, there may be variations in standards administered from one state to another, so your state must be used as a source of information. To verify the standards for which you are responsible, work with your own administrator or IDT, and ask for copies of the standards. Also be aware that the CMS website (www.cms.gov) provides information and clarification. One of its features allows users to

4. Your facility is going through TJC accreditation process. What steps would you take to help your staff prepare?

request clarification about specific standards and to review questions and answers from others. An entire section specifically addresses the "kitchen/food service observations."

CMS standards address many basic requirements, such as the need to establish menus, to assure that required nutrients are provided, and that food is palatable and safe. They also emphasize honoring the needs of individual clients and providing substitutions or alternates when requested. In addition, they stipulate a maximum time that may elapse from dinner to breakfast. They address staffing, dining room environment, and more. Like TJC standards, the CMS survey protocol includes a section about food service, as well as information in other sections that is pertinent to food service. Consider the following examples:

- Clients' rights and the right to refuse care apply to dietary choices and the right to refuse nutritional support.
- Confidentiality procedures relate toe everyone handling client information, which of course includes foodservice staff.
  > HIPAA is the federal Health Insurance Portability and Accountability Act of 1996 with the goal to protect the confidentiality and security of healthcare information.
- Standards relating to infection control have cross-over implications for sanitation and food safety in a foodservice operation.
- Many standards relating to nutritional status, hydration, and feeding assistance (if required) are truly interdepartmental issues.
  > For example, in complying with a diet order for thick liquids, both nursing and dining services staff need to work together to assure this is carried through.
  > In tracking weight changes or malnutrition, the staff must also work together closely to monitor progress and implement therapeutic plans.

In a long-term care environment, it is easy to understand that clients' clinical needs may change over time. So, CMS documentation requirements stipulate a schedule for assessing clients. For example, an admission assessment must be completed within a resident's first five days in the facility. Another assessment is required at approximately a two-week point, and then approximately monthly afterwards. Any major clinical change also signals the need for an assessment.

Certification, Surveys, and Quality Management

While all of these activities serve to ensure critical reimbursements to an institution, it also has an important bearing on quality management. A protocol for assessment serves as a type of quality management tool, and a way of ensuring that services are (dynamically) geared towards what each client needs. Clinical assessments are client-specific, proactive quality management tools.

CMS also uses quality indicators for tracking and benchmarking care. Quality indicators highlight issues relating to clinical care. Several quality indicators are

> **GLOSSARY**
>
> **HIPAA**
> The Health Insurance Portability and Accountability Act of 1996 is a law protecting the confidentiality and security of healthcare information

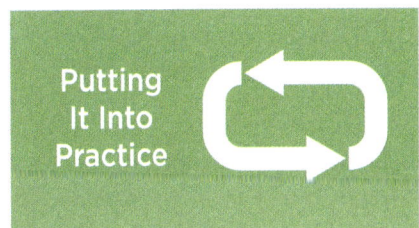

5. Your nursing home's community food services is not meeting the requirements for food safety. How would you use the PDCA worksheet from Figure 8.1 in the Supplemental Material and the steps outlined in Figure 8.2 to meet quality standards for the CMS five star rating?

very specific to nutritional care, as implemented by the healthcare team. For more information about quality indicators and CMS standards for clinical nutritional care and documentation, please check *Nutrition Fundamentals and Medical Nutrition Therapy* (ANFP, 2020) or the CMS website. As a CDM, CFPP, you can include this in your routine quality management procedures and evaluate this information as you would any other quality data.

The Centers for Medicare & Medicaid Services (CMS) initiated a five-star quality rating system for nursing homes in December 2008 that resembles the "star" rating system that measures quality in hotel chains. Clarity and public awareness is what CMS is hoping to provide from this initiative. Giving consumers a recognizable scale to search for quality elder care is what prompted the creation of the five-star quality ratings. The ratings are based on these three separate categories:

1. Health Inspections
2. Quality Measures
3. Staffing Levels

Each category is assigned from one to five stars, with one star being the lowest rating and five stars the highest. CMS includes this statement when describing the rating's merits.

> *"Nursing homes with five stars are considered to have above average quality compared to other nursing homes in that state. Nursing homes with one star have quality much below the average in that state (but the nursing home still meets Medicare's minimum requirements)."*

Legal Implications

The surveyors look at what you do for quality assurance and how you are using the data for performance improvement. CMS has language in both the hospital and long-term care regulations that facilities must:

- Develop, implement, and maintain an effective, ongoing, facility-wide, data-driven quality assessment and performance improvement program.
- Involve all departments and services.
- Focus on indicators related to improved health outcomes.

At the time of a survey, a CDM, CFPP may be asked to provide documentation and pertinent information. Surveyors will focus on quality indicators. They will review medical records and interview clients. Part of the survey may include a detailed tour of foodservice areas. A manager should accompany a surveyor and cooperate fully. When the survey concludes, the survey team will state any deficiencies noted and reference F-Tag numbers.

A deficiency is a finding that the facility is not in compliance with CMS Guidelines. The facility is cited and instructed to correct the deficiency. Deficiencies are categorized by the level of risk/harm that may occur. If a problem is identified, the manager and other members of the interdisciplinary team need to follow up promptly and effectively to correct them. If deficiencies are not corrected within a reasonable amount of time, the facility may be shut down.

In all, a Certified Dietary Manager, Certified Food Protection Professional plays a critical role in assuring that quality of dining services meets the needs of the clients and that the end results of care are excellent.

Chapter References

RESOURCES	
Centers for Medicare & Medicaid Services	cms.gov/center/provider-type/hospital-center
FDA Food Code	https://www.fda.gov/food/fda-food-code/food-code-2017
Food for Fifty	Molt, Mary, Pearson Education, Inc.
Hospital Consumer Assessment of Healthcare Providers and Systems (HCAHPS)	cm .gov/Medicare/Quality-Initiatives-Patient-Assessment-Instruments
IHI Model for Improvement	http://www.ihi.org/resources/Pages/HowtoImprove/default.aspx
Learning to Self-Survey and applying QAPI Principles	https://www.dhs.wisconsin.gov/regulations/training/c5-d8-ppt.pdf
QAPI Description and Background	https://www.cms.gov/Medicare/Provider-Enrollment-and-Certification/QAPI/qapidefinition
Quality of Patient Care Star Ratings	https://www.cms.gov/Medicare/Provider-Enrollment-and-Certification/CertificationandComplianc/FSQRS
The Joint Commission	https://www.jointcommission.org/en/standards/

Labor Analysis and Staffing Needs

Overview and Objectives

Planning for staffing needs involves anticipating the future, and what it will require in personnel. Tools such as job descriptions and job analyses help define the staffing needs in the facility. Calculating the number of full-time equivalents, planning for appropriate staff in response to changes in census, and the impact on the budget are all functions of human resource planning. After completing this chapter, you should be able to:

- Assess the staffing needs of a department
- Calculate FTEs and employee turnover rates
- Develop job analysis, gantt Charts, and job descriptions
- Prepare an organization chart for the department
- Understand hierarchy chain of command, and delegation in an organization

Staffing is one of the major functions of a Certified Dietary Manager®, Certified Food Protection Professional® (CDM®, CFPP®) and is defined as the selection, training, management, and development of employees to fulfill the dining services department needs. Determining the current and future personnel demands is done through a needs analysis by reviewing the staffing history data and trends. In many dining services departments with long-term staff, it is especially important to consider future hiring needs. When conducting a personnel needs analysis there are several factors to consider.

Strategic Plan

Most facilities today have some type of strategic plan in place that outlines the goals and objectives for the future. Your personnel needs analysis must fit within that strategic plan. For instance, one objective of the facility's strategic plan is to *expand the community outreach*. One way to implement that would be to enlarge your cafeteria to serve the community residents. This would impact the dining services personnel needs analysis as your requirement for human resources/staffing would likely increase.

Full-Time Equivalents (FTEs)

As part of the job of organizing work, a manager must coordinate job descriptions, staffing plans, and **full-time equivalents (FTEs)**. The FTEs, discussed in greater detail in Chapter 12, are a means of measuring how many hours of work go into an overall labor budget. One person working full-time translates into one FTE. The definition of how many hours constitutes a full-time employee can vary from organization to organization.

Typically, the benchmark of one FTE is 40 hours per week, times 52 weeks for a total of 2,080 paid time in a year. The calculation of full-time equivalent (FTE) is an employee's scheduled hours divided by the employer's hours for a full-time workweek. When an employer has a 40-hour workweek, employees who are scheduled to work 40 hours per week are 1.0 FTEs. Employees scheduled to work 20 hours per week are 0.5 FTEs. An employer with a 35-hour workweek would simply divide the employee's scheduled hours by 35 to determine the FTE. For example, an employee scheduled to work 21 hours per week would be 0.6 FTE when the full-time workweek is 35 hours.

FTE calculations are about hours worked rather than number of employees. You could have four employees and only one FTE. Four 0.25 employees would be 1.0 FTE. Amir, Mark, Phyllis, and Sue could each work 10 hours per week and the total would be 40 hours worked, or one FTE based on a 40-hour workweek. Employers may use the FTE calculation for different purposes, such as benchmarking revenues or profits per employee. Converting hours worked by part-time employees into full-time equivalents can be helpful when calculating these metrics.

> **GLOSSARY**
>
> **Full-Time Equivalents (FTEs)**
> One person working full time translates into one FTE. The number of hours that constitutes full time can vary. The most common definition is 40 hours per week or 2,080 per year

View the Supplemental Material for this chapter for FTE calculations.

1. Thirty (30) employees work 40 hours a week, 10 employees work 24 hours a week, and 15 employees work 16 hours a week. How many FTEs do you have based on a 40-hour work week?

Budget

As you analyze your personnel requirements, keep in mind that whatever staffing needs you determine must be consistent with the budget. One way to minimize adding staff is by analyzing the tasks that each employee in a position performs. Many of these tasks may work well with utilizing cross-trained staff from other departments, such as those from the environmental department who may also be able to assist with dining room services. Cross-training your staff can allow you to more efficiently use your labor budget.

Trends and Forecasting

As part of the budget planning process related to labor and staffing, the CDM, CFPP should be flexible as staffing needs develop. Today's fast-changing dining services may foster personnel concerns of which you are not even aware. Participating on a work team that is comprised of human resource department representatives, top dining services department staff, and other management staff within the department is useful. As you look at trends and forecasting future staffing needs, use the data that either your department or human resources department should have, such as:

- Turnover rate
- Staffing levels
- Retirement eligibility

If your human resource department does not calculate the **employee turnover rate**, you can easily calculate that for your own department. Decide what length of time you want to consider, although six months or a year is typically used. Determine the average number of employees over that time. Take the total number of employees who left your employment during the same time. Divide the number of employees who left by the average number of employees to obtain your turnover rate.

> January 1 - December 31 Average number of employees = 16
>
> January 1 - December 31 Number who left employment = 2
>
> Turnover rate: 2 ÷ 16 = .125 x 100 = 12.5%

A 12.5% turnover rate is considered very low in comparison to the restaurant industry where turnover rate can be as high as 80%.

Forecasting the staffing needs allows you to plan for recruiting, hiring, and training before the issue becomes a crisis. You should, therefore:

- Anticipate the number of staff retirements in the coming year.
- Recognize long-term illness or surgical concerns.
- Identify the number of employees returning to school in September.
- Calculate the turnover rate.
- Define the labor impact of planned new services or reductions in services (i.e. third floor is scheduled for four months of renovation starting in May).

> **GLOSSARY**
>
> **Employee Turnover Rate**
> This is calculated by dividing the number of employees who left the company by the average number of employees in a certain period of time. This number is then multiplied by 100 to get a percentage

External Environment

Employment laws also affect your staffing levels. The CDM, CFPP must make sure that all policies regarding staffing and human resources are developed within the framework of the employment laws. If you have a human resources (HR) department, work with it to develop goals and developmental programs for the staff members who are new, in training, or in career advancement modes. If you do not have an HR department, work with your administrator to ensure that you are following the employment laws.

Another external influence on your staffing will be the Centers for Medicare & Medicaid Services (CMS) regulations. Both state and federal regulations may address staffing in your department. It will be very important to pay attention to these considerations as you analyze your personnel needs. The basic steps are shown in Figure 9.1.

In staffing, the bottom line is that planning is the only effective way to ensure that the number of surprises will be minimal. While no one can predict what will happen in the future, a great deal of your human resources requirement can, in fact, be predicted. By planning and taking appropriate action, you help to ensure that your operation will continue to function smoothly now and in the future. A CDM, CFPP is perpetually thinking about these steps daily in order to meet the ongoing staffing needs.

In contrast to the broad issue of staffing, a manager must also consider the finer detail involved in scheduling, or planning the employees' specific activities and day-to-day assignments. Tools that can help a manager with scheduling include a staffing pattern, a job analysis, and a job description.

Figure 9.1
Steps in Personnel Needs Analysis

1. Forecast future personnel needs—The forecasting of future needs should be in harmony with growth.
2. Determine base staffing pattern needs—What are the minimum positions and hours needed on a daily basis?
3. Conduct inventory of current staff—What are the skills, abilities, interests, and needs of currently employed staff members?
4. Assess staff planning needs—Consider planned vacancies or changes.
5. Develop internal training/education activities—Depending upon your needs, retain staff. *OR*
6. Plan for new recruitments, selection and training procedures—Recruit, select, and train new staff.
7. Design program monitoring system—Develop a way to monitor your progress (how many staff were hired, trained, etc.?).
8. Control and evaluate planning systems—Evaluate how your analysis is working and make adjustments if necessary.

Putting It Into Practice

2. Your department has a staff of 55. If your turnover rate has been about 15%, your staffing level is 95% and you know of four employees who will retire next year. Forecast your hiring needs for next year.

Staffing Pattern

The **staffing pattern** defines what positions are needed each day of the week. Employee names and tasks are not included. It is based on the optimal number of positions to meet the production and meal service needs. Generally, on Saturdays and Sundays, there is less staff than during the typical five-day work week, so that some positions may be covered only five days a week instead of every day.

The staffing pattern may also be adjusted for increased labor needs on the scheduled foodservice vendor delivery days. Evaluation of the menu may indicate that a staff person is needed on Mondays only. Likewise, coverage of a position needs does not always require an 8-hour shift.

The sample staffing pattern shown in Figure 9.2 of the Supplemental Material is for an organization with a cafeteria that is open for breakfast and lunch only on the weekends. Note how the staffing needs change from day-to-day which in turn can affect the number of employees scheduled each day.

Comparing the desired staffing pattern to your current schedule can help identify where the plan does not match the reality. Consider the following questions:

- How well does the staffing pattern compare to the actual number of positions you schedule and the total hours paid each week?
- Are you correct or do you find that there are some days when you have enough coverage and others that you do not?
- Do you have the right number of staff to cover positions needed or do you need more staff?
- If you need to make some changes and rearrange the employee schedule to better meet the staffing pattern, where and how will you do that?
- Often labor and staffing is the target of expense reduction. Can you reduce your staffing based on the schedule?

All of these questions are wrapped up in the Job Analysis or Position Workflow. What position is assigned to complete the specific tasks, and are all needed tasks assigned to some position?

Workflow and Job Analysis

A **job analysis** is a process used to collect information about the duties, responsibilities, necessary skills, outcomes, and work environment of a job. You need as much data as possible to put together a job description, which is the frequent output result of the job analysis. Tasks are assigned to the position, not the person. The tasks are individual events sorted into a logical workflow for the day. By reducing a lot of backtracking and by creating a workflow of related tasks, a job analysis can improve the assigned daily tasks to flow more logically throughout the workday. The job analysis is useful in providing an overview of the fundamental requirements of any position.

Below is a summary of an individual job analysis for a Hot Foods Cook. Note that it divides the job of preparing food into individual tasks. A job analysis summary lists tasks specifically and concretely, but does not clarify the procedures for doing the work. For example, if you are writing a job analysis for a receiving clerk, it is appropriate to list tasks such as: "Checks food deliveries against invoice" or "Rejects food deliveries that do not meet established standards for quality and sanitation."

> ### GLOSSARY
>
> **Staffing Pattern**
> The base schedule of positions needed each day
>
> **Job Analysis**
> Identifying the content of a job in terms of activities involved and attributes or job requirements needed to perform the activities

View the Supplemental Material for this chapter for Figure 9.2, Sample Staffing Pattern Example.

Job Analysis for a Hot Foods Cook

- Take out the ingredients from food stores and document on requisition form.
- Use food production sheet and standardized recipes to measure ingredients per standard procedures.
- Complete food preparation of all assigned hot food items per standardized recipe instructions.
- Create pureed versions of assigned products per procedures.
- Complete HACCP records for food prepared.
- Arrange presentation and garnish food per recipe.
- Cover and label food products; take foods to hot holding area.
- Clean up work area.
- Complete pre-prep for next day.
- Complete leftover records after meal service.
- Discard or label and store leftovers per procedures.

A good job analysis workflow identifies what each position is assigned to do and confirms how many positions are needed to complete the assigned tasks. If large blocks of unassigned times are identified, the workflow can be used to develop a position link and reduce hours on the schedule. Likewise, if there are a number of unassigned tasks with no open labor time available, the workflow can help justify the need for an added position in the department. The easiest way to see the whole day's work is to lay it out in what is called a **Gantt Chart** or a timeline.

> **GLOSSARY**
>
> **Gantt Chart**
> A spreadsheet with a timeline to design task assignments by staff position

Figure 9.3 in the Supplemental Material is an example of a Gantt Chart being developed. Note that:

- Each position is listed with start & stop times.
- Time sensitive deadlines (meal service times) are highlighted.
- Major tasks to be completed by the different positions are entered.
- The planned time needed to complete the task is blocked out.

Once the staffing pattern is defined and the workflow has been completed, you need to consider the skill sets required of each position. A potential employee's skills and knowledge must match the requirements of the job. For example, an upscale catering service will require the expertise of someone trained in culinary arts. The job of serving clients in the dining room will require excellent customer service and people skills, along with an ability to work in an organized and efficient manner. It is important to identify what skills would be considered essential for each type of staff position based on the type and style of facility you manage.

View the Supplemental Material for this chapter for Figure 9.3, Gantt Chart examples.

Job Descriptions

The word "job" or "position" describes the tasks for which an employee is responsible and accountable. Positions have titles to help you refer to them. Titles are shown on organization charts, on schedules, and in descriptions of the job themselves. Jobs are not the same thing as individual people.

For example, you may have a job titled Morning Cashier. This is a position with a set of assigned responsibilities. One day, an employee named Mary may fill this position. The next day, a different employee, named Carlos, may fill it. The job title simply refers to the scope of assigned work.

Tasks are the individual activities that, together, comprise a job. For example, the morning cashier job may involve tasks such as:
- Setting up the cash register or point of sale system
- Counting the bank and verifying that it is accurate
- Checking out clients; and many others

The job of a trayline employee may involve tasks such as:
- Transporting food and supplies to the trayline
- Portioning food
- Cleaning the tray assembly line and work area after other tasks have been completed

Tasks such as these are outlined in a **job description**. A job description is the official, written account of an employment position. It includes the job responsibilities of the employee and defines whom the employee reports to. It specifies the typical working hours of the job and generally where the person works (such as dining room, receiving dock, trayline, dishroom, etc.).

A job description also documents the qualifications a person must have for the job and it includes the salary range for the position. It forms the basis for evaluating an employee's performance. Duties and expectations defined in the job description help the managers structure their coaching activities and will help in the discipline or termination of an employee.

> **GLOSSARY**
>
> **Job Description**
> The official, written account of an employment position. It includes hours, location, salary range and what the employee is responsible for doing

What to Include in the Job Descriptions

The job description is a written document of the general responsibilities and duties of a job. A well-written job description defines for the employee and the employer what is expected of them. A job description should be written for each type of position in the dining services operation. For example, there should be a job description for the Cook with a list of the tasks and responsibilities which could include the morning cook, main line cook, late cook, patient cook, and possibly even the grill cook. The different positions represent all the locations that the Cook may be assigned to, but they have the same job descriptions. Likewise, a Dining Services Worker may be assigned to the trayline, passing trays, the dishroom, or the "cut & plate" in the cold food area. While these are very different tasks, they typically do not have different job descriptions.

View the Supplemental Material for this chapter for a sample job description.

The exact format of a job description is usually set by your organization, and may include most or all of the following:
- Job title
- Section or department
- Supervisor's title
- Brief summary of basic responsibilities
- Description of duties

Putting It Into Practice

3. Complete a job analysis for a cafeteria cashier and write out a job description for the position using the Sample Job Description found in the Supplemental Material for this chapter, as an example.

- Working conditions (e.g., heavy lifting involved)
- Employment qualifications or minimum job requirements
- Education and experience requirements
- Conditions of employment (e.g., health and drug screening)
- Wage scale
- Date developed or last revised

Job descriptions answer several questions, such as: What are the tasks an employee in this position must perform? Who supervises an employee in this position? What knowledge and skills must a candidate possess to qualify for this position? What is the pay scale for anyone in this position?

Managers use job descriptions as tools because they clarify who is responsible for a job, e.g., who receives food deliveries—the dining services supervisor or the cook?

Occasionally, a manager may need to reference job descriptions with employees to clarify disagreements. Also, most managers use job descriptions as a communication tool to help define expectations of employees during job interviews, new employee orientation, and later, in performance evaluations.

Job descriptions also indicate how each position relates to other positions in the dining services department. As such, they lay the foundation for the flow of communication, authority, and responsibility throughout the organization. They help a manager organize positions into work sections to form a basis for developing effective labor control systems.

Note that many organizations end a list of duties in a job description with this point: "Other duties as assigned." This addresses the fact that some flexibility is required. There may be one day when your department has an unexpected need to serve coffee and breakfast rolls to an ad hoc board of directors meeting in your building. To whom will you assign the work of providing this food? It may not fall under anyone's job description. There may be another day when two employees call you early in the morning and say they are unable to report to work. You may have to divide their responsibilities among other employees who are working that day.

These are just examples of why flexibility is important. From a management perspective, it is best to communicate your expectation of flexibility from the beginning with every employee. This minimizes surprises and possible resistance down the line. Another benefit of the job analysis and a well-written job description, is that it helps identify what standard operating procedures you should develop. The performance expectations also help determine what the audit monitors should track for the Quality Improvement Process.

You should maintain a reference of all job descriptions in your department. As jobs change, it is important to review, and if needed, update job descriptions. The survey process and Quality Assurance Plans often specify annual dated and signed reviews to ensure that job descriptions are current.

Organization Chart

As you write job routines for new positions you should also add them to your organization chart. An organization chart is a fundamental management tool representing task groupings and responsibilities in a graphical form. An **organization chart** (often referred to as the "org chart") shows the names of task groupings as departments or something similar. In a few words, it defines responsibilities.

Boxes representing groupings and/or positions (managers) are connected with solid lines signifying responsibility, authority, and accountability. In a traditional organization chart, authority flows from the top of the chart to the bottom. While this tool does not include everything, it provides a useful framework for organizing the structure of a facility. An organization chart may show an entire facility or a close-up view of a given area, such as a dining services department.

Figure 9.5 (see Supplemental Material for this chapter) shows a sample organization chart for a hospital. In this example, the departments are named in boxes. These include Admitting, Information Services, Human Resources, Medical Records, Quality Assurance, Public Relations, Audiology, Clinical Labs, and more. You can see that the hospital is organized into two main sections: administrative and medical. You can also see that there are three assistant administrators responsible for the groups of departments. The dining services department falls under one of these assistant administrators. Another, more detailed chart would show the divisions and relationships within the dining services department.

The flow of formal power may go through several hierarchies or levels. An organization chart graphically illustrates a concept called **chain of command**, which means the flow of formal power through organizational lines. The chain of command must be clearly defined in any organization. As you look at an organization chart, you should be able to trace the chain of command for any area from top to bottom or from bottom to top. If you are in charge of the dining services department in this hospital, you know that your supervisor is the Assistant Administrator of Support Services. That person's supervisor is the Administrator. Furthermore, the Administrator reports to the Board of Trustees.

Another key management term is **delegation**. Delegation means passing authority downward through the organization. The ability to delegate is one of the essential features of a manager. Delegating means that you do not and cannot do everything yourself. For example, if you manage the dining services department, you cannot cook all the food for all the meals. You delegate the authority downward through the chain of command to a group of cooks. Along with the job, you delegate responsibility and accountability to the cooks.

So, the lines on the organization chart designate responsibility, authority, and accountability throughout the organization. You are responsible for the department and have the authority and formal power to make things happen. You are also accountable to the Assistant Administrator of Support Services for the work performed

> **GLOSSARY**
>
> **Organization Chart**
> A graphical management tool that shows job relationships in a facility
>
> **Chain of Command**
> The flow of formal power through organizational lines
>
> **Delegation**
> Passing authority for tasks or assigning duties downward through the organization chart

View the Supplemental Material for this chapter for sample organizational charts.

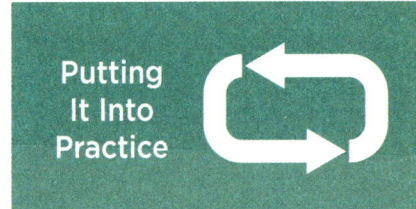

Putting It Into Practice

4. Using the Sample Organization Chart found in the Supplemental Material for this chapter, develop an organization chart for a small hospital dietary service department.

in dining services. Meanwhile, this Assistant Administrator is accountable to the Administrator for the dining services, and so on. In any organization, people are expected to respect and follow the chain of command. In this hospital, it would be professionally inappropriate for you to call the Administrator directly to discuss your new idea for the employee cafeteria or to complain about a problem you are having with the purchasing department. Instead, you should be discussing these matters with your own supervisor, the Assistant Administrator of Support Services. It is up to him/her to work through the next level up in the organization as needed.

You also notice in an organization chart that each person has only one supervisor. This is called unity of command, which means each person reports to only one superior. Management experts suggest that this is a sound idea since having more than one supervisor can lead to conflicting commands and a breakdown in the operation of the department.

Now, let's take a closer look at the organization chart of a dining services department. The Supplemental Material for this chapter shows a sample of a dining services department for a retirement community serving about 165 people In this example, you can see that the person in charge of dining services reports directly to the administrator of the organization. Furthermore, the dining services department is split into two areas, which represent two main purposes. First, there is a dining services section. This group clearly purchases and produces food for the residents of the retirement community. There are several levels of supervision, and there is an established chain of command.

Secondly, there is a Nutrition Services section. This section addresses the nutritional needs of residents (beyond food itself). Notice that within this area, there is also a Consultant Dietitian who reports to the Director of Dining Services, but does not directly supervise anyone. This type of relationship is sometimes called a staff relationship.

> **GLOSSARY**
>
> **Staff Position**
> Provides advisory or consulting support but is not in the chain of command

A **staff position** provides advisory or consulting support to a manager who is in the chain of command. This person is not a supervisor and is not in the chain of command, but provides valuable expertise that the manager needs. In this example, the Consultant Dietitian provides expertise in nutrition on a periodic basis to assist with evaluating the individual needs of residents. Typically, a Consultant Dietitian in this setting may assist with planning menus to assure that the nutritional needs of the residents are met and with planning, monitoring, and reviewing the nutritional care of individual residents. A staff position may be filled by an outside consultant or even by an employee of the organization. The important point is that someone in a staff position supports a manager.

A hospital foodservices organization, much like the retirement community, delivers clinical nutrition services in addition to dining services. The dietitians delivering this service may report directly to the Director of Dining Services or report to the Chief Clinical Dietitian, depending on the number of dietitians and the size of the department.

The structure of the university dining services (sample found in the Supplemental Material for this chapter) is significantly different from that of a hospital. Clearly, the organization chart has been developed differently to reflect the purposes and tasks of this university dining services operation. Notice that Dining Services fall in with a cluster of activities that relate to residence halls. Why is dining services bundled with sanitation employees and a building supervisor? In this environment, all of these functions relate closely to a single purpose of providing housing for students.

You might also imagine that employees throughout this chart will need to coordinate their efforts, interact with one another, and work as a team to achieve the purposes of the residence halls department. A manager shown at the top of this chart bears responsibility for assuring that the sum total of tasks related to housing are accomplished.

Some facilities and corporations are utilizing a circular organization chart. While it is more difficult to represent distinct reporting relationships, it encourages the integration of all employees on the chart and can be useful for representing team-based organizations. While it might appear drastically different from the conventional organizational structure, the circular structure still relies on hierarchy, with higher-level employees occupying the inner rings of the circle and lower-level employees occupying the outer rings. The leaders or executives in a circular organization aren't seen as sitting atop the organization, sending directives down the chain of command. Instead, they're at the center of the organization, spreading their vision outward.

However, in each of these examples, you can see that organization follows a logical task list that varies from one facility to another. It bundles related tasks. It pulls together similar resources and skills. It defines the responsibility, accountability, authority, legal power, and chain of command.

Consult with your facility administration for assistance in editing, or if need be, in developing the organization chart for the dining services department. All department staff members should know how their position relates to the activities of the department and how the department relates to the other departments in the organization. The organization chart clarifies the chain of command and reporting structure, which is also part of the written job description.

Once staffing needs are identified and met, the Certified Dietary Manager, Certified Food Protection Professional should be proactive in hiring, training, and retaining employees, which will be discussed in the subsequent chapters.

Chapter References

RESOURCES

Brown, Robert Douglas; Henkel, Shri (2007). The Non-Commercial Food Service Manager's Handbook	
Gregoire, Mary (2013). Foodservice Organizations, A managerial and systems approach, 8th ed. Upper Saddle River, NJ: Pearson Prentice Hall	
New CMS Long-Term Care Requirements	https://www.anfponline.org/docs/default-source/legacy-docs/docs/nc112016

The Employment Process

Overview and Objectives

Because of high employee turnover rates, effective recruitment and interviewing becomes an important staffing tool. After initial recruitment efforts, you may be able to predict how well candidates will perform through a structured interview process. This chapter will review employment laws, interviewing, and hiring techniques. After completing this chapter you should be able to:

- Identify laws impacting human resource management
- Understand discrimination and lawful questions in the pre-employment inquiry
- Successfully recruit applicants for an open position
- Plan and prepare for the interview process
- Design an orientation checklist for new employees

Before establishing policies and practices related to human resources management, it is important to be aware of the legal environment that surrounds the organization.

These take the form of federal and state employment laws that affect what a manager can and cannot do. In addition to government legislation, union contracts may also influence human resources planning. In this chapter, several federal regulations will be explored. State regulations vary by location, so it is important to investigate these in your own state. In addition, the human resources department and/or legal counsel of a facility can serve as an excellent resource for understanding the obligations regarding personnel management.

Federal Equal Employment Opportunity (EEO) Laws

The U.S. **Equal Employment Opportunity Commission (EEOC)** provides the oversight and coordination of all federal equal employment opportunity regulations, practices, and policies. Figure 10.1 shows some of the important employment legislation that has been passed making it illegal to discriminate in hiring based on a person's race, color, religion, sex (including pregnancy), national origin, age (40 or older), disability, or genetic information. Note that the EEOC does not enforce the protections that prohibit discrimination and harassment based on sexual orientation, status as a parent, marital status, and political affiliation. However, other federal agencies and many states as well as municipalities do. An organization may be held liable for the discriminatory acts of its employees, even if administrators were unaware of these acts. Not only does a Certified Dietary Manager®, Certified Food Protection Professional® (CDM®, CFPP®) need to be aware of the legislation contained in Figure 10.1, but the employees also must realize that they are under a legal obligation not to discriminate. If there is a human resources department, work with it whenever there are employment concerns or questions.

Discrimination

Discrimination is the prejudicial treatment or unfair consideration based on class or category, rather than on individual merit. In essence, discrimination places people in categories based on personal factors, and treating everyone within a category the same. Since this conduct is based on an ignorance of the individuality of the employees, it can generate unjust managerial policies, decisions, and actions based on stereotyping and prejudices.

Discrimination based on age, gender, race, color, religion, national origin, physical or mental disability is illegal in the workplace. There are certain questions that may not be asked on an employment application or during an interview. Care, therefore, is important in structuring questions included in application forms. Figure 10.2 summarizes what a potential employer may and may not ask of a job applicant.

Individual departments or managers should not set conflicting dress codes. Exceptions in requirements may be needed for specific departments, such as hair restraints in food service, jewelry restrictions in surgery, and others. The same general dress code standards apply to men and women. These standards must be reasonable, appropriate, and consistent.

Religious discrimination must be avoided. Employees must be scheduled so that their work requirements will not conflict with their religious commitments/beliefs. It is, therefore, necessary to make whatever schedule and other adjustments to meet these special requirements. For example, if an employee's personal appearance reflects a religious heritage such as length of hair, human resources must accommodate this through its policies.

GLOSSARY

Equal Employment Opportunity Commission (EEOC)
An organization that provides the oversight for federal employment legislation

Discrimination
Treatment or consideration based on class or category, rather than individual merit

Figure 10.1
Federal Laws Affecting Employment Management

1963 Equal Pay Act	This law makes it illegal to pay different wages to men and women if they perform equal work in the same workplace.
1964 Title VII of the Civil Rights Act (amended in 1974)	Protects against employment discrimination based on race, color, religion, gender, or national origin. The law also requires that employers reasonably accommodate applicants' and employees' sincerely held religious practices, unless doing so would impose an undue hardship on the operation of the employer's business. Formed the basis for establishing the EEOC.
1967 Age Discrimination in Employment Act (ADEA)	Protects individuals who are 40 years of age or older from discrimination because of age.
1973 Rehabilitation Act	This law makes it illegal to discriminate against a qualified person with a disability in the federal government.
1978 Pregnancy Discrimination Act	This law amended Title VII to make it illegal to discriminate against a woman because of pregnancy, childbirth, or a medical condition related to pregnancy or childbirth.
1990 Americans with Disabilities Act (ADA)	Prohibits employment discrimination against qualified individuals with disabilities in the private sector, and in state and local governments.
1991 Civil Rights Act, amended	Provides monetary damages in cases of intentional employment discrimination; established glass ceiling.
1993 Family and Medical Leave Act (FMLA)	Provides up to 12 weeks leave, unpaid and job-protected, per year to an employee for birth or adoption; or to care for a spouse, parent, or child with a serious health condition.
1994 Uniformed Services Employment and Reemployment Act	Protects individuals who leave work to fulfill their military service obligation.
1996 Health Insurance Portability and Accountability Act (HIPAA)	Protects confidentiality of medical records and provides for transfer of medical coverage of existing illnesses to another employer's insurance plan.
1996 Illegal Immigration Reform and Immigrant Responsibility Act	Provides for severe restrictions on persons who remain in the United States longer than permitted by their visa and/or who violate their nonimmigrant status.
2008 Genetic Information Nondiscrimination Act (GINA)	Prohibits employment discrimination based on genetic information about an applicant, employee, or former employee.

Source: https://www.eeoc.gov/laws/statutes/index.cfm

GLOSSARY

Bona Fide Occupational Qualifications (BFOQ)
Allowed personal or physical characteristic normally considered discriminating

Privacy Act
Protects employees against invasion of their privacy in the workplace

Americans With Disabilities Act (ADA)
Requires reasonable accommodation for disabled persons

Disability
A physical or mental impairment that substantially limits one or more major life activities of such individuals; a record of such an impairment; or being regarded as having such an impairment

Three exceptions to discrimination are: **bona fide occupational qualifications (BFOQ)**, seniority and merit systems, and education requirements. A bonafide occupational qualification is an essential attribute required for performing a task. For example, a CDM, CFPP may ask if an employee is able to lift heavy boxes or a case of canned goods if the job requires it. Seniority refers to the length of employment and allows for employee rights and benefits based on length of employment. Education requirements, if used as a selection criteria, must be related to the job.

Privacy Act

Federal and state laws also protect employees against invasion of their privacy. The **Privacy Act** covers employee records, locker and personal inspections, background investigations, and other areas. Normally, employees are entitled to a reasonable expectation of privacy and, if this is denied, legal liability may result.

Disabilities

The **Americans With Disabilities Act (ADA)**, passed in 1990, requires covered organizations to take steps to accommodate disabled persons, including employees, and to employ qualified disabled job applicants.

The law's definition of **disability** is important: "A physical or mental impairment that substantially limits one or more major life activities of such individuals; a record of such an impairment; or being regarded as having such an impairment." This definition includes persons with a wide range of disabling conditions, such as blindness, hearing impairments, arthritis, heart conditions, emphysema, shortness of stature, amputation, and others.

Regulations state that organizations must make "reasonable accommodations" as long as doing so does not create an "undue burden." Issues such as costs, financial resources of the facility, and its relationship, if any, with a parent corporation are all taken into account as these and related issues are assessed.

Generally, public accommodations must remove architectural barriers in existing facilities if such removal is readily achievable (easily carried out without too much difficulty or expense). Each public accommodation must evaluate its facilities and determine what can be done. If a problem exists, the organization typically must provide goods, services, facilities, and accommodations through alternative methods.

In regard to the facility itself, there are several priorities:

- The first priority is the actual access to the public accommodation (doorways, entrance ramps, etc.).
- The second priority is the access to goods and services. (For example, do all disabled visitors have access to the cafeteria?)
- The third priority is the access to restroom facilities.
- The fourth priority is the access to any other services, goods, or facilities offered by the organization.

1. You are interviewing a prospective employee who is visibly limping. During the interview, your head cook asks, "Can you tell me what happened to your leg?" Is this a legal question? Why or why not?

Figure 10.2
EEOC Guide to Pre-Employment Inquiries

	QUESTION CATEGORIES	QUESTIONS ALLOWED	EXAMPLES OF POTENTIAL DISCRIMINATORY QUESTIONS
1.	Arrest records	None (*for convictions, see No. 5*)	Number and kinds of arrests
2.	Availability for work on weekends, evenings	If asked of all applicants and it is a business necessity for persons to be available to work weekends and/or evenings	Any inquiry about religious observance
3.	Child care	None, unless asked of all applicants	Inquiry into child care arrangements of only female applicants
4.	Citizenship, birthplace, and national origin	The only legitimate concern here is whether the applicant is eligible to work in the United States, under the terms of the Immigration Reform and Control Act of 1986. There is a fair and advisable way to obtain information. The best approach is to ask: Are you either a U.S. citizen or an alien authorized to work in the United States? The Yes or No answer that follows provides all needed information while not disclosing which (citizen or alien) the applicant is.	Birthplace, national origin, ancestry, or lineage of applicant, applicant's parents or applicant's spouse
5.	Conviction records	Inquiry into convictions if job-related	Any inquiry about conviction, unrelated to job requirements
6.	Creed or religion	None, except where religion is a bona fide occupational qualification	Applicant's religious affiliation, church, parish, or religious holidays observed
7.	Credit records	None, unless job-related	Inquiries about charge accounts, bank accounts, etc.
8.	Family status	Whether applicant has responsibilities or commitments that will prevent meeting work schedules, if asked of all applicants regardless of sex	Marital status, number and age of children, spouse's job
9.	Height and weight	None, unless job-related	Any inquiry unrelated to job requirements
10.	Language	Language applicant speaks or writes fluently, if job-related	Applicant's other tongue, language used by applicant at home, or how applicant acquired the ability to read, write, or speak a foreign language
11.	Marital status	None	Whether applicant is married, single, divorced, separated, engaged, or widowed

(*Continued*)

Figure 10.2
EEOC Guide to Pre-Employment Inquiries *(Continued)*

	QUESTION CATEGORIES	QUESTIONS ALLOWED	EXAMPLES OF POTENTIAL DISCRIMINATORY QUESTIONS
12.	Military status	Military experience or training	Type or condition of discharge
13.	Name	Whether applicant has worked under a different name	The original name of an applicant whose name has been legally changed or the national origin of an applicant's name
14.	Organizations	Applicant's membership in professional organizations if job-related	All clubs, social fraternities, societies, lodges, or organizations to which applicant belongs
15.	Photographs	None except after hiring	Photographs with application or after interview but before hiring
16.	Pregnancy	None	Any inquiry into pregnancy, medical history of pregnancy, or family plans
17.	Race or color	None	Applicant's race or color of applicant's skin
18.	References	Names of character references	Name of applicant's pastor or religious leader
19.	Relatives/friends	Names of applicant's relatives already employed by your organization or a competitor, but you may not give preference if women and minorities are underrepresented in workforce	Names of friends working for the company or relatives other than those working for the company
20.	Sex	None, except where sex is a bona fide occupational qualification	Any inquiry except where a bona fide occupational qualification
21.	Workers' compensation	None	Past workers' compensation claims

A wide range of regulations apply when there is new construction or alteration to existing facilities. Likewise, enforcement provisions include opportunities for victims of discrimination to go to court.

Most healthcare facilities have been designed to accommodate persons with disabilities and, in fact, exist to provide health services for them. However, healthcare facilities may be confronted with the same types of issues as other organizations relative to the employment of persons with disabilities.

Figure 10.3 reviews major concerns that must be addressed in the personnel policies and procedures of most employers.

Harassment

Today, **sexual harassment** in the workplace receives significant attention and is one of the most frequent reasons for employee litigation (lawsuits). In March 1980, the Equal Employment Opportunity Commission (EEOC) issued specific guidelines dealing with sexual harassment. Sexual harassment is a violation of Title VII of the

---

GLOSSARY

Sexual Harassment
Workplace conduct that is:
1. Sexual in nature and
2. Unwelcomed

Figure 10.3
Americans with Disabilities Act Requirements (ADAR) Fact Sheet: Employment

- Employers may not discriminate against an individual with a disability in hiring or promotion if the person is otherwise qualified for the job.
- Employers can ask about one's ability to perform a job, but cannot inquire if someone has a disability or subject a person to tests that tend to screen out people with disabilities.

- Employers need to provide "reasonable accommodation" to individuals with disabilities. This includes taking steps such as job restructuring and modification of equipment.
- Employers do not need to provide accommodations that impose an "undue hardship" on business operations.
- All employers with 15 or more employees must comply to this ADAR.

Civil Rights Act of 1964. Simply stated, in order for a conduct to be considered sexual harassment:

- The conduct must be sexual in nature.
- The conduct must be unwelcome.

Sexual harassment may be physical, verbal (including suggestive comments), or visual (for example, displaying pornographic photographs).

While the laws and their interpretations may vary, some principles are well established. The CDM, CFPP and/or employer may be held liable for sexual harassment if an employee is deprived of a tangible job benefit (e.g., promotion) because of a refusal to provide sexual favors. If an employee's work environment is negatively affected (in the employee's opinion) by the sexual harassment of a supervisor or co-worker, and if the employer knows or should have known of this conduct and does not take immediate action, the employer will probably be held liable. The manager and the facility can also be found liable for the harassment of employees by clients or their guests if unwanted activities occurred, and the facility personnel were aware of them, yet no immediate corrective actions were taken.

A facility must exercise reasonable care to prevent sexual harassment. In the event that a manager is informed that an employee is being sexually harassed, the EEOC Guidelines on Discrimination Because of Sex mandates that the following steps must be taken:

1. Notify your own superior.
2. Investigate the situation according to your organization's policy.
3. Seek legal advice before further action is taken.
4. Confront the accused party and get the accused party's side of the story.
5. Take any necessary disciplinary action(s).

2. Your male cook has a habit of putting his arm around the female cashier. Is this a violation of the sexual harassment law? How would you deal with a complaint from the cashier?

To deal effectively with the issue of sexual harassment:

- The facility or organization should have a formal written policy specifically addressing the step-by-step procedures to be followed regarding sexual harassments. As a corporate or system-based policy, the approving signature is typically that of the senior administrator and a lawyer or the facility's Risk Manager.
- All managers should be familiar with the sexual harassment policy. This should include disciplinary guidelines for both the individual who is guilty and guidelines for harassers who retaliate against those who report them. The policy should include a formal complaint procedure for employees to use if they think they have been victims of sexual harassment. Provisions for immediate investigation and prompt disciplinary action when appropriate must be taken.
- Employees should be instructed on how to recognize sexual harassment, how to report it when it occurs, and the steps that shall be taken if an employee is guilty. All cases of possible sexual harassment must be investigated according to this policy.
- Follow-up needs to be provided after all instances of sexual harassment. Victims must be contacted and witnesses asked if the sexual harassment has indeed stopped and that no retaliation is taking place.

Fair Labor Standards Act (FLSA)

The **Fair Labor Standards Act (FLSA)** addresses the idea that an employee deserves to be paid fairly. It defines the:

- Minimum wage
- 40-hour work week
- Requirements for overtime
- Restrictions on child labor

Individual states also have provisions relating to these standards. What is legally acceptable varies from state to state. The FLSA specifically includes state and local hospitals, as well as educational institutions. Among other things, the law requires that employees exceeding a 40-hour work week receive overtime pay.

The overtime pay requirement does not apply to an exempt employee. An **exempt employee** is on salary (as opposed to receiving an hourly wage). An exempt employee does not receive overtime compensation. In a facility where employees belong to a union, an exempt employee may have a broader definition. Employees who meet the following criteria can be exempt from the overtime provisions of the Wage and Hour Law because as executives:

They supervise two or more other employees.

- Their salary is the minimum amount determined by the Wage and Hour Division (which changes periodically).
- They have the power to hire and fire, or their recommendations must carry significant weight.
- Their primary duty is management. They cannot do non-exempt work (substitute for employees) more than 40 percent of the time in any given work week. Generally, they cannot do the work of the people they supervise.
- They are able to exercise discretionary powers and set policies on the job.

Often only the department manager can set policies within that department, and all others follow these policies. Therefore, only one person in a department is considered

GLOSSARY

Fair Labor Standards Act (FLSA)
Addresses the idea that an employee deserves to be paid fairly

Exempt Employee
An employee who is salaried and does not qualify for overtime compensation

exempt as an executive. However, the Wage and Hour Division has been interpreting this rule to allow an assistant manager who is working on an entirely different shift from the manager to be exempt if the other requirements are met.

Definitions regarding what determines full-time versus part-time status, eligibility for benefits and "paid time off" are not specifically defined by FLSA or other federal regulation.

Workers Compensation

The concept of workers compensation is to limit the liability of the employer if an employee becomes injured while on the job. It also provides income to an employee who is unable to work due to an injury on the job. The federal government has laid the groundwork for workers compensation through the **Federal Employment Compensation Act (FECA)**, which is administered by state governments. Each state has its own policies and legislation and administers the program.

Unemployment

Another form of protection provided by law is the financial protection awarded to employees in case they become unemployed through no fault of their own. The law providing this protection is the **Federal Unemployment Tax Act (FUTA)**. FUTA provides a right to unemployment compensation to protect the income of former employees while they seek new employment. It does not apply to an employee who was terminated through a disciplinary process.

For example, if a facility determines that it needs to eliminate a set of jobs, the employees who lose their jobs may be eligible to receive unemployment compensation. How much and for how long depends on a number of factors. State entities are involved in administering the legislation, and employers pay a tax to help provide funding for this program.

These are some examples of employment regulations, although this section does not present an exhaustive list. For information about federal employment regulations, visit the U.S. Department of Labor website Compliance Assistance section (www.dol.gov) to review regulations by name or topic. Furthermore, the human resources department is the best authority on all the employment laws (federal and state) that may affect your actions as a manager.

Reviewing the human resources policies and procedures of the organization assists a CDM, CFPP in understanding the standards for the department. These policies affect how to recruit new employees and manage existing team members.

Selecting Employees

The best employees start with the hiring process!

Selecting employees involves several steps: recruitment, screening, checking references, interviewing and making a hiring decision. Some facilities may use their human resources department to coordinate the selection process. It is important to have standardized procedures for each of these steps, as they are covered by the EEOC. The government provides free guidelines for the selection process titled, Uniform Guidelines on Employee Selection Procedures. If there is no HR department, be sure and consult these guidelines, including the questions and answers found on the website.

GLOSSARY

Federal Employment Compensation Act (FECA)
Establishes workers compensation for employees injured on the job

Federal Unemployment Tax Act (FUTA)
Provides a right to unemployment compensation to employees who become unemployed through no fault of their own

GLOSSARY

Recruitment
Process of locating potential applicants for a job opening

Screening
Process of comparing applicants on the basis of their skill level, knowledge and abilities, and choosing the most qualified for the job

Pre-Employment Testing
Aptitude, personality, or skills testing conducted prior to employment as part of the screening process

The Recruitment Process

The **recruitment** process helps to build a pool of applicants for open positions. The CDM, CFPP will need to decide if they are going to recruit from within the facility or search outside the facility. The human resources department can assist in the recruitment process, based on the open positions and the availability of qualified candidates in the facility. If outside recruitment is needed, the human resources department can assist in obtaining candidates via newspapers or online job sites.

After initial recruitment efforts, the manager is faced with the task of predicting how well the candidates will perform on the job. Much of the information for a final decision is gathered during a structured screening and interview process. This determines who is selected as the new employee.

The Selection Process

Many businesses now use a screening process to select the applicants to be interviewed. This means comparing each applicant's qualifications to the job description. To be protected by the EEOC and to follow the Uniform Guidelines for Employee Selection, you should use a screening committee that compares each applicant in the same way to the job description. Some facilities have a written form for the screening process which is used for each applicant, such as shown in Figure 10.4. Using the same template with each applicant helps to reduce discrimination.

Figure 10.4
Screening Template for Foodservice Employees

QUALIFICATIONS	EDUCATION	EXPERIENCE					OTHER
		Sanitation	Record Keeping	Food Protection	Customer/ Client Service	Notification	
Applicant #1							
Applicant #2							

Some organizations have implemented a **pre-employment testing** process consisting of some or all of the following:

- Aptitude testing: Evaluates a candidate's critical thinking and problem-solving skills.
- Personality questionnaire: Tests for behavioral characteristics related to customer service and other workplace performance.
- Skills testing: Checks for basic competencies needed in the workplace or specific skills required for the position.

The testing may be a general evaluation of candidates required for all positions within the organization or highly specific to individual job descriptions. When there are too many applicants for consideration, use of both the paper screening process (match to the job description and results of pre-employment testing) and a formal interview should be considered.

The Interview Process

Much information about job applicants can be gained from application forms, reference checks, selection tests, and medical examinations.

- Reference Checks—Without a human resources department, use a standard form for all candidates that asks for: dates of employment, relationship to applicant, reason for leaving.
- Pre-employment Selection Tests—If used for any applicants, it should be used for each applicant.
- Medical Examinations—The Americans with Disabilities Act requires that this be directly related to employment and cannot be required until employment is offered.

This may not be enough information for determining whether an applicant will be suitable for the available position. One or more pre-employment job interviews may also be essential to match a candidate with a job vacancy.

A second manager that has not been part of the preliminary interview may also want to conduct a second meeting with the candidate prior to the selection process. The purpose of the interview is to assess the abilities, attitudes, and compatibility of the applicant for the position. It is very important, therefore, that the immediate supervisor be involved in the applicant selection process. Figure 10.5 identifies some basic questions that may be useful during an interview.

An interview is really a planned conversation and provides a structured discussion of relevant topics for both parties. Generally, an interviewer works from a pre-determined list of questions in order to assure fairness in assessing candidates. However, the best interview process puts the candidates at ease and allows them to open up and provide more needed information. Figure 10.6 provides additional interviewing information.

3. Your chief clinical dietitian is an exempt employee and recently put in extra hours to help for an audit. Is she entitled to overtime pay?

Figure 10.5
Frequently Asked Interview Questions

- Why do you choose to be with our organization?
- Describe your ideal job.
- What can you offer us?
- What skills have you developed?
- What did you enjoy most about your last employment?
- What did you enjoy least about your last employment?
- Have you ever quit a job? Why?
- Why should we hire you rather than another candidate?
- What do you consider to be your greatest strengths?
- Would you be successful working on a team?
- What do you know about our organization?
- Have you worked under deadline pressure? When?
- How do you feel about working in a structured environment?
- How do you feel about working overtime?
- How did you get along with your former co-workers?
- What are your expectations for rate of pay?
- What can you tell us about yourself?
- What type of computer experience do you have?
- Would you be willing to take a drug test?
- How does your past experience apply to this position?
- How does this job match your interests?
- What skills do you have which will help in this job?
- What are your main strengths for this job?
- What major weaknesses will need to be overcome for you to do this job effectively?
- Will you have any problems getting to work?
- What other information can you provide which will help me to understand your capabilities for this work?
- What questions do you have about the job?
- When would you be able to begin work?

When interviewing a prospective employee, you are indirectly setting the tone for the relationship that may follow if that individual is hired. The interview can ultimately be construed as a legally binding description of both the job opportunity and the company's value system (or lack of it).

Types of Interview Questions

There are three basic types of interview questions: directive, non-directive, and situational. **Directive interview questions** are specific questions formulated in advance and asked in a checklist fashion. Questions asked should solicit important information. Examples of directive interview questions include:

- What did you do in your last job?
- Why did you leave your last position?

Directive interview questions solicit facts and do not seek opinions. All topics of directive questions should directly impact on how well the applicant can perform the job. Any other questions may be in violation of EEOC or other laws. When directive interview questions are used, it is important that the job applicant be given time to ask questions and that the interviewer provides basic information about the job. Generally, the interviewer should record responses to questions as they are provided.

The second type of questions are **non-directive interview questions**. While these questions are also planned and perhaps written down in advance, they are less structured and more non-directive so that the interviewee can provide creative responses. Examples of non-directive questions include:

- Why do you think you'll like this job?
- What elements do you regard as important when you consider a new position?

GLOSSARY

Directive Interview Questions
Pre-planned interview questions seeking specific information

Non-Directive Interview Questions
Pre-planned open-ended interview questions seeking more expansive responses

Figure 10.6
Interviewing Tips

- Respect a candidate's feelings and self-esteem at all times. Strive to put the candidate at ease.
- Begin with a pleasant, professional introduction and appropriate light conversation.
- Remember that to the candidate, you are the organization.
- Don't give excessive encouragement, verbally or nonverbally, at any point.
- Examine candidate evidence in areas of past performance and achievement, as well as work philosophies and beliefs.
- Use verbal rejoinders to trigger additional response in crucial areas, such as "Tell me more…," "Give me another example," etc.
- Use nonverbal reminders, such as nodding, facial gestures, etc. to maintain a steady flow of information.
- Take notes as needed and in a natural sequence. Don't make a final appraisal of notes until the interview is concluded.
- If you don't see a desired characteristic, ask for it specifically. If it is still not apparent, score the applicant accordingly.
- Make yourself thoroughly knowledgeable about the candidate prior to the interview and use that knowledge throughout the meeting.
- Portray the available position adequately and accurately; question candidate to determine specific qualifications.
- Have a set questioning process prepared prior to the interview; seek specific data to match against the job description.
- Don't wander into EEOC-sensitive information unless you are seeking BFOQ—Bona Fide Occupational Qualifications. Avoid areas such as age, race, marital status, and any other sensitive areas unless information is volunteered by candidate.
- Let the candidate do the majority of the talking.
- Listen attentively, accurately, and actively.
- Postpone all final judgments until after the interview.
- Interrupt the candidate only when necessary, and then with tact and brevity.
- Ask candidate for permission to take notes, or merely inform candidate you will do so.
- Control excessive applicant rambling by introducing the next question or a rejoinder.
- Ensure the candidate answers a question at hand completely before moving on to another area.

Many interviewers like to use responses to non-directive questions as springboards for additional questions formulated on-the-fly. With this approach, the interviewer can go on in depth and learn more about the applicant. Applicants who are encouraged to speak on their own will usually provide much more information than they will in response to closed-ended yes-or-no questions.

The use of **situational interview questions** is an excellent way to further evaluate how well a candidate will fit in with the department. These questions ask a candidate to describe a type of situation and related decisions and/or actions. Here are some examples of situational questions:

- Tell me about a time when you knew a co-worker was not following work procedures. What happened, and what did you do?
- Describe a personal conflict that you had with a co-worker. What happened, and how did you respond?
- If you knew someone was stealing, what would you do?
- Can you think of a time when you disagreed with a company policy? Tell me what you decided to do.
- If you saw an unsafe situation, what would you do?

GLOSSARY

Situational Interview Questions
Questions designed to describe an event or situation

During an interview, a CDM, CFPP can combine directive, non-directive, and situational questions to help build an understanding of the candidate's suitability for a job. To encourage the applicant to tell you as much as possible, avoid leading questions.

Leading questions can also influence a candidate's response and interfere with receiving valid information. Here are some examples of leading questions to avoid:

- "You would like to work here, wouldn't you?"
- "You wouldn't argue with a client, would you?"

Preparing For and Conducting An Interview

Needless to say, there is much more to an interview than just asking questions. The interviewer must properly prepare for it. The following are essential in the interviewing process:

- Choose a private environment free from interruptions.
- Set a beginning time and stick to it.
- Read over the application form and any other information available about the applicant.
- Provide enough time so that information can be solicited without the need to rush.
- Review the checklist of questions and be sure that all questions are relevant to the selection decision.

Some basic principles help develop good interview techniques. It is essential to put the applicant at ease. Candidates are likely to be nervous, so some friendly, opening conversation can be helpful in developing the rapport necessary for a good interview. A friendly handshake, a hospitable greeting, and perhaps a cup of coffee are always good ways to start.

Once the interview begins:

- Ask simple questions first.
- Be aware of the time and don't allow yourself to feel rushed.
- Listen to what is being said.
- Concentrate rather than thinking ahead when the interviewee is speaking.
- Strive to maintain excellent eye contact and observe the candidate's nonverbal behavior.
- Listen open-mindedly.

Recognize that the candidate is probably very eager to learn about the position and the facility. A rule of thumb is to listen for about 75 percent of the interview, and talk for about 25 percent. Most of the facility information can wait until the late stage of the interview. Again, relating the details of your philosophy and standards may influence an applicant to simply say what he thinks you want to hear.

4. You are preparing to interview candidates for the cook's position. What techniques would you use during the interview?

Follow-up after the interview is necessary. If there is no human resources staff assisting, it is a considerate gesture to notify the applicant that they are not being considered for the position. Perhaps there is another vacant position for which the interviewee will be eligible. Put yourself in the interviewee's place. Wouldn't you like to know about the interview results as soon as possible?

If you believe the applicant is qualified but want to interview others, it is fair to inform the interviewee. Name a time by which you will relate the selection decision. Adhere to the schedule or apprise the interviewee of any changes in the timetable. If the interviewee is qualified and there are no other applicants to consider, you may inform the interviewee that a job offer will be extended.

If working with a human resources department, each interview team member may be asked to rank the candidates based on the selection criteria. The human resources department will follow up with the candidate after the interview.

The Hiring Decision

To make a **hiring** decision, review the notes from interviews and weigh them carefully. In certain cases, you may have picked up son ome red flags indicating a candidate may not be able to take direction, or work with others, or perform in a reliable manner. You will probably want to remove these candidates from the list.

At the same time, there may be a list of multiple candidates who seem to be well qualified and may fit in well with the job requirements. Who should be offered the position?

Typically, this decision is made by reviewing applicant information, considering the relevance of training, experience, education, assessing how well the candidate is likely to work with others on the team, and making a prediction of how likely the candidate is to become a successful long-term employee. Checking references at this point may provide additional decision information.

Sometimes, you may feel that there are no qualified candidates for an open job. While there may be pressure to fill a job, it is usually worth waiting to make a good match. Bringing in the wrong person may seem easy and expedient for the moment, but it is likely to create more work down the line. In fact, if the candidate does not work out, you will find yourself again at the point of recruiting. A better approach is not to hire the applicant and immediately increase your recruitment efforts to find more candidates.

All information developed from the recruitment and selection process should be maintained on file in the new employee's personnel record. Sometimes the reasons applicants were not selected may also be important. Documentation of applicant information is very important and must be emphasized as permanent files are developed.

The Onboarding and Orientation Process

All employees need to complete an initial orientation process as new hires. This may include required tuberculosis screening, fitting for respirator masks, and completion of a formal training period regarding facility and department policies. Often, the orientation program conducted by the human resources department addresses the system-wide policies required by the regulatory agencies, but does not refer to the policies specific to food handling and service.

> **GLOSSARY**
>
> **Hiring**
> Selecting the candidate for the job and offering the position to the candidate

GLOSSARY

Orientation
Formal process of familiarizing new employees with the organization, department, and job

Onboarding
The process designed to educate new employees about the department's expectations and standards

View the Supplemental Material for Figure 10.7, Orientation Checklist for Food and Nutrition Services for Skilled Nursing.

Orientation is an important step in the employment process because new employees may make costly mistakes if not oriented properly. Orientation can also help create realistic job expectations. Three types of information are generally included in orientation:

1. Review of the organization, its structure, mission and objectives
2. Specific information on policies, work rules, and benefits
3. General information about the daily work routine

Development of your own **onboarding** process helps ensure that the departmental expectations and standards are communicated to all staff members. Consistent, clear expectations minimize the confusion of "I'm not sure how I am supposed to do this task" or "I don't know if I am doing a good job," which is a common reason for losing new employees. The onboarding process may last throughout the probationary period, and may include multiple learning tasks and/or on-the-job training sessions.

The onboarding and orientation process should be clearly defined in both the human resources and the dining services policies. Documented success, or failure, to complete the tasks may determine whether employment will be continued.

Documentation in the employee's personnel file verifies the training provided and proficiency achieved by the staff member. These documents can also support you in the event of future performance issues.

A comprehensive orientation and step-by-step onboarding process will improve your employee retention and increase their job performance from the first day.

In the Supplemental Material for this chapter is an example of an orientation checklist for food and nutrition services unit of a skilled nursing facility.

Chapter References

RESOURCES	
A Guide to Disability Rights Laws	https://www.ada.gov/cguide.htm
Casco, W.F,. &Aguinis, H (2011). Applied Psychology in Human Resource Management (7th ed.) Upper Saddle River: Prentice Hall	
Department of Labor	https://www.dol.gov/
National Labor Relations Board	https://nlrb.gov/
U.S. Equal Employment Opportunity Commission	https://www.eeoc.gov/laws/index.cfm
U.S. Equal Employment Opportunity Commission Religious Discrimination	https://www.eeoc.gov/religious-discrimination
Uniform Guidelines for Recruiting Employees	http://www.uniformguidelines.com

Ongoing Employee Education

Overview and Objectives

A key part of developing personnel is education and training. Training builds the value of people in the facility through motivation, positive morale, and superior performance. Planned and focused education is designed to achieve results and behaviors that align with the facility's needs and objectives. After completing this chapter you should be able to:

- Orient new employees to facility procedures
- Develop and implement training programs
- Identify training resources and needs
- Conduct and arrange in-service and on-the-job training with a focus on food and dining services activities, such as:
  - Safe food preparation practices
  - HIPAA guidelines
  - Hospitality and customer service
  - Physical and workplace safety
- Document completion of training and orientation

> **GLOSSARY**
>
> **Training**
> Ongoing process of updating skills of an employee

Career development of employees involves continued training to increase their skills and knowledge for the job. The success of an organization depends on its workforce. **Training** improves all aspects of the foodservice department. It is important to remember as you review this material that training is not a one-time event, it is an ongoing process.

Onboarding and Orientation

As discussed in Chapter 10, onboarding of new employees often starts with human resources-developed education and orientation requirements. This, however, may not include information specific to the dining services department.

Federal, state, and local guidelines often stipulate specific training programs on food safety and sanitation, medical confidentiality, equipment usage, disaster preparedness, as well as foodservice fire and safety training. Remember that new employees do not know where the fire pull box is located, or the safest route for evacuation of residents from the dining room. Developing a dining services orientation program, with a comprehensive checklist, will help ensure that all staff members are fully aware of policies and expectations that affect them.

The following is all of the information a new employee needs to get through on Day 1, and then what they need to know generally to do their job.

- Introduction to supervisors and co-workers
- Tour of the department and all relevant areas of the facility
- Map of the department with fire pulls, extinguishers, exits, break room, and locker room
- First day policies
  > Fire and weather safety
  > All needed phone numbers
  > Attendance/call-in/tardiness policy/etc.
  > Schedule locations and shift swap process
  > Relevant job routines
  > Dress code
  > Reference HR department policies
  > Foodservice sanitation and health code policies
- Review of their specific job description
  > Temporary or probationary limitations
- Employee health sign-off for tuberculosis (TB) testing, mask fitting, and any physical restrictions

1. Prepare a sample onboarding training for a new diet clerk at a long-term care facility.

As discussed in the earlier chapter, it is helpful to use an orientation checklist to organize the content, to ensure that everything is covered, and to develop documentation of the orientation. Some facilities require two sets of initials next to each item on a checklist: the supervisor's initials to verify that this content has been covered, and the employee's initials as a way of accepting responsibility for having learned this content. The orientation also includes the training and skills testing essential for the specific tasks they will be performing. For example, a diet clerk does not need to be approved for use and cleaning of the meat slicer, but a new cook needs that skill validation plus demonstrated proficiency with the fryer, char-broiler, and knife safety, etc.

- Equipment competency checklist
- Skills testing

The onboarding process is the sum of all the orientation activities, and is often planned to cover the first 30-90 days of employment (the typical probationary period). Completion of the different activities frequently includes a signed checklist and often a test of some kind. Documentation validates that each employee has been given the information they need to appropriately perform their assigned tasks.

Many managers have developed a New Hire Training Manual or three-ring binder system that employees can build during their onboarding process. This may include copies of all relevant policies, department and facility maps, schedules, contact information, job descriptions, etc. Retaining the employee-signed receipt for the materials and training post-tests verifies the completion of each step in the process.

An additional scheduling consideration relates to the length of time for orientation. Working with content in smaller segments gives the employee time to process new information and improves retention. An additional advantage of this approach is that as an employee begins working, familiarity grows. The employee develops a context in which to understand and store this new information. The employee may also come across questions and curiosities that enhance learning.

On the first day, cover some basic elements related to timeclock procedures, uniforms, and department layout.

- As follow-up on the next day, cover work procedures and routines.
- At yet another time, review safety policies.

The dining services-specific onboarding process record should be kept in the employee's department file for easy reference.

> Some managers have used a color-coded system to make recordkeeping easier. The Onboarding Process record is on blue paper, Fire and Safety are on pink paper, Sanitation is on yellow paper, Diet Information is on green paper, etc. By looking in a file, they can quickly see if an employee has a signed checklist or post-test for the different training programs.

Training Beyond the Orientation Period

Mastering new skills and realizing his or her own potential are tremendous motivators. Training can meet employees' basic needs and foster good morale. (Maslow A. H. 1954) It also serves other purposes. For a facility, effective training can:

- Reduce the occurrence of injuries, accidents, and mistakes.
- Improve quality of services and/or products.
- Improve productivity.
- Reduce turnover rate and recruitment expenses.
- Bring about better management of resources often with associated cost reductions.
- Improve compliance with regulations and standards.
- Support implementation of new procedures or techniques, new systems, or new equipment.

All foodservice employees, those new on the job as well as those with years of experience, can benefit from effective training programs. The Joint Commission (TJC), the Occupational Safety and Health Administration (OSHA), most state licensing laws, and many health department regulations require specific ongoing employee training programs for foodservice employees, which may specify training on topics, such as:

- Sanitation practices
- Employee illness reporting
- Safety and disaster preparedness
- Role in medical nutrition therapy
- Confidentiality
- Safe operation of equipment
- Injury/accident prevention and reporting
- Safe use of chemicals
- Risk management
- Sexual harassment
- Labor laws and employees' rights

A number of regulations and standards stipulate that orientation and training must be provided to all employees from all shifts, and must be planned and conducted for all foodservice personnel. Check with members of the facility to determine specific guidelines that apply to the situation. As new procedures are implemented and new equipment is purchased, there is a need for ongoing in-service (on-the-job) training.

Furthermore, long-standing employees need periodic (some annual) updates and refreshers, even for information they have learned in the past, to increase motivation and reinforce work practices.

All training should be documented. Documentation may be required by health inspectors or surveyors. It also helps in keeping track of what has been completed and what training is outstanding. One way to do this is to ask each attendee to sign an attendance sheet and file this along with the outline of the training session.

Developing and implementing effective training programs is not difficult, but it does require time. Figure 11.1 provides the steps to effective training.

Figure 11.1
Steps in Training

1. Determine the need—who and what should be offered.

2. Develop the training content. How do you determine what content to cover in training? To identify the content, you can:
   - Check standards that specify content.
   - Identify changes in the operation that require training.
   - Review quality studies and identify areas that require training for improvement.
   - Talk with employees during performance reviews and ask them what they need and want to learn.
   - Observe operations and make notes of skills that need to be developed.
   - Check with colleagues for new ideas about training content.

   As training content is defined, try to focus on specifics. For example, a session about all aspects of safety may be too much. A session about appropriate knife handling and another session about lifting objects safely are likely to generate better outcomes.

3. Decide on the objectives/outcomes of the training. To write an objective, start with thinking about what the employees need to do after the training. If a task has been documented as a performance standard, then these tasks are the training objectives. A well-written objective begins with an action verb and should fit the S.M.A.R.T. principle: **S**pecific. **M**easurable. **A**chievable. **R**elevant. **T**imely (https://www.smart-goals-guide.com/). Examples of S.M.A.R.T. training objectives for foodservice employees are:
   - Describe the importance of and access to Safety Data Sheets (SDS).
   - Use proper protective equipment when using chemicals in the kitchen.
   - Document food waste using appropriate forms.
   - Compute cost of menu items.
   - Demonstrate proper handwashing procedures.
   - Use proper portion control utensils.
   - Define proper cooling procedures for soup.

   As you can see, these all begin with a verb and are outcomes of the training session.

4. Once there is an objective, it is time to gather the materials needed for teaching the objective. The materials will depend upon the objectives. For example, when training on how to use SDS forms, having actual forms available will improve the training.

   Use of proper portion control utensils will require having various portioning utensils and perhaps some food items to practice portioning. Use posters and reminder signs in your department to reinforce training content. Many training resources are available through trade and industry websites.

5. Decide where to hold the training.
   - Does the facility have a conference room where you can be undisturbed and comfortable?
   - Consider using the kitchen if there will be equipment demonstrations.
   - Make sure to reserve any rooms needed ahead of time.
   - Plan to use a stand-up meeting to quickly cover one or two points, or as a reminder of specific activities.
   - Consider a roving in-service to briefly meet with staff in small groups throughout the department or facility.

6. Promote the training. Post the date, place, and time far enough in advance for every shift to see the information. If it is a facility-wide training, confirm that the staff has received the information.

7. Conduct the training. (See the section later in this chapter on training techniques.)

8. Evaluate the training.

Who Should Train?

As with every other task on the job, a motivated individual can develop and refine his or her training skills. As a Certified Dietary Manager®, Certified Food Protection Professional (CDM®, CFPP®), expect to deliver a great deal of training. At the same time, plan to enlist the help of staff members who are showing excellent performance, positive attitudes, and motivation to lead others. This provides recognition to qualified staff members and creates new opportunities for them. In addition, you may find that a staff member who is particularly skillful at a certain task is the best teacher.

Since the person selected to train is critical to the ultimate success of the program, the characteristics of effective trainers must be applied in the selection of a trainer. Among the attributes of a good trainer are:

- An interest in training
- Extensive knowledge of the subject matter
- An ability to communicate effectively
- Strong interpersonal skills
- Patience
- A sense of humor
- Respect for trainees
- Confidence in the ability of others to learn
- An enthusiasm for the training assignment

Beyond the dining services staff, there may be others in the facility and community who can provide training about specific topics. For example, a social worker in your facility may be an excellent resource for providing a training session about dealing with angry clients, or a financial expert might be willing to deliver a session about cost control. A local college or university may be able to provide training about almost any topic. A consulting dietitian can provide training about special diets or tube feedings, or many other topics. Vendors and others may also offer training.

When delegating the training to others, be sure that he or she is aware of the objectives or outcomes. Discuss the content, and review the outline together before finalizing the program. If applicable, check any handouts in advance to ensure that they complement the internal policies and procedures.

Training Techniques

Several principles of learning should be incorporated into the training programs. Educational material, particularly the required annual safety and sanitations programs, can become very repetitive year-after-year. Mixing up the material and trying different techniques can help make the content more interesting.

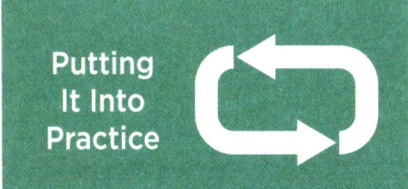

2. Plan a training for a group of hospital food service staff following Figure 11.1. Who would be the trainer for the training and what techniques would be best for optimal retention of information?

Typically, employees want to take an active role in the training activities. Everyone learns best by doing, not just by passively reading or listening. The more staff members can be involved and active in training, the more effective training will be.

Training should focus on real-world problems which employees face and solve on the job. Trainees can then see how the training activities will apply directly to their own work. Perhaps the most important aspect of adult education is the idea of knowledge transfer. This means relating the training content to the job where participants apply it in actual practice.

People learn differently. For instance, some people are auditory learners (they learn by hearing the information). Some people are visual learners (they learn by reading or seeing a diagram). Many people learn by doing (this is known as kinesthetic learning). When training techniques combine listening, reading, and doing, trainees will learn more (Visual, Auditory, and Kinesthetic Learning Styles (VAK). 2015). It may be important to determine the literacy level of the employees. If employees have low reading skills, use more pictures in the training. With a diverse group of employees, language may also be a barrier that pictures can help overcome.

Lectures, online videos, and PowerPoint presentations are examples of one-way flow of information from the trainer to the trainees. Although these methods are inexpensive and require little preparation time, they require the learner to be passive. To use these aids effectively, follow up with activities that help participants transfer the information, such as problem solving, hands-on practice, or role playing. Another option is the use of case studies that present a problem or situation. Trainees analyze and discuss the problem and devise a set of solutions. Have them work in small groups.

For any procedure requiring a series of steps, demonstration is a very useful technique. An effective demonstration breaks a task into clear steps, and walks trainees through the steps at a comfortable pace. Following a demonstration, each trainee needs to practice the procedure with feedback from the trainer. Then, the trainee should do it again. On the job, the trainee should repeat the process with intermittent feedback and support from the CDM, CFPP.

Types of Training

One type of training is called **on-the-job training (OJT)**. This technique is common in many dining services departments because it is practical and easy to use. It involves simply teaching an employee how to do a job while the employee is on location and actually on the job.

To conduct OJT, break down the job into parts, just as you would for a demonstration. In the training, address each part and provide the procedures, performance standards, safety information, and all relevant components. Then, demonstrate and allow the employee to practice.

Repetition is important both to make sure that the trainee knows how to do the work and to allow them to build confidence and speed. Coaching, an integral part of training, is also important while the trainee practices. The trainer can observe and make friendly suggestions about the work. The trainer should frequently compliment the trainee for performance that meets quality standards.

The final step in OJT is the follow-up. After the training has been completed, the trainee should be able to do the work without constant supervision. However, the

> **GLOSSARY**
>
> **On-the-job Training (OJT)**
> Involves teaching an employee how to do a job while the employee is on location and actually on the job

trainer should continue to observe the trainee to ensure that no problems arise. At this time, reinforcement and feedback become important. Figure 11.2 lists the steps for on-the-job training.

In-Service Training

In-service training is the professional development for the employees to improve or update their specific skills. It takes place after the employees have started working.

In-service training should follow the training steps outlined earlier in this chapter. (See Figure 11.3 for an in-service outline for a HIPAA presentation.)

There are many topics that can be included in the in-service training plans. Some are:
- Coping with emergencies
- Dealing with difficult clients
- Professional and ethical expectations for foodservice employees
- Security and confidentiality (HIPAA guidelines)
- Client/customer service

It is extremely important to maintain a record of each in-service training session to include:
- The objective and lesson plan
- Sign-in attendance record with date
- Results of a post-test to verify understanding
- If appropriate, a color-coded post-test to be placed in each employee's file

Figure 11.2
Four Steps for On-the-Job Training

Organize the work area to allow the trainer to stand next to the trainee. Collect any needed tools and remove distractions, if possible.

Reduce the trainee's anxiety and assure him/her that you are there to help. Encourage the trainee to ask questions if he/she doesn't understand any directions.

Demonstrate the job function to the trainee and allow him/her to observe you. If the trainee desires, he/she may take notes during this phase.

Explain key points of the task to the trainee, while demonstrating. Attempt to answer the questions: who, what, when, where, why, and how.

Repeat the demonstration as the trainee observes. This reinforcement increases the likelihood that the trainee will retain the new information.

Let the trainee attempt parts of the job. After he/she attempts to do part of the job, provide constructive feedback, coaching, and suggestions.

Let the trainee perform the entire job under observation. The trainer now provides feedback periodically rather than frequently and encourages the trainee to begin acting independently.

Conduct periodic progress checks. The trainer should step back and only spot check the trainee's progress.

Allow the trainee to work independently. At this point, the trainee has formally completed the training topic, but is encouraged to seek out the trainer if assistance is needed. Complete the training checklist.

Figure 11.3
HIPAA In-Service Training

Intended Audience: All Foodservice Employees

Content to Cover:
Health Insurance Portability and Accountability Act (HIPAA) was made into law in 1996. The Privacy Rule took effect in 2003 with updates in 2006 and 2013. The primary goal is for everyone to keep all health information confidential and to help the healthcare industry control administrative costs. This in-service identifies how HIPAA is applied in the foodservice department.

Resources:
Additional information on the law is found at the Health & Human Services website (www.hhs.gov). General information on HIPAA is available at the following links: (http://www.cms.gov/Regulations-and-Guidance/HIPAA-Administrative-Simplification/HIPAAGenInfo/). Health information privacy. U.S. Department of Health and Human Services website (http://www.hhs.gov/ocr/privacy/) (http://optimalhealthcareinc.com/wp-content/uploads/2012/12/HIPAA-online-in-service.pdf).

Objectives:
- The ability of the staff to describe which parts of HIPAA affect their work.
- The protection of private client information.

Outline:
1. What is Health Insurance Portability and Accountability Act (HIPAA)?
   - Protects the privacy of all personal and health information about clients, including written, spoken, and electronic.
   - Identifies clients' rights to their medical information.
   - Limits access to client-protected information.
   - Clients can request that no information be shared without specific permission.
2. What does the medical facility have to do?
   - Develop privacy policies and procedures.
   - Train staff on the procedures.
   - Define disciplinary action if information is inappropriately released.
3. How does HIPAA affect the Foodservice Department? What is confidential information?
   - Computerized diet information includes name, DOB, diet, medical record number, and often diagnosis.
   - Meal identification menus or cards include name, DOB, diet, and medical record number.
   - Meal delivery sheets include identifiers on all clients on the unit.
   - Clinical and diet office staff can access more detailed information via the medical record.
4. How to manage the privacy of clients:
   - Do not discuss client information with anyone other than those needing the specifics.
   - Do not discuss client information with family members or friends without the client's permission.
   - Keep client information closed, covered, or out of sight.
   - Do not access the electronic medical record for information other than what you need to do your job.
   - Discard client-related materials in the shredding boxes.
5. Review the HIPAA facility and department policy.

Activity:
As a group create a poster that can be put up in the department, of areas where client information is located and procedures for what they should do with the information.

Evaluation:
Administer the post-test to determine the level of understanding.

Source: dk Foodservice Solutions, LLC. Used with permission.

Sanitation and Safety Training

This is listed as a type of training because safety and sanitation training is a mandatory program. According to the 2011 CDC findings,

> CDC estimates 48 million people get sick, 128,000 are hospitalized, and 3,000 die from foodborne diseases each year in the United States.

These numbers give us a reason to pause since most foodborne illnesses are preventable. CDM, CFPPs have an obligation to train every member of the foodservice team in food protection. In fact, the 2017 FDA Food Code stipulates that managers must train employees on such topics as:

- The risks of bare-hand contact with food
- When and where to wash hands
- How to wash hands
- How to maintain fingernails
- Prohibition of jewelry
- Basic hygiene

The FDA Food Code also notes that managers must document sanitation training. Many managers document training with attendance sign-in sheets, along with a summary of each training meeting. (A good tool is the color-coded post-test placed in the employee file which verifies the successful completion of the training.)

Training improves the likelihood of compliance with food handling policies and practices, reduces the need for constant supervision, and improves employee self-esteem and job satisfaction. Training for food safety should include topics such as:

- Personal hygiene
- Restrictions and precautions for illness
- Why, when, and how to take the temperatures of food, refrigerators, freezers, ovens, etc.
- Safe thawing and preparation practices; sanitation techniques
- Other food protection practices that relate to the employees' job responsibilities

Particularly because of the health and safety consequences, trainers should be carefully selected based on job knowledge and ability to facilitate learning. Training strategies appropriate for sanitation training include new employee orientation, on-the-job training, and group training (in-services). Each of these approaches is important for improving and maintaining the sanitation skills and knowledge of foodservice employees.

3. Following Figure 11.3, prepare an outline for an in-service training on handwashing. Indicate the training techniques used.

For instance, the OJT program for a new dishmachine focuses on the proper steps in manual and automatic dishwashing. The new employee learns how to perform these job tasks by working with an experienced employee. The training is accomplished through observation of the work, thereafter by the new employee. The experienced employee continues to provide coaching and feedback.

Instructional Materials

The CDM, CFPP may need instructional materials to assist in providing food safety training to staff. A variety of online web resources are available from groups and organizations such as:

- Professional associations in the foodservice and hospitality industry.
- State and local health departments.
- Federal agencies such as the Food and Drug Administration, United States Department of Agriculture, and Centers for Disease Control and Prevention.
- Universities and technical schools.
- Vendors and suppliers to the foodservice industry.

Many free posters, handouts, and interactive resources about food safety are available on reliable websites, such as those from the U.S. government and county extension agencies. Many are available in various languages, and some may even rely on graphics to support the message. All these can be useful in training employees who speak English as a second language or have language barriers.

Evaluating Training

Remember that training is a process and that involves evaluation. Two ways of evaluating this are measuring the knowledge gained or satisfaction obtained by the employees through the use of a written evaluation and by providing feedback.

Written Evaluation

Some standards applying to non-commercial foodservice operations specify that employees' knowledge should be measured both before and after training. So, the CDM, CFPP may use a pre-test and a post-test to measure knowledge. A sample pre-test that doubles as a post-test appears in Figure 11.4. A test such as this does not measure transfer of learning, but it does tell whether employees have grasped the prerequisite information.

Employees should also evaluate the training session. Find out whether participants felt the training was useful, what questions were left unanswered, and how participants rate their own confidence in being able to do something differently on the job. Ask them what they will do differently as a result of training. Ask them what else they would like to learn. A sample in-service training session evaluation appears in Figure 11.5.

4. You are training employees on the temperature danger zone and optimal temperatures for cooking, holding, and refrigerating food. How would you incorporate the three major styles of learning (auditory, verbal, and kinesthetic)?

Figure 11.4
HIPAA In-Service Training Post-Test

Name: _____ Date: _____

1. **True or False:** When approached by a visiting family member, the dietitian should explain the reason for a cardiac diet to the client's son.

2. What could happen if an employee leaves the unit's diet sheet on the counter?
    a. The employee could lose their job
    b. The patient could sue the facility
    c. Both of the above
    d. Neither of the above

3. How should confidential paperwork be managed?
    a. Dispose of expired or unneeded paperwork in the shredder boxes
    b. Keep active information nearby on the desk
    c. Maintain current client information filed in drawers
    d. A and C above

4. **True or False:** Diet Office staff need to know a client's diagnosis and should look up test results.

5. **True or False:** HIPAA really only affects medical and nursing staff in a medical facility.

ANSWER KEY: 1. False 2. c. Both of the above 3. d. A and C above 4. False 5. False

Source: dk Foodservice Solutions, LLC. Used with permission.

Figure 11.5
Sample In-Service Evaluation Form (Measuring Satisfaction)

In-Service Session Title: _____ Date: _____

Please answer the following questions to help us improve our training programs.

1. Please rate how well this session relates to your own job:
    ○ Excellent match   ○ Fair match   ○ Poor match

2. Was this material:
    ○ Too complex   ○ Too simple   ○ Just right

3. Please rate the audio-visuals used:
    ○ Excellent   ○ Fair   ○ Poor

4. Please rate the learning activities used:
    ○ Excellent   ○ Fair   ○ Poor

5. Please rate the handouts used:
    ○ Excellent   ○ Fair   ○ Poor

6. What did you like most about this training session?

7. What did you like least about this training session?

8. What topics would you like to see covered in future training?

The best way to assess the training efforts is to work with the list of objectives and to note what the employees are actually doing. If objectives have been met, the training has been successful. If not, it is time to analyze further.

Giving Feedback

Feedback is the information on what an employee is doing. It provides perspective, direction, and recognition. During orientation, and in later training activities, it is important to provide the staff with relevant and prompt feedback on how well they have mastered a task. An encouraging word or early correction of a misstep may be all that is needed.

Everyone enjoys receiving positive feedback, such as praise for a task well done. At the same time, though, constructive feedback about something that did not go perfectly conveys a critical message. The critical message is: *Your work matters. What you do is important.* All forms of feedback, when handled well, can improve an employee's performance and boost their self-esteem.

Often, CDM, CFPPs expect training to solve all problems; however, it does not. When an employee performs poorly, most think the employee needs training. This may or may not be true. An employee may know how to do something, but fails to do it because of:

- Poor motivation
- Peer pressure
- Obstacles in the workplace
- Lack of resources (such as time or supplies)
- Malfunctioning equipment
- Poorly designed systems

Whenever an employee's performance does not reflect the training provided, talk with the employee. Listen, and determine the need. Decide what interventions can be provided and then try them out.

Training and education should be a lifelong expectation in the workplace. Technologies change, staffing patterns change, basic systems change, and we need to continuously update and train all staff members to the current trends. New views and knowledge reflect on the skills and qualifications of the dining services staff.

> **GLOSSARY**
>
> **Feedback**
> Information about what an employee is doing. It provides perspective, direction, and recognition

Chapter References

RESOURCES	
4 Different Learning Styles You Should Know: The VARK Model	https://educationonline.ku.edu/community/4-different-learning-styles-to-know#:~:text=The%20acronym%20%E2%80%9CVARK%E2%80%9D%20is%20used,Mills.&text=These%20different%20learning%20styles%E2%80%94visual,of%20hours%20of%20classroom%20observation
15-Minute Training Topics for School Food Service Employees	https://childnutrition.ncpublicschools.gov/information-resources/haccp-food-safety/haccp-continuing-education/15-minute-training-topics
Be SMART: Setting Measurable Restaurant Goals for 2019	https://www.mondernrestaurantmanagement.com/be-smart-setting-measurable-restaurant-goals-for-2019/
FDA Food Code 2017	https://www.fda.gov/media/110822/download
Food Safety Training	https://www.extension.iastate.edu/foodsafety/foodservice-employee-training
Health Insurance Portability and Accountability Act (HIPAA) Inservice Training	http://dkfsolutions.net
How to Set & Achieve Your Goals. Smart Goal Guide	https://www.smart-goals-guide.com
International Association of Food Protection, Food Safety Training and Foodservice Employees' Knowledge and Behavior	https://krex.k-state.edu/dspace/bitstream/handle/2097/806/RobertsFPTApr2008.pdf?sequence=1
Maslow's Hierarchy of Needs	https://www.simplypsychology.org/maslow.html
UC San Diego Safety Training for Foodservice Employees	https://blink.ucsd.edu/safety/resources/training/food.html

Employee Scheduling and Assignments

Overview and Objectives

Well-planned schedules ensure that you have adequate staff at the right times to accomplish the work. They also control labor cost. Scheduling involves assessing the production and service needs, the volume of work or output, and how long it takes to fulfill the assigned duties. In this chapter, we will look at different types of schedules, time and attendance, and the documentation process. After completing this chapter, you should be able to:

- Prepare a time schedule
- Maintain time schedule chart/records
- Control overtime with effective scheduling

> **GLOSSARY**
>
> **Scheduling**
> Assigning employees to specific work days and hours
>
> **Staggered Scheduling**
> Scheduling staff so they come in at different times instead of coming in at the same time
>
> **Flex Scheduling**
> Designed to increase staffing as activity increases and reduce labor hours during slower periods

In foodservice operations, scheduling can be challenging because the set of job routines may not be the same every day. In many operations, the volume of work and level of services declines on weekends, while in others weekends may be the busiest times. The number of employee dining services provided also varies. Additionally, holidays may change the staffing requirements.

Scheduling is an important function in any foodservice operation to have sufficient staff for busy meal periods without having excess staff between meals or on slower days. The work performed in many positions in the operation should be adjustable to reflect the changes in number. Seasonal events or changes in the economy may lead to shifts in the client count or census, affecting the daily staffing needs. As client numbers reduce, being proactive by adjusting the employee schedules downward based on staffing needs creates sound management and financial control. Conversely, as the client numbers increase, it may be necessary to add to the staffing levels.

Goals for Scheduling

Once it is determined how many employees are needed in each position for the day-to-day operations, a schedule can be written. This is what most managers complete and post about a week before each new pay period begins. A schedule identifies when each employee will work during that pay period, as well as to what position(s) the employee will be assigned.

When developing a schedule, consider the following goals:

- Schedule staff to fit work needs.
- Use creative scheduling plans.
- Use the skills of your staff.
- Recognize employee schedule requests.
- Establish and use scheduling policies.
- Plan ahead for special events.

Schedule Staff to Fit Work Needs

It is generally not useful for all staff to begin and end their shifts at the same time. In reference to the Staffing Pattern discussed in Chapter 9, the staff should be scheduled at the times needed to meet the work required. This is called **staggered scheduling**.

For example, one employee working with the dishmachine might be scheduled to begin work an hour before the evening meal period. The time may be used to clean up any remaining dishes from lunch and take care of production pots and pans for the dinner period. A second service employee might be brought in 30 minutes before the time of service to perform other duties. Both employees will be ready for the evening rush period.

Likewise, other personnel can be scheduled to meet the need for the various positions at different times of the day. Typically, the first employee to arrive will be the first employee to leave. Staggered ending times also help maximize employee efficiency.

Flex scheduling is a concept used in some organizations to increase staffing as activity increases and reduce labor hours during slower periods. Hospitals may have a planned schedule based on their typical census resulting in defined reductions in shifts for weekends or declining client activity. Identifying the appropriate activity levels that trigger a change in staffing is the first step. Dovetailing responsibilities to reduce the labor hours and still maintain the needed quality of service is the second step. Finally, implementing the reduction, when appropriate, is the last step. Flexing the labor hours to reflect the census or level of activity can have a significant impact on the department budget.

Use Creative Scheduling Plans

Part-time staff can be hired to work short shifts, such as three, four, or five hour shifts. Sometimes, a job is designed as a **split shift**, or two short shifts in one day separated by some time off.

Temporary or "as-needed" employees can also be used. Many facilities maintain a list of people who are not interested in steady work, but who would like to work occasionally. If there is a special event, an employee illness, or another need for temporary assistance, these personnel can be very helpful.

In the continuous challenge to do more with less, Certified Dietary Manager®, Certified Food Protection Professionals® (CDM®, CFPPs®) are becoming quite creative in devising ways of providing essential human resources to the operation. One idea is the use of **cross-training**, which means training one employee to perform more than one job. To a certain degree, cross-training is a given in foodservice operations. Most employees are trained for several positions, which provides the manager with the flexibility to adjust staffing on a daily basis.

Branching out, some organizations even cross-train employees between departments. An employee of an environmental services or laundry department, for example, may also learn certain jobs in the foodservice department—and vice versa. Cross-trained employees then become part of a job pool, and can be assigned or reassigned as needed into various work areas. This flexibility helps managers in all affected departments use human resources very efficiently, and can result in full-time employment for the staff member.

Job sharing is a management tool that may assist in retaining employees. Job sharing is splitting one full-time position into two or more jobs. This often works better in positions that have a fair amount of flexibility in the scheduling, such as the clinical dietitian in healthcare facilities. Job sharing can be split on the day, by different days of the week, or alternating weeks. A drawback of job sharing is the potential for increased cost of benefits, such as medical insurance. (Note: Usually job sharing only provides the same benefits as one employee would receive. Often employees already know it will have less benefits but will allow the employee to have a flexible schedule that meets outside demands.)

Another idea used frequently, particularly in healthcare facilities, is to establish a volunteer program. This is done on a facility-wide basis, and an individual is assigned to manage volunteer services. Volunteers are available from all walks of life. Their help in a dining services department typically is limited to assisting clients with menu

GLOSSARY

Split Shift
Two short shifts separated by a period of time off in one day

Cross-Training
Training an employee to do more than one job

Job Sharing
Dividing a full-time position into two or more positions

1. Prepare a day's schedule for the kitchen staff made up of 2 dishwashers, 4 cooks, 3 cold prep workers, and 4 cashiers. Meal service starts at 7 am for breakfast and the cafeteria closes at 9 pm.

selections, the transport of items from one area to another, help with some clerical tasks, and other non-food contact activities.

Creative scheduling, job sharing, volunteer hours, and cross-training do not mean scheduling abuse. These are alternative scheduling options that may help the department and the employees, but they need to be managed carefully. Bouncing staff from one position to another, day-after-day, gets old quickly.

Use the Skills of Your Staff

Consider the skill sets of each staff member. If there is an employee with a pleasing smile and personality, he or she might enjoy helping in the dining room or serving in the cafeteria with high client contact. If an employee does not handle the demanding speed of the trayline, you can assign him or her to a less time-sensitive position.

Every department has skilled employees as well as those who are not as skilled or experienced. Plan to schedule the staff to create a balanced team each day. The goal is to get the job done with the best available staff. Cross-training staff for multiple positions allows the flexibility to maximize their value to the organization and raises the performance of the whole department.

Recognize Employee Schedule Requests

Consider personnel preferences whenever possible. Have a system for employees to communicate their special scheduling needs in advance of the time you prepare the schedule. All of the following are examples of when an employee needs to complete a request for time off or change in schedule:

- If Mary needs to be off on the first Tuesday of the pay period, she should let you know by completing a form.
- If Mark needs to leave by 2:00 p.m. to attend a wedding, he can request to work an early shift.
- If Juanita wishes to take a one-week vacation next month, she needs to request it in advance.

Request forms may be used by personnel to indicate in advance the days/shifts they wish to be off duty. It is a good management practice to honor employee requests whenever possible.

Establish and Use Scheduling Policies

The operation of a foodservice department typically requires staffing at times that many employees might not consider optimal work hours. The breakfast cook may start at 4:30 or 5:00 in the morning, and the night cashier may be working until 2:00 in the morning. Holidays and weekends are a normal part of the dining services schedule. When employees work weekends, they often do not enjoy having two other days off in a row. A day off might occur on a Tuesday in one week, and on a Friday in another week.

In addition, the number of employees who can take days off or schedule their vacation at any given time is limited. During peak vacation seasons, many employees may wish to take the same time off work. However, rarely can all requests be approved.

If there is no consistent method for requesting time off and making scheduling decisions, employees may feel that scheduling practices are not fair and equitable. (Scheduling preferences and task assignments are often the source of employee complaints about "favoritism.") Poorly planned schedules become a source of discontent among employees.

To manage these kinds of situations, you should establish policies relating to working hours, rotation of shifts, scheduling for weekends, holiday assignments, and decision-making regarding requests for time off. You need to make these policies known to all employees, and follow them consistently. Without clear and consistent policies, each scheduling decision can become a random or arbitrary action, subject to the scrutiny of all employees. (The Policies and Procedures are discussed in greater detail in Chapter 14.)

Several factors which may affect how you set policies include:

1. The first is employment law.
   a. There are limits to how many hours each employee is scheduled.
2. Next, if the department employees belong to a union, there may be stipulations in the union contract with which the policies must comply.
3. If the facility has human resources policies that relate to scheduling, you must comply with these also.

Beyond these constraints, you must develop your own workable guidelines. There may be a history of scheduling preferences or assumed "promises" extended by a prior manager that need to be clarified, in written policy format, with human resources and the employees.

Here are examples of practices CDM, CFPPs sometimes include in scheduling policies:

- Employees in _____ area are required to work weekends. The schedule is developed in such a way that each employee works every other weekend.
- An employee who works the night shift on one day is not scheduled for the early morning shift the very next day.
- For holiday scheduling, each employee completes a holiday request form, indicating a first, second, and third choice for holidays to be scheduled off duty.
  > The manager takes these requests in sequence, honoring as many requests as possible, and checking as to who worked the holiday the year before.
  > Regularly scheduled days off may need to be changed to accommodate holiday schedules. Consider the following real-life example:

   > *Hazel had worked at the hospital for 10 years making salads and desserts for both the patients and the cafeteria. Although she worked every other weekend, she had been consistently scheduled off on Thursdays.*

   > *When the holiday request schedule went up for Thanksgiving, Christmas, and New Year's, Hazel considered herself lucky because this year Christmas and New Year's fell on Thursday. She knew she would be off all three days and not have to take a single vacation or paid holiday because "Thursday was her day off."*

   > *Hazel was stunned when the manager reminded her to enter her preferred holiday off request. As a long-term employee with her schedule of having Thursdays off, she took her concerns to the Human Resources Director. To her surprise, Human Resources reminded Hazel that "per the hospital policy," there are no guaranteed days off and that in departments, where appropriate, all staff members would be scheduled to work holidays.*

   > *Hazel requested Christmas off and, as luck would have it, also got Thanksgiving off. She was scheduled to work New Year's Day and she volunteered to work the supper line on New Year's Eve as a swap for New Year's Day with another employee.*

- Requests for time off are granted on a first-come, first-served basis.
  - If two requests are received on the same day and only one can be granted, the request is granted to the employee with the longest tenure.
  - Establish a reasonable request period to eliminate 20 requests submitted on December 26th for the following Christmas off.
  - Accepting requests a couple of months out allows employees to make travel plans.

Plan Ahead for Special Events

Often, a two-week schedule can be copied and adapted to fit the next two-week pay period. Sometimes, special events and holidays require a totally different schedule. You can use past schedules as a reference.

Planning the staffing needed for the employee holiday dinner, the Foundation Annual Extravaganza, Mother's Day brunch, or even the monthly board of directors meeting can be a lot easier when you reference prior schedules. Keep a history of these events to help plan both the food needed and the staff to make it happen.

Schedules with the Union Contract

Typically, a significant portion of the union contract is focused on the scheduling of the union staff members. The contract may specify times, days, and frequency with which employees may be scheduled. Often, the contract will specify how the replacement staff will be scheduled to cover for vacation, holiday, and sick time.

Remember that the union contract is another version of the Policy and Procedure Manual. Read it, know it, and understand it. Work with the Human Resources Department and the Union Steward to make sure that management and the employees understand the guidelines and requirements of the contract as it relates to scheduling and task assignments.

Do not let the contract come between you, the staff, and the needs of the facility. Use the contract, and the Union Steward, to help set the scheduling policies and explain them to the department staff.

Schedules and Employee Relations

Work schedules directly affect employees' lives. Whether it is the day of the week, the start/stop times, or total hours scheduled, they are expected to adjust their personal lives to meet staffing needs. Few things cause disruption in the department faster than an inconsistent or frequently changed schedule.

Here are some "rule of thumb" scheduling courtesies that are not difficult to follow but are frequently overlooked.

- Post a written schedule at least one week prior to the start of the schedule.
  - Typically, schedules are based on the two week pay period; some start Sunday and others start Monday.
  - Post the schedule no later than the Monday prior.
- Covering the schedules is more than filling in the blanks.
  - Schedule qualified people into the positions.
  - A dining room server may be willing to make breakfast, but may not be qualified to do so.

- Try to establish regular days off for each staff member.
  - > As a 365-day operation, weekend and holiday coverage is essential.
  - > If employees consistently work every other weekend or one-in-three, although not always possible, try to give them the same day off in the week before and after working a weekend. (It is important to remind the staff that such is a courtesy and not mandatory. The schedule is developed for the needs of the department and clients and, as such, could change. Also, it is important to communicate these changes with the staff involved.)
- If there is a change to their regular day off to cover the schedule, make the employee aware of it before posting the schedule.
  - > They may have a doctor's appointment or family event planned for that regular day off and may not be available for the schedule.
- Try to accommodate employee requests for days off—both paid and unpaid.
  - > Although not always an option, when staff members know that you tried they often become a little more flexible in their requests.
- Avoid scheduling "double back" assignments or having too many work days in a row.
  - > Many jobs have early and late positions, but it is physically difficult to work a late shift one day followed by an early shift the next morning.
  - > Frequently scheduling more than five days in a row is very taxing for most staff members.
- Do not change a posted schedule without first talking to the affected staff members.
  - > Once the schedule is posted, they are responsible for what was posted—not what has been changed without their input.
- Be fair. Rotate weekends and holidays around to all qualified staff members.
  - > Unless there is an organizational policy, or it is written into a contract or job description, all employees within a given job description should experience an equal number of working weekends, holidays, and ease of access to vacation time.
  - > Post tentative schedules for Thanksgiving through the New Year's holidays in early November so all staff can plan for travel and family time.
  - > Often, when given the opportunity to work it out:
    - Older staff want Thanksgiving and Christmas Eve off for cooking and family time.
    - Younger staff often prefer New Year's Eve off, with New Year's Day to relax.
    - Staff with young children want Christmas Day morning off.
    - Schedule employees consistent with their employment status.
  - > Full-time employees expect to be scheduled 32-40 hours a week depending on your facility's definition of full-time.
  - > 30-, 24-, or 20-hour positions should be scheduled according to their hours and should not be consistently scheduled above those hours.

Employment Status Terminology

Full-time status is typically referenced as 40 hours of work per week and overtime eligible. Some employers define 32 or 35 hours per week as full time.

Part-time status is less than 40 (or 32-35) hours per week and with a consistent number of hours, i.e., 16 or 24 hours.

PRN or **pool status** refers to employees with no set schedule—they are scheduled "as needed."

Temporary, casual, agency, or **per diem status** refers to staff assigned from an outside agency on a per-day basis or as independent contractors.

Nonexempt status positions are paid on an hourly basis, covered by minimum wage and overtime guidelines (the majority of the employees in a facility).

Exempt status positions are paid a defined salary and excluded from minimum wage protection and overtime regulations (primarily the management and professional level employees).

Employees need to be able to anticipate how much they will earn in wages to pay their life expenses and, if needed, take on another job. A predictable schedule shows respect for the employee and allows them to better manage their time away from work.

Creating the Schedule

Scheduling can be a time-consuming task. Managers often develop a scheduling form that has standard details, such as the shift times, names of employees, and the hours of operation already completed.

Some facilities have computer programs for timecard/payroll management and scheduling employees. A typical **electronic scheduling** program allows for entry of facility-defined scheduling guidelines and current employee requests. It generates a schedule based on all available information, and allows for review and edits if necessary.

As with most software programs, the number and types of reports available can be overwhelming.

- Employee scheduling software usually allows you to establish desired staffing ratios that define the number of employees needed based on meal or client counts.
- Advanced reports help verify that the proposed schedule will meet the budget.
- Once the schedule information is set, there are several format options: a master schedule, a daily schedule, an employee's personal schedule, and so forth.
- e-Schedules can be sent to staff via company staff emails.

GLOSSARY

Electronic Scheduling
Computer-based program for scheduling and time and attendance tracking

Putting It Into Practice

2. What are some reports that can be generated using an electronic scheduling program?

- Programs can generate overtime reports, vacation and sick time reports that can be used when working with individual staff requests.
- FTE reports are based on budget and actual numbers.
- Most systems track attendance and tardiness within the program. Some systems may notify you when unscheduled absences and/or late work arrivals meet the criteria for disciplinary action.
- Employee records within a scheduling program may include contact information to make calling of replacement staff easier when there are unscheduled absences.
- Typically scheduling packages are available as part of a time-clock system, which then integrates with time-clocks and payroll reporting.
- The various scheduling programs offer different features and the manager may need to check the organization's particular software for specific tasks available.

Calculating Total Labor Hours and FTEs

The computer can easily calculate the number of Full Time Equivalents (FTEs) in the entire schedule or by individual job description. How to calculate FTEs and total hours based on the staffing pattern is covered in Chapter 9. The electronic scheduler makes the process easier and readily available for review by the year, the month, the pay period, or by the day.

If the organization functions under a **position control** structure, knowing how many FTEs are in each job description can be a major benefit. Position Control is a finance and human resources concept where each job description in the department is authorized a specific number of positions. This defines the number of hours approved in the budget for cooks or meal servers or supervisors. Each position is assigned a unique number in the human resources system that ties to the financial budget for the number of hours approved for the position.

Position control relates to the hours and number of positions approved in the budget, irrespective of how many staff members are actually on the payroll. When facilities do not implement the control side of position control, approved positions are not being filled while other positions are over-staffed. Following the position control for labor hours approved will keep you on the budget.

Using a Productivity Standard

Much of today's foodservice industry estimates staffing needs using a productivity standard, such as meals per labor hour or minutes per meal. If you know your **meals per labor hour** or **minutes per meal**, compare this figure to industry benchmarks. Many of the electronic schedulers will accept a productivity standard for tracking purposes.

For instance, imagine that you are a school foodservice manager and have calculated the meals per labor hour to be 9.7. The industry standard is 13-15 meals per labor hour (Hanna, 2008). This example means that the staff is not producing as many meals per labor hour as the benchmark. While that could mean that the number of meals served was not calculated correctly, in reality it probably means you are overstaffed. This information can help identify the opportunity to increase the number of meals served or areas for reduction in labor hours.

GLOSSARY

Position Control
A management system to control the number of positions for each job description

Meals Per Labor Hour
A productivity standard that is a calculation of the total meals served divided by the total number of department labor hours

Minutes Per Meal
A productivity standard that is a calculation of the total department labor minutes divided by the total number of meals served

Types of Schedules

There are generally three types of employee schedules which you can use to communicate with the staff: Master Schedule, Work Area Schedule, and Shift Schedule.

Master Schedule. The master schedule is for the entire department and includes days on and off, plus vacation days for all employees. The master schedule may be developed for a week, two weeks, or even a month.

Work Area Schedule. In larger departments, or departments where there are multiple managers or supervisors, a separate schedule may be posted specifically for those employees. For example, a schedule may be posted for the production staff while a different schedule is posted for the dining room or cafeteria staff.

Shift Schedule. The shift schedule shows the different shifts, when they begin and end for different positions. For instance, using a small hospital as an example, a shift schedule for the a.m. and p.m. cooks would look like the graph below, Figure 12.1. The shift schedule is useful when interviewing new employees to show them the position coverage.

The Gantt Chart developed in Chapter 9 is similar to the shift schedule. It displays the positions and the overlap of shifts, plus the work details related to the flow of the day.

Communicating the Schedule

Needless to say, a schedule works only if communicated clearly to all employees. Once the schedule has been developed, post it in a highly visible location for review by all employees. The policy on posted schedules should make it clear to each employee that it is his or her responsibility to review the schedule and comply with it.

It is the manager's responsibility to post the schedule far enough in advance so employees can review it and adjust their personal activities to coordinate with their work times (typically one week before the new pay period). For example, you cannot post a schedule on Saturday if it takes effect on Monday, as many employees may not be at work and would not know their schedules. Employees who are not at work before a new schedule goes into effect should be advised to call and confirm when they are working.

Figure 12.1
Staff Schedule for Cooks

3. Your tray line produces 3 meals per minute and serves 120 patients at breakfast, 140 patients at lunch, and 150 patients at dinner. There are 5 people on the tray line at each meal. How many labor hours are needed to staff the tray line?

A schedule should be clear and specific:

- When two employees have the same first name, it's important to use a last name or initial to avoid confusion.
- Each schedule should clearly identify the dates, so that employees do not confuse the schedule for one pay period with that of another.
- Only the supervisor or manager should have authority to edit a posted schedule, never the employees themselves.
- Any changes to a posted schedule should be entered in colored ink (red, green, purple, etc.) so each edit can be quickly seen.

Finally, the manager should keep an extra copy of the schedule in a secure location, in case the posted schedule disappears or becomes damaged.

After use, the actual edited copy of the schedules should be retained. You may need them for several purposes, such as reviewing and completing the records for payroll at the end of a pay period, reviewing past actions in order to enforce scheduling policies, and responding to inquires or complaints that may arise in the future. The actual posted copy of the schedule records which employees were absent from work, the days they missed, and any changes in other staff schedules to cover.

Scheduling Adjustments

As with all things, the best laid plans may go awry. The most common scheduling challenge concerns employee tardiness and absence. When a job needs to be covered, other employees may be called to see if they would be willing to come to work on short notice. (Due to privacy concerns, maintain a master list of employees with current contact information in a secure location available to managers. Your list may also identify what jobs each employee is trained to do.) Depending upon the policies and/or union contract, coverage for a missing staff member may be based on the most available employee or the most senior.

As part of the scheduling process, many managers maintain a call record posted in the office where all supervisors can access the information to plan their workflow for the day. A sample call record (see the Supplemental Material for this chapter) documents who has "called-out" and a general reason for the absence. In addition, it records who was contacted to cover the open shift and their response. This can be particularly important in a union-staffed department.

View the Supplemental Material for this chapter to see a Sample Call Record.

From here, adjustments may have to be made to the schedule to avoid incurring overtime for the employee who has just punched in. Or, an overtime may be authorized for this employee. An alternative method of dealing with employee absence is the re-assignment of duties among existing staff. Sometimes, it is possible to divide the duties of an absent employee among staff members who are present. This requires careful planning, fairness, and tact.

4. Your staff serves a total of 500 meals in 1.75 hours. How many meals per hour do they serve?

To minimize the disruption and difficulty associated with finding coverage for jobs or re-working assignments, every facility develops and enforces some basic policies regarding unscheduled absences and tardiness. Most likely, these policies will come from the human resources department of the facility.

For example, an attendance policy might specify that any employee should not exceed a total of six occurrences of unscheduled absence or tardiness over the past 12-month period. It may specify how far in advance a supervisor must be notified if an employee will be unable to come to work or will be late. It may specify that non-compliance with this policy is cause for corrective action.

A specific policy may also address what is known as no-call, no-show. In this situation, an employee does not come to work, and does not call to notify the manager. This is a serious situation that makes it especially difficult for a manager to direct and control the activities of the department. In some facilities, two occurrences of no-call, no-show may be considered job abandonment and grounds for immediate dismissal.

Reports and Documents

As a CDM, CFPP you will most likely be responsible for ensuring that all documents and paperwork related to scheduling and payroll are maintained in a complete and accurate fashion. Typically, the manager is required to initial timesheets and authorize any overtime and check time records against the schedule to ensure there are no discrepancies.

Depending on the system in the organization, time records may be automated through an electronic timeclock or computer-generated payroll reports. For example, the review of the payroll time and attendance records allows the manager to monitor the employee timeclock patterns. The manager would know who clocks in early, who leaves a few minutes late resulting in overtime, who is frequently absent on Fridays, who picks up extra shifts, and who never does.

Often, an electronic scheduling program has the capability to notify the manager of the absences and tardiness an employee has accumulated in the past 12 months. Within the department's personnel filing system, the manager should also maintain accurate and timely records indicating when employees have come to work tardy and/or had unscheduled absences. Routine monitoring can help provide timely feedback and, if need be, initiate disciplinary actions.

If budget information is contained in these reports, labor usage for each time period can be checked against the financial records. This will verify good labor controls. Payroll reporting documents reflect the number of **productive hours** to be paid for time worked, training, and education plus **non-productive hours** paid for holidays, sick, and vacation time (unpaid leave of absence should be recorded). Also, hours paid should be monitored in addition to the dollar cost of the labor.

Often, the payroll reports include the pay scale and dollars paid to each employee for the pay period. This personal and sensitive information should be treated as confidential data.

> **GLOSSARY**
>
> **Productive Hours**
> Time paid for hours worked, training, and education
>
> **Non-Productive Hours**
> Employee hours paid (or tracked) for not working: vacation, holiday, sick time, and leave of absence

Controlling Overtime

What is overtime? **Overtime** refers to time worked in excess of the number of hours beyond which laws require payment of one-and-one-half times the hourly rate for every hour worked. There is more than one definition of when overtime must be paid.

- The most common guideline is the 40 hour work week.
  - > Based on the federal **Fair Labor Standards Act**: "Under the FLSA, "overtime" means "time actually worked beyond a prescribed threshold." The normal FLSA work period is the work week—7 consecutive days—and the normal FLSA overtime threshold is 40 hours per work week." (http://www.flsa.com/overtime.html)
  - > A 40-hour work week allows employees to be scheduled with variable hours, such as 10 hours on Tuesday and only 6 hours on Friday, but no more than 40 hours in the 7-day work week.
  - > If employees work a consistent 8-hour shift each, they can work no more than 5 shifts a week.
- An alternative used in some medical care settings is called "8/80" or "8 and 80":
  - > Based on the federal Fair Labor Standards Act: "Nonexempt medical care providers working at medical care facilities may be paid based either on the standard 40 hour work week or on so-called "8/80" systems. If the medical employer chooses, it may pay these employees FLSA overtime for actual time worked in excess of 8 hours per day, or 80 hours every two weeks (whichever is better for the employee), instead of for hours worked in excess of 40 hours per work week." (http://www.flsa.com/overtime.html)
  - > Overtime is paid on anything over eight hours per day or over 80 hours in a two week period.
  - > This allows employees to work six days in one week and four days in the second week, with every other weekend off.
  - > This is not a common work status, but it is an option in some healthcare settings.
- States, union contracts, and even individual employers may develop additional criteria for overtime:

  > Union contracts may specify anything over 8 hours within 24 consecutive hours.
- 10:00-6:30 on Tuesday plus 8:00–4:30 on Wednesday equals two hours of overtime for the 8:00–10:00 time on Wednesday.
  - > Nevada has a similar requirement for employees who earn less than one-and-one-half times the current minimum wage.
- The state defined minimum wage in 2020 was $9.00 (with no employer paid health benefits).
- If an employee is paid less than $13.50 an hour (1.5 x $9.00 = $13.50), then any time over 8.00 hours within 24 hours is paid overtime.

GLOSSARY

Overtime
Time worked by nonexempt employees in excess of the allowable amount, typically 40 hours per week, resulting in one-and-one-half times the hourly rate

Fair Labor Standards Act
This Act of 1938, also referred to as the Wages and Hours Bill, is a federal statute of the United States

5. An employee is paid $8 per hour and has worked for 45 hours this week. How much overtime would the employee receive? What is the total amount the employee would be paid for this

Clearly, overtime is very expensive and should be minimized to remain within budget. In some facilities, it may not be permitted at all. If overtime occurs frequently, look for factors that may be contributing to this situation, such as:

- Ineffective or unrealistic scheduling.
- Inaccurate estimation of the volume of work or failure to adjust staffing according to an increase in volume.
- Poor compliance with performance standards or poor work habits.

A Certified Dietary Manager, Certified Food Protection Professional can generally contain overtime through sound supervision. The key is to establish a policy of requiring advance authorization for overtime. Prior approval requires the employee to check with the manager or supervisor, who must approve the overtime. This gives the manager an opportunity to review why the need for overtime is arising and address any issues that require intervention. It also gives the manager a chance to use an alternate method of meeting the need, such as assigning another employee on a regular shift to pick up certain tasks.

Chapter References

RESOURCES	
Fair Labor Standards Act, Controlling Overtime	Dol.gov/whd/flsa
Hanna, Elizabeth Northway, "An Assessment of Performance Measures in Child Nutrition Programs" (2008). Retrospective Theses and Dissertations.	https://lib.dr.iastate.edu/rtd/15678
Predictive Scheduling Laws	https://www.workforce.com/news/predictive-scheduling-laws-what-are-they-where-do-they-exist-and-employers-reaction

Manage Department Personnel

Overview and Objectives

A productive workforce is important for the success of any organization. Ensuring that employees perform the job well and are motivated to work and improve is the responsibility of the Certified Dietary Manager®, Certified Food Protection Professional® (CDM®, CFPP®) Having standards in place to compare with and evaluate the employee on a regular basis and to offer positive feedback is extremely important. Another valuable aspect in managing department personnel is having procedures in place for disciplinary action so that workers learn to adhere to work rules. After completing this chapter, you should be able to:

- Develop and implement performance standards
- Conduct a performance review and appraisal
- Follow disciplinary procedures to correct problems (e.g., coaching, performance improvement plan)
- Conduct exit interviews and work on employee satisfaction
- Value diversity in the workplace

Performance Standards

Performance standards specify what the task is, how it is to be completed, and how well it has to be done. To ensure that the work is "done well," you need to define what "well" means. The definition should be objective and specific, and allow a quality measurement in a definable manner.

One type of standard that serves as an essential management tool is a **performance standard**. Some simple examples are:

- A trayline employee is responsible for portioning food on trays.
    - Items served match the list of food ordered, as specified on each tray ticket. In this example, the:
        - "What" is *items served*;
        - "How" is *match portions*;
        - "How well" is as *specified on each tray ticket*.
    - Food portions on the tray should match the portions specified on each tray ticket. In this example, the:
        - "What" is *food portions* on tray;
        - "How" is *match portions*;
        - "How well" is as *specified on each tray ticket*.

A performance standard for a food production position might specify that the:

- Employee prepares food in accordance with standardized recipes.
- Employee prepares food in the quantity specified on the daily food production schedule.
- Employee delivers food to the service area according to the time stated on the daily food production schedule.
- Endpoint cooking temperatures meet the standards specified on each recipe, and are accurately documented on the temperature log.

To develop meaningful performance standards, the manager should include these three criteria:

- The standard addresses the outcome in specific, clear, complete, and accurate terms.
    - It should let the employee know exactly what is expected. There should not be anything confusing or easily misunderstood.
- The standard describes how the outcome will be measured through observation:
    - An objective standard to assure fairness is used to evaluate the employee's work performance. ("Good" and "well" are subjective terms to avoid.)
- The standard explains the action verb used.
    - For example, if the action verb is "document," the performance standard would require the employee to document.

GLOSSARY

Performance Standards
Specific statements describing the outcomes of the work performed

1. Develop a performance standard for a dishwasher on washing utensils in a 3 compartment sink.

An effective performance standard is within the physical and mental capabilities of the employees and is realistic in the working environment. Unrealistic expectations will result in employees failing to meet them. If a particular standard is not being met on a consistent basis, you need to re-examine the validity of the standard before proceeding with other interventions.

When reasonable, involve employees in developing fair and realistic standards for their own work. Needless to say, each standard must adhere to company policies, company goals, and applicable legal and moral constraints.

While we all want the performance to be perfect, we realize that this is not possible. It is not realistic to expect 100% compliance with every performance standard. What we can do, though, is to specify a realistic and acceptable gauge of performance, often expressed in terms of numbers. It may be speed, quantity, or rate. For example:

- A number as an accuracy rating:
  > Food is portioned correctly, as specified on each tray ticket, at a rate of 99% accuracy.

Another example might measure rate of output, or productivity, such as:

- Employee accurately sets up the snack assembly station within a period of 15 minutes.

Developing Performance Standards. The steps for developing a performance standard are as follows:

Step 1: Using the organization chart or the staffing pattern, list all the job titles in the department. For example, the list may include buffet server, receiving clerk, morning cook, afternoon cook, pot washer, and others.

Step 2: Review the job analysis workflow (Gantt Chart) for each position and list the tasks or sets of tasks that will need a performance standard. For example, the task of "sanitizing pots" will require a performance standard.

Step 3: Write a performance standard for each task, seeking employee input.

Step 4: Train employees.

Step 5: Evaluate performance (ongoing).

Performance standards as a communications tool. In the process of interviewing prospective employees, explain that the operation uses performance standards. This prepares a candidate for the commitment to quality that will be expected. You may choose to show a candidate a sample performance standard that relates to the position for which the candidate is applying.

Training for employees follows the job analysis, the job description and the performance standards. Whatever the procedures and standards are, specify what must be included in both new employee orientation and ongoing employee training. For example, if performance standards have been developed on documenting information for HACCP records, then training must include the details of how to do this (the procedure), as well as the description of how an employee will know it has been done effectively (the performance standard).

Once training has been completed, ongoing evaluation and feedback of outcomes must be based on the performance standards. If employees are consistently not meeting a standard, find out the reason. They may need more or different training. The performance standard may have to be revised to be clearer and realistic. If a particular employee is not meeting the standard but others are, this may be a sign that the employee needs coaching and direction, or even a disciplinary action.

It can be easy just to assume that all employees know what is expected of them. However, this simply is not true. It is not fair to evaluate employees based on unwritten rules or a judgment call of what constitutes good work. Instead, clarify the expectations through performance standards. Clear and fair performance standards improve consistency, accountability, and quality because everyone knows what the outcome should be.

Performance Review

Performance standards are essential points of reference used during a performance review. The **performance review** is a structured and scheduled component of nearly every organization. A performance review, performance appraisal, or evaluation is a formal, structured meeting between the employee and his or her supervisor/manager that encourages an exchange about the individual employee's performance on the job.

The process should account for how the quality and quantity of an employee's work compares with the performance standards that have already been established for the position.

As part of the ongoing responsibility to provide feedback to employees, a CDM, CFPP must comply with the organizational policies and procedures. At times, the manager must also take corrective action to help improve the employee's performance. Both of these are documented activities which become part of an employee's personnel file.

A performance review does several of the following:
- Ensures that the supervisor/manager speaks with the employee about performance, and provides extensive feedback.
- Identifies needs for improvement and growth.
- Serves as a formal basis for wage increases related to performance.
- Provides an opportunity for an employee to set personal work objectives that relate to the departmental objectives.
- Provides an opportunity for the employee to raise needs related to the work, and for the supervisor/manager to help.
- Provides documentation for the employee's personnel record.
- May be used to help evaluate eligibility for promotion.

How often a performance review occurs is generally dictated by the policy of the facility. For example, one facility may conduct performance reviews for every person employed at three months, six months, and annually thereafter. The review is typically documented on a form that is standardized for the facility, signed by both employee and supervisor, and retained as part of the personnel file. The department manager typically signs every performance review before forwarding them to Human Resources.

Employee performance review programs can benefit the employee, the CDM, CFPP, and the organization itself. For example, a manager who recognizes individual staff members through a formal review process may obtain ideas from employees about how the work procedures can be improved. As strengths and weaknesses of each employee

> **GLOSSARY**
>
> **Performance Review**
> A formal, structured meeting between the employee and supervisor to evaluate the employee's performance

are identified, the employee and manager together can develop action plans to improve performance.

The groundwork for motivation can be laid out during a performance review as well. This occurs when employees understand that the CDM, CFPP is concerned about them and is interested in learning about their needs. Coaching, counseling, training, orientation, and many other ongoing programs can be strengthened as the result of information learned during performance appraisals.

It also becomes easier to justify job actions such as promotions, transfers or demotions, when formalized evaluation sessions have been completed and documented. If the CDM, CFPP can show that performance is consistently inadequate and the employee has agreed that a problem exists, improvements are expected. However, employee failure to make these improvements may provide justification for disciplinary actions.

The performance evaluation can help improve the relationship between the CDM, CFPP and the employee. An effective manager asks for feedback during a review and sometimes learns more about how to lead and motivate employees through this process. As the manager and employees work together as partners in the performance review process, a relationship can be built which helps each gain mutual understanding and respect.

Types of Performance Reviews

There are several basic types of performance reviews. Some of these include a review that uses absolute standards, an open-ended summary, an objectives-based evaluation, and a 360 review. Performance reviews may be a printed form to be manually completed, or an electronic version to be completed online. The latter is often used now.

Typically, performance reviews are designed to reference the general characteristics of a position without addressing the specific tasks of the job. The evaluation likely has questions about communication skills, safety, accountability, attendance, quality of work, and other general work performance terms. Specific job tasks are usually addressed in the comment section of the evaluation.

A CDM, CFPP may keep a catalog of commonly used evaluation comments for easy referral of appropriate commentary. The online versions of a performance review often include a drop-down list of relevant comments, both positive and negative, that can be added to an evaluation.

Absolute Standards Performance Review

In this type of performance review, the work performance of an individual staff member is considered as a stand-alone function without comparison to others. One popular example of the absolute standard type of performance review is the **critical incident method**. Using this technique, the CDM, CFPP keeps a log of incidents that represent both effective and ineffective job performances. The log is then used to measure the employee's performance. The manager simply lists any activity observed on the job that he or she judges to be critical to the job performance and compares the

> **GLOSSARY**
>
> **Critical Incident Method**
> A log of incidents that represent both effective and ineffective job performance

observations with established performance standards. This way an employee is receiving both reinforcement and coaching about observed behaviors.

Certain events are called critical because they illustrate the key behaviors that define (or violate) standards for performance. For example:

> A CDM, CFPP observes an employee arguing with a client. The manager may record this as a critical incident because it represents failure to meet a performance standard about providing friendly service.
>
> In another event, the same employee may check and record food temperatures of hot and cold foods before service with 100% accuracy. This may relate to another performance standard about documenting food temperatures accurately before serving trays. The manager may record this too, as a critical incident on the performance review form.

View the Supplemental Material for this chapter to see a sample:
- Checklist Performance Review Form
- Forced Choice Review Form
- Open-Ended Performance Review Form

In today's digital world, a CDM, CFPP may have an electronic file for each employee. An efficient way to record a critical incident is to send yourself a brief email with the details that provide the date and information regarding the incident. When time allows, move this email into the employee's file.

Another type of absolute standards review is an evaluation checklist developed by the manager or the facility. The evaluation lists important performance items and provides a numeric rating scale. The supervisor/manager completing the evaluation selects a number to rate the performance of the employee related to each item.

Another example of the absolute standards approach is a forced-choice plan, which requires a CDM, CFPP to select a statement which is most accurate in describing how an employee performs on the job. The manager first lists factors which are important to successful job performance in the left-hand column, then he or she must indicate how the work performance of the employee meets each of the criteria. In some facilities, both the employee and the manager mark separate forms and then compare their answers during the performance review.

Open-Ended Summary Performance Review

A review based on free text allows the manager to note strengths and weaknesses of the employee's performance and to indicate suggestions and support for improvement.

Objectives-Based Performance Review

This is based on individualized objectives; developed with input from both the CDM, CFPP and the employee.

First, the two develop a mutually-defined set of job-related objectives. Later, during a performance review session, the two assess how well these objectives have been met. They also develop a new set of objectives. This system is also called **management by objectives (MBO)**.

Basic steps in an objectives-based evaluation plan include:
- The manager and employee set measurable behavioral objectives. The employee commits to attaining these objectives by the time of the next review.
- The employee is given assistance on the job through training, coaching, and/or

GLOSSARY

Management by Objectives (MBO)
The process of setting objectives through participative goal setting by management and employee

other developmental activities.

- Employee and supervisor separately prepare a reflection on how each feels the employee met the objectives.
- At the time of the performance review, the actual level of performance is measured against the level defined by the objectives and any progress is discussed.
- The supervisor and staff member work together to develop new objectives and plan strategies for attaining them before the next performance review session.

The **360 review** has been gaining acceptance at the manager and professional level. In a traditional evaluation, the performance review tends to focus on how well the employee performs his or her assigned tasks. While the manager may seek input from co-workers, their comments are not the basis of the evaluation. In a 360 review, the emphasis is more on how the employee contributes to the organization.

Peer review of the employee's leadership skills, work habits, accountability, effective communication, and level of teamwork make up the core of a 360 review. Managers will seek feedback from the employee's peers and representatives from the other departments that the employee regularly interacts with, such as nursing directors and administrative or medical staff. The objective is to provide the employee with both positive and constructive feedback based on how well they function within the organization.

Performance Review Process

The exact type of performance review forms used will likely depend on the facility. In using the forms and method defined by administration or Human Resources, you may need to customize the feedback somewhat for a food production or dining services employees. For example, if the standard form lists "quality of work" as a factor for evaluation, the manager should edit the indicators to reflect the specific tasks related to the employees' positions.

As with any feedback, a performance review should be specific. The more an employee knows what the criteria are for evaluation, the more readily an employee can meet these criteria. Some CDM, CFPPs provide a blank copy of the evaluation form to a new employee during orientation. This is one way to define the expectations for the employee and clarify what is needed for him or her to succeed.

Before conducting a review, take the time to complete the form and give the review some thought. If multiple supervisors work with one employee, talk to each of them about the performance review and obtain specific feedback and comments to include.

To conduct a performance review, schedule a time with the employee. Find the time when both the employee and you will not be rushed to allow for a meaningful discussion.

> **GLOSSARY**
>
> **360 Review**
> A review where the emphasis is on how the employee contributes to the organization, peer review of the employee's leadership skills, and work habits

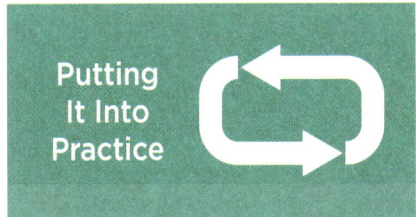

2. You need to conduct performance reviews for your kitchen staff. What type of review process would you select and why?

Then set aside a private place to talk. A performance review should not be held in a high-traffic area or in any place where others are likely to overhear the conversation. A performance review is a confidential exchange between the manager and the employee.

During the review, explain each item—what is being measured, what standard is being used, and what specific observations have been made about the employee's performance. Throughout the review, provide the employee with the time to react, respond, and ask questions. As with other types of feedback, a performance review gives the CDM, CFPP time to listen to the employees.

Often, the manager can learn how to remove obstacles on the job, provide training and support, and help the employee solve problems. Let this review be an exploration in which both parties walk away with greater understanding. As the review concludes, design a plan for on-the-job employee development. It may include items such as additional training for the employee, practice of certain skills, and more.

Both the employee and the manager should sign and date the form. This will indicate that the employee has received this feedback (not that the employee agrees with everything it says). If the employee disagrees with parts in the evaluation, these should be discussed. A typical procedure allows an employee to add comments. If an employee refuses to sign the form, write "refused to sign," and date and initial the note.

The time for the performance review is often when an employee shares personal development needs in more detail. One employee may state that he would really like to train for a cook's position, or another may share that she wants to sign up for the CDM, CFPP education program. These aspirations are important and should be considered for the staff development plans. By encouraging staff to expand their skills, advance their education, or even pursue a different job opportunity, you raise the quality of staff in the department and become an employer of choice.

Finally, the paperwork should follow the procedure defined for the facility to assure that a pay raise, if indicated, is processed, and that the form is filed in the employee's personnel record.

Several common pitfalls can occur during the employee performance review process. These may include:

- Surprising employees with negative feedback:
  - > If there has been an ongoing problem, the employee should know this well before a performance review. The manager should be giving feedback on a regular basis so that there are no surprises.
  - > The same is true for positive feedback.
  - > An effective performance review becomes a summary of items that have already been discussed.
- Using reviews for corrective action:
  - > Sometimes performance reviews are used only to reprimand employees rather than to assess where, if at all, employees can improve.
- Using ineffective review forms:
  - > If review forms do not correctly summarize factors important for an effective job performance, the evaluation process will be inadequate. A CDM, CFPP should, therefore, identify the specific, job-related criteria for review.

- Failing to use or keep up with performance reviews:
  - Some managers may procrastinate due to busy schedules. Although it can be difficult to schedule time, a manager must give this process high priority.
  - On occasion, an employee whose review has been postponed or overlooked begins to experience poor morale. If a pay raise is associated with the review, the situation may become compounded.
  - The employee needs to know that their performance is important to the organization.
- Comparing employees:
  - The objective of performance reviews should be to compare an employee's performance with defined performance standards, not with that of other employees.
- Failing to use performance review information:
  - Some managers may perform reviews—but then fail to make use of information gained, or neglect to follow through with commitments to support an employee's development.
  - The best action is to follow through with plans and commitments.
- Failing to be thoroughly familiar with the union contract:
  - If employees are represented by a union, the contract will outline the performance review process.
  - Ensure, as the manager, that you know this and follow it.

The basic elements of a functioning employee review program are shown in Figure 13.1. Be familiar with, and follow, the specific procedures established for the facility.

Figure 13.1
Elements for a Performance Review System

- Objectives for conducting performance reviews are defined.
- Performance standards are in place and have been communicated to employees.
- Employees are aware of the performance review process, criteria, and timetable from the time of the initial employment.
- Employees have received relevant training.
- The schedule for completing performance reviews has been established and is being followed.
- The manager applies a consistent and fair review process to all employees.
- The manager provides objective, specific feedback during the review process, describing observed behaviors.
- The manager uses methods to solicit employee participation and comments during a review.
- The manager listens attentively.
- The manager and employee work together during a review to solve performance-related problems, as appropriate.
- The manager seeks to resolve any misunderstandings and clarify expectations as needed during a review.
- The manager and employee agree upon areas for improvement and growth.
- If needed, the manager and employee create follow-up plans.
- The manager asks for the employee's commitment to achieving objectives.
- The manager completes required documentation and obtains the employee's signature as well. Documentation is placed in the personnel file.

Legal Implications

If you work with a union contract that covers transfers, promotions, and discharges, make sure you read and follow the union contract when disciplining, transferring, or promoting staff. Many of the government regulations from Chapter 8 also impact performance reviews such as the Civil Rights Act of 1991 and the Americans with Disabilities Act (ADA). If there is a human resources office, they can help navigate the legal implications of employee relations. If not, be aware of the legislation that can impact performance reviews.

Diversity in the Workplace

According to the Bureau of Labor Statistics (BLS) data from 2018 showed that 17.4% of the U.S. workforce is foreign-born. Hispanics accounted for nearly half of the foreign-born labor force in 2018, and Asians accounted for one-quarter. Beyond national origin, the U.S. population is a melting pot in many different respects. People come to the workplace of a dining services department with different languages and with various levels of literacy in written English. Differences in customs, values, lifestyles, sexual preferences, religious beliefs, style of dress, age, and communication styles could impact their interactions with co-workers and clients.

Diversity is a term that describes the many ways in which people differ from each other. Diversity means that CDM, CFPPs cannot assume all employees respond to the same style of communication, coaching or reward. Managing diversity is essential for promoting teamwork and accomplishing department objectives.

Every facility should have a clearly stated diversity policy which may say, for example, that the organization is committed to respecting the diversity of the work team. A policy may also explicitly prohibit derogatory comments about cultural groups. As a manager, you need to communicate this policy clearly, make it part of the employee orientation, and enforce it.

When recruiting employees, some recruitment avenues may seek out various groups. For example, consider recruiting through neighborhood newspapers in addition to the traditional ads to include members of the local community in an equitable manner. During the interview process, ensure that you are not filtering the applicant's responses through your own cultural background. Instead, appreciate how individuals may be different and seek to hire people who represent the community in which the facility is located.

Multicultural management does not mean that there are no rules. However, be alert to differences in nonverbal behavior and how it is interpreted, which can vary among cultures. For example, if a male employee comes from a cultural background in which men do not accept orders from women—and the employee has a female supervisor—it is not the employer's responsibility to give the employee a male supervisor. Conflicts that result in behavioral or performance issues need to be addressed. Discussion of cultural differences may help improve the employee interaction with others. Ultimately, an agreement of the job expectations is essential for the department to accomplish its mission. By recognizing the cultural differences, you can make the process much easier than it would be otherwise.

> **GLOSSARY**
>
> **Diversity**
> The many ways in which people differ from each other

Diversity in the Workforce

There is more than one meaning for the term diversity in the workplace. The above discussion refers to the characteristics commonly associated with human resources and diversity. Additionally, diversity is based on education, experiences, and "life lessons," all of which define one's perspective of an issue. Diversity is often the key resource that can help a work team meet its objectives. Why? It is because each member of the team has something unique to contribute. Diversity means having multiple perspectives and many points of view. Managers need to recognize and appreciate what is unique in every person on the team, including themselves. While this may take effort, it is worth it.

Today, many facilities offer diversity training, to help CDM, CFPPs with their own internal biases and to teach skills for managing diversity. This can be a great resource. After all, a non-judgmental attitude of openness and acceptance can go a long way towards managing a diverse work team.

Within your department, it is not enough to examine only yourself and your own practices. As a CDM, CFPP, you also need to observe the behaviors within your work team, listen to employees, and express an interest in others. A manager can encourage employees to share their backgrounds through involvement in cultural theme days, for example.

Disputes and Consensus

A work team is comprised of many individuals with unique cultural backgrounds and values, which can lead to occasional disputes. To maintain an effective work team, a manager should be alert to any conflict situations and intervene in a timely manner to resolve disputes.

To be successful as a group, employees must be encouraged to share one needed value, which is respect for themselves and for one another. Based on a respectful relationship, many disputes and conflicts can be resolved. Often, the steps are as simple as hearing the issue from everyone's perspective and helping everyone involved reach an understanding or consensus. A **consensus** is a general agreement within a group. It may not reflect the first choice of every individual member of the group. However, it reflects a plan that has been developed through some type of group process to represent the best, acceptable middle ground for everyone.

A process such as this can help resolve conflicts between or among employees; conflicts between a union and an employer; conflicts that arise from the presence of a diverse workforce, and many other situations. The steps are as follows:

1. Always base the process on respect. (Do not let anything change this.)
2. Recognize the importance of relationships among employees and protect these relationships.
3. Establish what the outcome of the process must be, such as having a policy that everyone will honor, or an agreement to which everyone will commit.
4. Discuss and clarify the issues from multiple perspectives.
5. Assure that every member of the group participates.
6. Work creatively and fairly as a group to come up with solutions.
7. Select a solution that meets the defined needs of everyone involved as closely as possible. Apply a sense of fairness and balance during this process.
8. Ask each member of the group to commit to this solution.

> **GLOSSARY**
>
> **Consensus**
> A general agreement within a group

> **GLOSSARY**
>
> **Corrective Action**
> An action taken by a manager to correct an employee performance problem

View the Supplemental Material for this chapter to see a sample Corrective Action Form.

Employee Discipline

Corrective action is a move taken by a manager to correct an employee's performance problem. The goal is always to correct or improve performance. Despite how it sometimes may be viewed, corrective action is neither negative nor punitive. It is one of the basic tasks of management required to control the activities of the employees in the department.

As defined by the human resources policies of the facility, corrective action is generally a formal, documented process. As such, it becomes part of an employee's personnel record. The form, like a performance review, is dated and signed by both the manager and the employee. Also, as in a performance review, the employee's signature represents acknowledgment that the employee has seen it, not that the employee agrees with the action. The corrective action form shows that an employee has been asked to make a specific behavioral change. In some organizations, this may be called a written warning or something similar. An example of a corrective action form appears in the Supplemental Material for this chapter.

As a CDM, CFPP, when you become aware of a performance problem, there are a few questions to be asked right away. These are:

- Have the relevant expectations and performance standards been previously communicated to the employee?
- Has appropriate training to support the employee's success been provided?
- Has constructive feedback been previously given to the employee?

When the answers to these three questions are "YES," it is generally time to take corrective action.

Formal corrective action, which may also be called discipline or disciplinary action, is a serious matter. In the extreme situation, it may provide documentation for termination of employment. Here are some examples of continued behavior that may require a formal, documented corrective action.

- Absenteeism/tardiness:
  > An employee who is habitually late or absent disrupts operations. Feedback regarding attendance should be based upon clearly established standards and policies that are uniformly administered. For example, a facility may have a policy that states an employee may not be absent or late to work more than six times in a 12-month period. In some facilities, an event of "no-call, no-show" (not calling in and not showing up for work) may be cause for immediate suspension or discharge.
- Violation of timeclock policies:
  > Punching in too early, leaving early, not clocking out for lunch, or incurring unauthorized overtime can all be examples in this category.
- Repeated failure to meet work standards:
  > If an employee's performance does not improve with ongoing feedback and provision of all required support, a manager may need to take formal corrective action.

- Violation of critical rules:
  > Most facilities have defined a set of higher level rules, the violation of which may be cause for immediate corrective action, suspension from work, or even termination. As a manager, become familiar with the policies in the facility. In some facilities, any of the following might be considered cause for serious disciplinary action or immediate termination:
    » Theft
    » Violation of confidentiality policies
    » Sleeping on duty
    » Violating safety rules or willfully endangering others
    » Willful injury to another person (employee or client)
    » **Insubordination**, direct refusal to do what the supervisor asks

Most facilities also have specific policies governing corrective action related to using drugs, drinking on duty, sexual harassment, possession of weapons on facility property, immoral, indecent conduct on duty, falsification of records, and punching someone else's time card. In some cases, such as drug use, a facility policy may define a series of steps for helping the employee address the problem, rather than dismissing the employee.

An **Employee Assistance Program (EAP)** may be designed for this purpose. An employee assistance program provides support to employees in solving personal problems that may be interfering with work. These may include drug use, alcohol abuse, family problems, and others. Some EAPs may provide assistance in identifying those who have, or are at risk of, alcohol and drug problems.

> **GLOSSARY**
>
> **Insubordination**
> A direct refusal to do what the supervisor asks
>
> **Employee Assistance Program (EAP)**
> Provides support to employees in solving personal problems that may be interfering with work such as drug and alcohol abuse, family problems, and teamwork problems

To take the appropriate course of action, a CDM, CFPP should know the facility's policy and the proper corrective action procedure. In serious situations, the manager needs to secure the input from the human resources and/or other managers. He or she needs to gather the facts and impose action only after a fair hearing of all sides from all persons involved. When practical, action should occur as soon as possible after a problem has occurred.

To prepare for a corrective action meeting with an employee, the CDM, CFPP should:

- Carefully investigate and gather facts.
- Prepare a corrective action document, describing the problem and the subsequent steps for improvement. Write in factual and objective terms. (Avoid using "hearsay" or behavior described only by others.)
- Set aside a private time and location and ask the employee to meet.
- Request the presence of a supervisor or representative from Human Resources to avoid a one-on-one meeting with the employee. (This will provide a third party witness.)
- Explain to the employee the reason for the meeting, and that this corrective action will become part of the employee's record.
- Explain the corrective action process and the policies related to it.
  > For example, let the employee know that documentation of this meeting will become part of the personnel record.
  > Outline the flow and timeframe of the corrective action process, as defined by the facility.

- State the objective, e.g., "I would like you to know that your performance is not acceptable and I want to support you in correcting it immediately."
- Describe the performance problem to the employee. Be calm and objective. Using the document as a reference, describe what you have observed.
- Firmly and clearly state why this behavior is not acceptable. Describe the established standard or applicable policy.
- Give a reason why this is a concern.
- Ask the employee for input. Ask him or her why this behavior is happening.
- Ask the employee what he or she can do to correct this situation. As warranted, discuss with the employee and seek to solve the problem together.
- Agree on a plan of action, which may be very simple. If the plan requires action on the manager's part, identify the steps to follow through.
- Specifically ask for the employee's commitment to improving performance.
- Sign and ask the employee to sign the document, adding comments. Provide a copy to the employee.
- File the document according to the policies and procedures.
- If the manager anticipates that the employee may disagree with the written documentation, meet with a senior staff member first to review the write up.
- Work with Human Resources when corrective actions result in suspension or termination of employment.
- Advise security of pending terminations.

While CDM, CFPPs may feel stressed and anxious about corrective action, it is helpful to keep in mind that the performance comes from the employee. As a manager, provide the proper direction and support. Ultimately, the manager does not control the employee's behavior. During a corrective action meeting, keep the responsibility for action where it rightfully belongs—in the employee's area. When an employee is asked, "What can you do to correct this situation?" the manager is asking the employee to accept the responsibility and to take action. Managers who do this find that this question removes a lot of pressure, and also builds a framework for successful performance improvement.

After taking a corrective action, continue to be positive and optimistic in your interactions with the employee. Recognize that the employee may feel embarrassed or even angry. As follow-up, continue to observe his or her performance. As soon as corrected behavior is demonstrated, be sure to call it to the employee's attention and provide a positive reinforcement. This helps an employee make a positive change in behavior.

Human resources policies and procedures should also specify a process for an employee to appeal a corrective action. In other words, if an employee feels that the action is not justified, the employee can go to a union steward, a department or division head,

3. How would you best prepare for a disciplinary action meeting with your employee?

or another person higher in the organization chart, as designated in the policy and procedure. See Figure 13.2 for basic prerequisites in a corrective action form.

Corrective action falls within the realm of **progressive discipline**, which is a series of defined steps a CDM, CFPP takes to correct ongoing employee performance problems. The exact set of steps is defined by the human resources policies and procedures. Generally, each step in the progressive disciplinary process becomes more severe. For example, one progressive discipline policy might state the following:

Step 1: The initial step is a verbal warning resulting in a dated note in the file.

Step 2: The first time a manager takes documented corrective action, it references the prior verbal warning, such as "on June 19th we discussed…" and is reviewed with the employee, signed, and placed in the personnel file as a "first written warning."

Step 3: If the problem continues, a second corrective action is taken and classified as a "second written warning."

Step 4: If the problem continues, the employee is suspended without pay, (e.g., for three days).

Step 5: If the problem continues, the employee is terminated.

> **GLOSSARY**
>
> **Progressive Discipline**
> A series of defined steps taken to correct ongoing employee performance problems

Figure 13.2
Basic Prerequisites for Effective Corrective Action

- Policies, rules, and procedures must be developed for all areas in the facility.
- Rules and policies must be explained to employees—and also provided in written form. For example, they can be included in employee handbooks and can be explained during orientation, training, and other activities.
- Policies, rules, and procedures must be reasonable, fair, and just from the perspective of both the employees and the CDM, CFPP.
- Policies, rules, and procedures must be enforced in a consistent, fair, and equitable manner. Thus, if one employee receives a formal written warning for missing three days of work during the past month, another employee who has the same attendance record should receive a written warning as well.
- Specific situations must be taken into account. The supervisor must determine whether observed problems were within or beyond the employee's control.
- The manager must use objective judgment.
- Supervisors must prepare for corrective action and make an effort to understand why the behavior is occurring and how the employee is motivated.
- Affected employees must be informed of any changes in policies, rules, and procedures before they are implemented.
- Corrective action programs should be administered objectively, without any bias.
- The supervisor should not threaten, argue, and/or display anger.
- Corrective action should be done in private.
- A manager must keep corrective action a confidential exchange and refrain from discussing it with other employees. (A manager may need to discuss the action confidentially with an immediate supervisor, a human resources staff member, or others who also commit to this confidentiality.)
- The corrective action should spell out exactly what the employee needs to do to improve his or her behavior on the job. Both the manager and the employee must discuss this.
- A manager who is newly promoted or new to an organization must begin to apply consistent performance standards from the start. Waiting and letting things slide becomes a set up for poor success of corrective action.

Why Don't Employees Perform?

The toughest problem that can arise is the situation in which an employee simply does not perform well. An employee is asked to comply with performance standards and it does not happen. Another employee is directed to follow a specific procedure, but he does not. Why does this occur?

Needless to say, there is no easy answer to this troubling question. A CDM, CFPP must understand that certain aspects of employee performance are beyond immediate control. A good leader motivates and influences employees. However, excellent performance comes from within the employee. Some individuals are more able or ready to perform than others, even the first day on the job.

What can the CDM, CFPP do when the employee has the drive and talent to perform well but is not meeting the performance standards? Re-evaluate the Performance Standards. Check if they are realistic for this employee. Find out if there is a supervisory problem or personality clash. Is there an alternative approach that could be used? In addition, seek the advice of other managers, their experience and observations may help. Figure 13.3 identifies some questions to pinpoint areas that may be a target for action.

Sometimes employees appear to have all of the trained skills and experience to perform a job well but still struggle to meet expectations. Their performance may not be a direct violation of the job but more of a chronic problem of not measuring up. A **Performance Improvement Plan (PIP)** is a way to assist an employee through additional training and clarification of expectations.

The intent of a PIP is not to document poor performance for the termination of the employee, although that is how it is frequently used, but rather to provide the employee with a developmental plan to suceeed in his or her job. A PIP should include the following:

1. The observed problem or concern.
2. Action plan:
   a. What needs to be done, by when, and to what reasonable level of expectation.
3. Interim follow-up steps:
   a. Scheduled meetings, review dates, defined points of progress.
4. Conclusion:
   a. If the employee is successful close the PIP.
   b. Partial success may lead to extended time for completion or adjustment of the action plan.
   c. Failure to meet expectations should result in termination or reassignment to an alternative position.

> **GLOSSARY**
>
> **Performance Improvement Plan (PIP)**
> A method to assist an employee through additional training and clarification of expectations

4. Your receiving clerk has been coming in tardy every day for the past week. What steps would you take in the progressive discipline process?

Figure 13.3
What to Check When Employees Don't Perform Well

- Does the employee know what you expect? How can you be sure?
- Are your expectations and standards attainable? Measurable?
- Does the employee know how to do the work to the established standards of quality/quantity?
- Are there any obstacles to the employee's performance that relate to systems, procedures, resources, or interference? If so, identify them and intervene.
- What social relationships in the workplace may be affecting the employee's work? (For example, is the employee following an informal leader whose direction conflicts with yours?)
- Have you provided feedback to the employee? If so, how many times? How close to the event? How specific has your feedback been?
- Are you interacting with the employee on a fair and objective basis?
- What does the employee say is causing the problem you have identified?
- Is the employee capable of doing this particular job? If not, is there an alternate job in the organization that might be a better fit?
- What is the employee's attitude towards the job, and where is this attitude coming from? Can you influence it?
- Have you examined the employee's needs and sources of motivation?

Termination

The questions listed in Figure 13.3 will not solve every problem. In the final analysis, a few situations may come to a dead end, when there appears to be nothing further that will change the situation. First of all, it is important to acknowledge that there are no reasonable alternatives. Here are some examples of situations that cannot be resolved:

- The employee's performance issue relates to an attitude that you are not able to influence.
- The employee simply lacks the ability to perform the job as defined, even with training. The employee is in the wrong job.

A situation such as this may have two options. If the employee is willing and motivated but simply is not suited to the job, the supervisor may explore whether a transfer to a different position and/or different department may be a positive resolution.

If the employee is essentially unwilling to improve, **termination** of employment may be the best course of action. Before terminating an employee, however, review the situation with the human resources and/or senior management, as defined by the policy. Ensure that each step of a progressive disciplinary process with an employee has been completed, and that termination is the next step.

Finally, meet with the employee to complete the termination. This does not have to be a hostile interaction and should not be a surprise, if progressive disciplinary actions have been taken. It is best to approach it matter-of-factly, reviewing the events that led to this decision. If a union represents the employee, invite the union steward to this meeting. As with a formal corrective action, avoid conducting a termination without a third party witness present. Termination can generate anger and unexpected responses. Assess the situation before beginning a termination meeting, and be prepared with some assistance, should it be required.

A termination must be documented according to the established policies. Like other paperwork, it becomes part of the employee's record. If the employee files for

> **GLOSSARY**
>
> **Termination**
> The dismissal of an employee by the employer

unemployment compensation, or a grievance with the Equal Employment Opportunity Commission, the documentation becomes an essential paper trail. Accurate and complete employment records will determine the outcome.

Following a termination, some members of the work team may feel distressed. Verify that the employee is no longer with the organization. Do not violate confidentiality, however, by discussing the termination and the factors that led up to it. Many employees will understand the action through their own observations. Sometimes, termination of an employee who has been disruptive to the work of the team brings about an unexpected, positive shift in morale.

An exception to the above discussion of progressive discipline is the probationary period for new employees, such as his or her first three months at work. During a probationary period, unique policies may apply. An employee may be working on a trial basis, and termination during this time period may not require all steps outlined in the progressive disciplinary action.

Employee Turnover

Employee turnover is common in foodservice operations. Many of the employees view their position as a transition to their "real" job. Work institute reported that in 2019, three of every four workers that left their job did so voluntarily (2020 Retention Report, State of the Workforce). Some employees leave the job for explainable reasons such as relocation, graduation, and retirement. Some leave for better pay.

Often, turnover results in significant expense for a foodservice operation. The cost of turnover to replace an employee is about 16% of the annual wages for the position (www. americanprogress.org/wp-content/uploads/2012/11/CostofTurnover.pdf) This expense takes the form of:

- Managerial time required to recruit, interview, and select new employees.
- Advertising expenses related to recruitment.
- Managerial time required to orient and train new employees.
- Temporary setbacks in productivity and/or quality during transitional phases.
- The stress of adjustment for existing staff.

Chapter 9 discussed calculating turnover rates to anticipate staffing needs, Turnover rates can and should be calculated by the manager. **Turnover rate** is used as a measure of stability in the foodservice department.

Clearly, a good CDM, CFPP strives to retain valuable employees in order to minimize the burden and expense of ongoing recruitment. Several factors can contribute to employee turnover. These include:

- Lack of opportunities for professional growth and development
- Lack of effective supervision

GLOSSARY

Turnover Rate
The number of employees who left the department divided by the number of positions in the department

5. The cook that was hired a year ago has shown up to work under the influence of alcohol a few times already. How would you handle this matter?

- Inadequate levels of trust between the employee and the supervisor
- Lack of participative opportunities
- Perceived inequality regarding how employees are treated
- Poor compensation, such as wages and/or benefits
- Lack of rewards
- Competitive offers elsewhere
- Personal reasons

Surprisingly, when asked about what makes employees want to stay on the job, many rate pay as relatively unimportant. Some employees in the service industry stay because of the rewards of working with others and serving people. Good relationships with peers, supervisors, and even clients—along with a positive work environment—also rank very high.

One approach that is helpful in employee retention is participative management. This can take many forms, but the basic idea is to involve employees in the facility.

Empowerment provides a form of participative management. Employee teams assigned to develop improvements, standards, procedures, or systems can be another form of participative management. These actions all encourage employees to be more engaged in their jobs and the workplace.

Exit Interview

When an employee does leave, it is important to conduct an **exit interview**. Depending on the organizational policy, it may be conducted for employees who voluntarily leave or for all departing employees, including those who are terminated. It may be conducted by the CDM, CFPP, or by a designated member of the Human Resources staff.

An exit interview often provides valuable information which the organization can use to improve employee retention. Sometimes an exit interview can provide surprises, and it becomes apparent that without this process, managers may never learn what they needed to know. Questions that are typically asked during an exit interview appear in Figure 13.4.

As a matter of policy, information gathered through exit interviews should be routinely reviewed and assessed by human resources staff. The manager should also review this information and seek to learn from it to improve retention.

GLOSSARY

Exit Interview
An interview with an employee who is leaving the organization

View the Supplemental Material for this chapter to see the Focus on Formulas video on Calculating Turnover Rate.

Figure 13.4
Sample Exit Interview Questions

- Why are you leaving the organization?*
- What did you enjoy most about working here?
- What did you enjoy least about working here?
- How would you describe your relationship with your supervisor?
- How would you describe the working environment?
- Is there anything that would have changed your decision to leave?*

* Omit these questions if the employee is not leaving voluntarily.

Labor Unions

It is not uncommon to work as a CDM, CFPP in an environment where food production and dining services staff belongs to a labor union (an organization representing employees and designed to advance the needs and interests of its members). The union's focus generally relates to wages, benefits, working conditions, employee safety, and other aspects of human resources management. Unionization provides certain advantages to employees. It also defines certain guidelines for the manager related to employee scheduling and assignments.

Once employees are represented by a union, the policies and procedures related to those employees must agree with the union contract. Some union guidelines, such as seniority, may become a factor in matters affecting personnel-related decisions. While all employees should be treated fairly and equally, a union contract may identify fair and equal differently.

A CDM, CFPP should be familiar with the provisions of any existing agreement between a union and the facility. When the union representatives and senior management (CDM, CFPP to Chief Executive Officer) work together, through effective management practices, it can benefit both the employees and the organization.

Employee Recognition

Many studies have been conducted to determine why employees leave their place of employment. Managers frequently believe it is because the employees want higher pay. In reality, it is often because employees want recognition for what they do and they want to feel appreciated. There are three management strategies that will help retain your employees:

- Treat employees like clients—with respect and dignity.
- Provide an atmosphere of trust and support.
- Reward employees for a good job and deal fairly with those who don't perform well.

Treat Your Employees Like Your Clients

One of the main reasons clients leave is because their needs are not being met. The same can be said for employees. Most often, they leave because their needs are not being met. Treating employees with respect and dignity is demonstrated by:

- Treating each employee fairly regardless of the type of decisions made or required.
- Demonstrating integrity by doing what you say you are going to do.
- Providing regular feedback to each employee.
    > Communicate to each employee what is required of them, how they are doing, and what the rewards are.
    > Remember that communication goes two ways, so make sure you ask the employees for feedback on what is required of them, what their rewards are, and how they think they are doing.

Provide an Atmosphere of Trust and Support

Communication is also the key to providing an atmosphere of trust and support. Communicate with employees about the direction of the department. Develop a consistent habit of communicating with each employee in person. Get to know about their lives outside of work by listening to them. Encourage and support their growth. Establish a relationship of trust and respect, both outside and inside the workplace. Keep your relationship friendly, but always professional.

Reward Employees for a Good Job

Rewarding employees for good work doesn't mean waiting until performance evaluation time. When you "catch them in the act of doing a good job," let them know it right then. One manager carried bite-sized candy bars with her, and any time she caught an employee doing a good job, she would give him or her a candy bar.

Rewards do not have to be monetary. In fact in today's economy, it probably will not be. Employees appreciate a simple thank you or a personal note. Ask during a staff meeting, "What went well this week?" then acknowledge the successes. There are many resources available to get ideas about rewarding employees. Also, do not forget to ask the employees how they want to be rewarded.

The Association of Nutrition & Foodservice Professionals (ANFP) promotes Pride in Foodservice Week in early February. This can be an opportunity to call attention to the contribution foodservice employees make to the facility.

Along with rewarding employees is treating each person fairly. There will be some employees who are liked better than others, but that should not interfere with fair treatment for all employees. For example, if there are staff layoffs due to a declining census, make sure the layoff decisions are based on the job duties, not the employee. Treating each person fairly also means taking the responsibility to address those who are not carrying their load. When this is not addressed, the positive performers are penalized with more work.

Employee Satisfaction Surveys

One way to gather feedback from the staff is through formal or informal employee satisfaction surveys. Some facilities have satisfaction surveys for the staff of the entire facility. Satisfied staff usually means satisfied clients.

The satisfaction surveys help identify areas where employees are motivated. They encourage all staff to become more engaged in the workplace. A motivated employee works to reach a goal and the related reward, whereas the **engaged employee** works to complete the task because it "is the right thing to do" to improve the organization. The engaged employees bring new ideas, ownership, and commitment to the mission.

> **GLOSSARY**
>
> **Engaged Employee**
> An employee fully invested in their work brings new ideas, ownership, and commitment to the mission

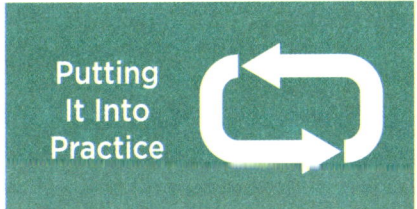

6. Employee satisfaction surveys show that employee morale is low at your workplace. What would you do to increase employee satisfaction?

If employees have the opportunity to express their feelings and beliefs about their job, they may be more engaged in the workplace. There are a number of corporate programs, such as Gallup and Press Ganey, that conduct formal employee satisfaction surveys.

Promotion, Development, and Succession Planning

An often overlooked role of the v is the importance of training and developing staff for the future. Part of the performance appraisal process is identifying the staff members with aspirations and capabilities for promotion. It is short sighted to keep the best employees in their current positions. Investing in their training through actively assigning them to new tasks or formally supporting their educational training has long-term benefits for the department and the organization.

Cross-training staff gives the facility a multifaceted employee with skills in many areas. Exposing employees to new areas of service prepares them for a lateral move to a different position, promotion, or even transfer to other departments. Encouraging staff to complete their education, become a CDM, CFOO, or pursue a college degree builds bench strength for the department.

Transfer to other departments, resignation to take another job, or even promotion within create short-term staffing issues with lasting employee benefit. Providing access to a career path for their growth and development motivates the best of employees and positions the manager as the employer of choice, improving the quality of future job candidates. When you support and champion for the staff, they commit and support you as their manager.

The promotion and development of staff members also aids in **succession planning**, the identification and grooming of potential leaders of the department. Succession planning is a way for the organization to plan for replacement of leadership through training, goal setting, and progressive management experience. The planned training of potential leaders ensures a smooth transition when a leadership role becomes open.

GLOSSARY

Succession Planning
The identification and grooming of potential leaders in the department

Chapter References

RESOURCES	
2020 Retention Report, State of the Workforce	https://info.workinstitute.com/hubfs/2020%20Retention%20Report/Work%20Institutes%202020%20Retention%20Report.pdf
ANFP Pride in Foodservice Week	https://www.anfponline.org/events-community/pifsw
Gregoire, Mary (2013). Foodservice Organizations, A managerial and systems approach, 8th ed. Upper Saddle River, NJ: Pearson Prentice Hall	
HR Metrics. How and Why to Calculate Employee Turnover	https://www.talentlyft.com/en/blog/article/242/hr-metrics-how-and-why-to-calculate-employee-turnover-rate
Professional Standards for School Nutrition Professionals	https://www.fns.usda.gov/school-meals/professional-standards
The Workplace and Alcohol Problem Prevention	https://pubs.niaaa.nih.gov/publications/arh26-1/49-57.htm

Policies and Goal Setting in the Workplace

Overview and Objectives

The regulations related to providing meals for the public and managing labor issues require written processes. Policies and procedures (P&P) represent an essential tool for presenting work practices. The Certified Dietary Manager®, Certified Food Protection Professional® (CDM®, CFPP®) is expected to meet department goals and communicate those goals to employees. This communication will be important in helping motivate the employees to accomplish the department goals and objectives. After completing this chapter, you should be able to:

- Participate in developing policies and procedures
- Develop S.M.A.R.T. goals and objectives for the department
- Identify practices to motivate and empower employees
- Compare department goals against key performance indicators (KPIs)

GLOSSARY

Policy
Describes an organization's approach to a certain situation

Procedure
Details the steps in carrying out a policy

Policy & Procedure (P&P) Manual
Printed or electronic documentation that describes almost every activity in the department

Standard Operating Procedures (SOP)
A step-by-step, written instruction for completing specific tasks accurately and consistently

Policies and Procedures

In any organization, a set of documents called policies and procedures serve as an essential reference. A set of **policies** are principles, rules, and guidelines formulated or adopted by an organization to reach its long-term goals. **Procedures** are the specific methods employed to express policies in action in day-to-day operations of the organization. Together, policies and procedures ensure that a point of view held by the governing body of an organization is translated into steps that result in an outcome compatible with that view.

There are several reasons for maintaining a set of written department P&P. They are to serve as a:

- Reference for anyone unfamiliar with the work.
- Communication tool within the department when presenting procedural plans.
- Communication tool for people external to the department.
- Working document which may be required by inspectors or surveyors examining the practices in the facility.
- Reference for those who may succeed the manager.
- And ultimately, "if it isn't written down, then it did not happen," and no one is accountable.

When surveyors and reviewers come into the facility for license or accreditation renewal, they are evaluating the performance and compliance of the organization to their regulatory set of standards. If they observe events outside of the expected, they reference the facility's or the department's **Policy & Procedures (P&P) Manual** against what they have observed to verify that processes are being followed correctly. The regulatory guidelines are often the basis of written policies for dining services.

For the employees, the P&P Manual also defines what the department expects them to do, and often details how the task is to be performed. This is true for your employees as well.

Many organizations have a policy template set by administration with defined content and format guidelines. Often, departments have revised and maintained a P&P Manual that describes almost every activity in the departments, and the responsible

Figure 14.1
Policy and Procedure Manual Relationships

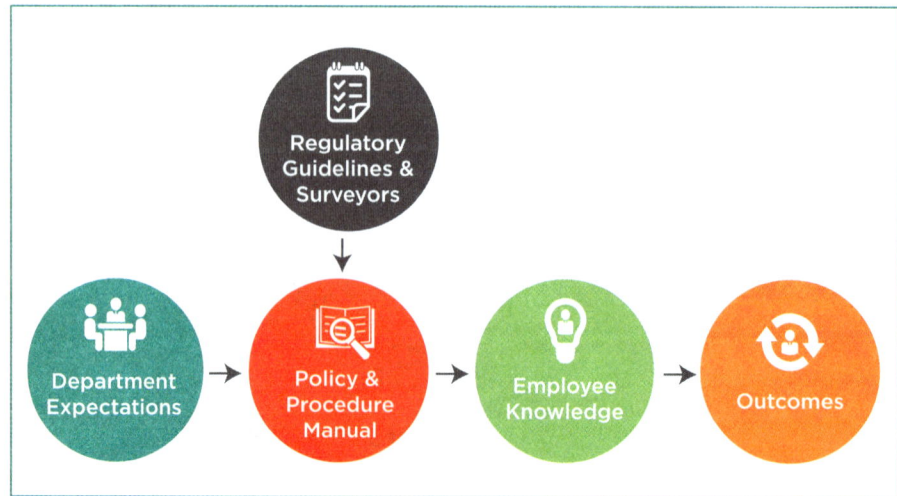

staff, as well as the expected outcomes. A printed, paper version of the P&P Manual, or an electronic version on the facility server, may have more than 100 different policies. **Standard operating procedures** (SOP) are also used to carry out the facility's mission. The SOP is separate from the P&P Manual as it is more of a step-by-step detailed written instruction to complete the specific tasks.

To make the P&P Manual easy to understand, present each one in a consistent, organized format. For example, the CDM, CFPP may maintain a notebook divided into sections with P&P Manual for:

- Departmental organization (including an organization chart)
- Menu planning
- Purchasing and inventory
- Food production
- Customer/client service
- Special services and catering
- Clinical services
- Client rights
- HIPAA compliance and confidentiality
- Scheduling and staffing
- Personnel issues
- Emergency contact information
- Disaster management

If the facility is part of a network or healthcare system, surveyors will expect to find that the P&P Manual is consistent across the system with variations specific to each facility. The Diet Manual (discussed in the companion textbook, *Nutrition Fundamentals and Medical Nutrition Therapy*) is approved by the medical staff and serves as the clinical support for the P&P.

Each P&P should be identified clearly with a title, a number, or both. Any time a procedure is changed, it should be dated. It needs to be filed and also dated in the document at each location. (This document or notebook is found in the department, the facility administrative offices, or the corporate shared file network.) And you need to include all the other departments that the policy may affect. For example: A procedure addressing how to order in-house catering services may be an essential reference in other departments. If this is the case, ensure that the revised procedures are distributed to those departments.

The manager is responsible for maintaining the policies on a regular basis, so that the P&P accurately reflects the activity of the department. Typically, the policies are reviewed on an annual basis, dated, and signed by the department manager.

If there is no P&P Manual for the department, or if new policies need to be written, the manager is responsible for developing them. Writing a new policy to document a change in a service is not difficult when you have a well-documented P&P Manual to use as a guideline. However, developing a comprehensive manual from scratch is a major undertaking.

There is an old saying "Don't reinvent the wheel. We already know that it is round." Instead of trying to develop all of the appropriate policies on your own, access what is already in the market. There are several electronic manuals available for healthcare and school food services. An Internet search for "healthcare foodservice policy manual" or "school foodservice policy manual" will pull in a number of options.

If you purchase a P&P Manual, verify that it has an editable electronic version that can be adapted to the facility without having to re-type the whole policy. Review each policy and determine if it applies to your operation. Skip any policy that does not apply. For example, if "Home Delivered Meals" is not a service provided, then the policies related to satellite meal services may not be relevant.

Refer to Figure 14.2 in Supplemental Material for a sample policy and procedure on social networking. (Even if this is not a corporate or organization-wide policy, it should be a department policy, as employees utilize social media to communicate with friends and family about their work experience.)

View the Supplemental Material for this chapter to see a Sample Policy and Procedure for Social Networking.

In designing policies and managing the daily activities in a foodservice department, consider some of the guidelines you must follow and use them as tools. For example, policies and procedures may need to support compliance with CMS regulations, OSHA requirements, health department codes, and other standards. Adapting these guidelines into policies for the organization is up to the manager. Therefore, base your decisions on the systems that function in the facility, the flow of work, the responsibility and accountability as detailed in the organization chart, and other practical factors. New or revised policies and procedures should be communicated to all employees using effective communication techniques.

Without a P&P Manual no one would know what is expected of him or her, therefore, it all becomes a matter of individual interpretation. For example, a new employee says "During orientation, this is the way that Tommy showed me how to deliver the meals to the unit." With no policies, there are no defined standards and no accountability for doing the job correctly or not.

When errors happen, and they will, how will the manager correct the issue without a policy? Based on what will you discipline the employee? From a surveyor's perspective and a legal liability perspective, how will you verify that there is a defined process and the staff know what the policy is? (Remember, if it is not in writing, it did not happen.)

P&Ps, SOPs, and the performance standards (discussed in Chapter 13) define the basis on which the department functions. These documents establish where the department is. Going beyond the standards and required activities are the department goals. Typically, new goals for the organization and for the department are written annually.

Goals Versus Objectives

Goals and **objectives** are closely related. Both describe purpose. However, a goal is a statement that outlines a broad direction or intention. An objective is a specific step that will help in accomplishing a goal. Here are some other comparisons:

- A goal is broad in focus while an objective is narrow.
- A goal is the aim. The objectives are how you get there.
- A goal may be abstract but an objective is concrete and measurable.
- A goal is more long-term, while an objective is short- to medium-term.
- A goal is the result we want. Objectives are the actions to get there.

GLOSSARY

Goal
A statement that outlines an outcome or result

Objective
The steps to achieve the goal or the actions that lead to the goal

Many facilities create master plans for growth that may describe the goals for the coming year, as well as the long-term ones for a five-year or even 10-year period. This kind of forward thinking helps to focus the direction a facility takes and keep it moving forward in a meaningful and effective manner. For example, an organization that operates skilled nursing facilities may establish a goal of expanding most of its properties into senior living communities, with assisted living and other services, over a period of five years. Or, a school system may establish a goal of centralizing most of its services, including foodservice operations, over the next two years.

Organizations set goals by looking into the future and predicting what will be necessary for success. Factors that may influence goal-setting include: financial constraints, regulatory changes, staffing needs, challenges faced by the industry, new opportunities, and client feedback as well as a review of available and needed resources. Goals align with the vision and mission of the organization, helping to fulfill them.

Setting Objectives

Once broad goals have been established in any facility, a number of related objectives must be developed. Every branch, department, and individual plays a role in helping the facility define its goals and achieve its objectives. A CDM, CFPP may play several key roles in managing objectives.

In some facilities, managers are involved in setting the objectives for the facility. In others, it may be less direct. Recognize that as the manager of a service-oriented department, you will have information and insights that can contribute to the formation of actionable objectives for the department and others.

Before customizing the goals and objectives to the department, first understand the big picture. Talk with your supervisor and peers to clarify the scope and intent of doing such. Then, extend these organizational objectives to be more specific to food production and dining services. For example, if a goal is to improve client satisfaction, an objective may be to improve their satisfaction with food temperatures.

Look for ways to make each objective clear and measurable. A meal satisfaction objective may be measured with ratings or percent changes. An example of a measurable objective is: *Client ratings about the temperature of food will improve by at least ten percent (10%) by December.*

There are a number of different goal setting systems used in business today. One is the Specific, Measurable, Achievable, Reasonable, Timely (S.M.A.R.T.) goal method which is a structured process to help identify the direction and plan the mid-point guideposts to achieve the intended goals. The use of the S.M.A.R.T. goal system process adds discipline to goal setting. Criteria for goals and objectives are summarized in Figure 14.3.

Plan of Action

Goals and objectives are good management techniques but accomplish little without an **action plan**. As a CDM, CFPP you should use the work team as a resource for developing a plan of action. Break the process down into parts: What objectives are needed to reach the goal? What steps are needed to accomplish the objective? In a plan of action, there may be a series of steps associated with each objective. Figure 14.4 provides an example of a sample action plan.

GLOSSARY

Action Plan
A process to accomplish specific goals and objectives

Figure 14.3
Criteria for Goals and Objectives

SMART GOALS

SPECIFIC: Answer questions such as: What precisely will happen? (Describe the outcome)

MEASURABLE: Answer questions such as: How will I determine if the goal is successful?

ACHIEVABLE: Answer questions such as: How can this be achieved with the resources available?

REASONABLE: Answer questions such as: What makes this possible to achieve?

TIMELY: Answer questions such as: When will this be accomplished?

EFFECTIVE OBJECTIVES

SPECIFIC: They describe what will be done, and by whom.

CHALLENGING: They represent growth rather than status quo, but are nevertheless practical.

OBSERVABLE: They describe a change that you as a CDM, CFPP can objectively observe.

MEASURABLE: They provide a form of a measure and time period you can use to evaluate achievement.

SIMPLE: They each cover one clear action item.

Source: https://www.smart-goals-guide.com

For goals and objectives to be successful, the involvement of supervisors and employees is necessary. Creating special teams focused on individual objectives, or even specific action plans, will improve the staff "buy-in" to the steps being taken. Participation of staff in the planning process and building the action plan increases their level of engagement in the department. Essentially, the manager's role becomes one of final approval, as well as the oversight and coordination of the different activities.

In virtually any facility, change is inevitable when carrying out the goals, objectives, and plan of action. It may come from external sources such as regulations and standards as they are revised, from within as a facility seeks to improve itself, or from personnel changes. Setting priorities, assessing available resources, and determining the timeline often define whether the manager will be able to successfully reach the goals.

Meeting Goals and Priorities for the Department

Once the organization's goals have been developed and communicated to all the directors, often at the annual planning meeting, time is set aside to relate them to the department goals. Start by listing the overall facility goals and have a second list of goals you think could or should be the focus of your department. How many of the potential department goals fit into one or more of the organizational goals? Some goals may fit in perfectly while others, although some good ideas, just do not fit with

Putting It Into Practice

1. A goal of your department is to increase cafeteria sales. How would you write this goal as a S.M.A.R.T. goal? List three possible objectives to achieve this goal.

Figure 14.4
Sample Goal With Action Plan

GOAL SETTING AND ACTION TASKS WORKSHEET

Writing an Effective Goal Statement

Rules for writing goal statements:
1. Use clear, specific language.
2. Start your goal statement with TO + a verb.
3. Write your goal statement using S.M.A.R.T. goal criteria.
4. Avoid using negative language. Think positive.

S.M.A.R.T. GOALS
- S Specific
- M Measurable
- A Achievable
- R Reasonable
- T Timely

Goal	Tasks	Target Date for Completion	Who's Responsible	Completed Date
Example: To review and revise the current menu to reflect the new or revised dining venue by (state the date).	1. Meet with Resident Food Council to brainstorm menu items.	Date	Foodservice Director	Date
	2. Prepare new menu for the new venue.	Date	FSD, Supervisor, Dietitian, and Consultants	Date
	3. Evaluate recipes and costing.	Date	Supervisor and Cooks	Date
	4. Create production sheets, including recipes.	Date	Supervisor	Date
	5. Educate staff on new menu.	Date	Foodservice Director and Supervisors	Date

the direction the organization is taking. Typically, those goals that best align with the facility goals take on a higher priority.

Assess the availability of resources to accomplish the goals. Some goals may be procedural and require little or no funding to be highly successful. Others may need major capital investment or the addition of labor hours, which may not be available. The resources can refer to dollars for investment, labor for completing implementation, or equipment and space to accommodate the planned changes. Demands on resources often determines whether the goal is a high or a low priority.

Determining department goals is the result of coordinating organizational goals and priorities, resources available, regulations, and appropriate fit with the services being provided. If the highest priority department goals do not align with the organizational goals, the manager should be prepared to advocate for his or her goals.

Departmental and facility goals may have a very high priority due to regulatory requirements. For example, the implementation of ICD-10 for medical record coding has consumed financial and labor resources for many facilities. This is done at the expense of completing other goals that would be nice, but are not required.

Likewise, a failing meal delivery system may need replacement within the next nine months, making it the department goal priority even though it does not match the organizational goals.

Once the goals and resources have been aligned, you should continue the planning process with a list of the tasks to be accomplished in the action plan. Assign staff members to the various tasks and identify measurable outcomes for each step. Schedule interim dates for progress reports to keep all staff on track with the goals. Working with and through staff members takes more effort on the part of the manager to support and mentor the work teams without taking over the process. The best planning will not succeed unless the manager motivates employees to help carry out the plan, then directs and coaches them in their actions.

Motivation

Motivation is an internal force that makes people want to do something in order to reach a goal. Motivation comes from within a person. A CDM, CFPP cannot force an employee to be motivated but he or she can encourage it. A manager can provide job conditions that help employees to attain their goals.

When a manager can match the employees' goals with those of the department, both benefit. Matching employee goals begins during the hiring interview process. Managers strive to hire people capable of doing the work assigned to them. If employees are not capable of doing the work, no amount of training or motivational support will make them effective.

Employees also need to be willing to do the work. They can have the ability to do the work, but if they don't really want to do it, they will not be effective. Finally, employees may be willing to work and are perfectly capable, but if they are not shown how to do the job correctly they still may not be effective. In-services and on-the-job training are useful techniques for developing employees' skills and aid in motivating staff.

Theories of Motivation

Several theories of motivation address the question of why people do things. Some approaches take the stance that most people strive to reach their full potential. Just how far they have advanced toward reaching their full potential will determine what motivates them. The idea is that if a manager knows what motivates employees, and that he or she can provide the appropriate incentives, their performance improvement will follow.

The best-known theory in this arena is the psychologist Abraham **Maslow's Hierarchy of Needs**. According to him, an individual's specific needs drive behavior. Maslow's Hierarchy of Needs represents the order in which these needs become motivators of human behavior. These are illustrated in Figure 14.5.

Maslow says that the physiological needs of survival, such as food and water, come first. When these needs are being met, an individual moves from focusing on survival to the second level of needs: Security and safety, such as stability, protection, and freedom from fear and chaos. The third level motivating behavior is social needs. These revolve around friendship, love, and the need to belong.

Self-esteem comprises the fourth level within the hierarchy. Starting with recognition and respect by others, esteem progresses to self-respect and self-worth. Public recognition and pride in a job well done or humiliation and personal shame in poor

---

GLOSSARY

Motivation
An internal force that makes people do something in order to reach a goal

Maslow's Hierarchy of Needs
The best known theory of human motivation

Figure 14.5
Maslow's Hierarchy of Needs, With Job Context Examples

Source: Adapted Maslow, 1954

performance are powerful motivators. The need for esteem gives rise in some people to the need for power as a way of commanding the esteem of others. Satisfaction of the need for self- esteem leads to feelings of self-confidence, strength, and worth. When these needs are unsatisfied, they produce feelings of inferiority, weakness, and helplessness.

The final level in Maslow's hierarchy is that of self-actualization or self-fulfillment. The drive to be all that we can be is a balance between meeting our other needs first and coming to accept "What a man can be, he must be." (Maslow, A. (1954). *Motivation and Personality*. New York, NY: Harper. pp. 91.) Maslow believed that to reach self-fulfillment, the person needed to not only meet the prior levels of needs but they needed to master them. Creative outlets might be as simple as a garden or painting. Or, creativity might be the fulfillment of a dream to teach as a second career in retirement.

It is important to recognize that not everyone is motivated by the same thing. A CDM, CFPP can use these ideas to help an employee meet his or her needs in the performance and commitment at work. Employee needs can be met, or supported on the job in a variety of ways:

- Physiological Needs: rest breaks, paychecks, bonuses.
- Safety/Security Needs: consistent application of work rules, policies, evaluation and performance feedback, non-threatening environment, proper working equipment, effective safety management programs.
- Social Needs: committee assignments, teamwork, friendship with fellow employees, sponsoring social activities such as bowling teams, employee picnics, newsletters.
- Esteem Needs: awards (e.g., employee of the month), attendance at seminars, recognition, promotions.
- Self-fulfillment Needs: support of personal development and/or tuition reimbursement; participation in planning of work area goals and objectives; encouraging creative projects.

It is generally true that:

- The staff member who is interested in the work is more likely to have internal motivation, which will benefit the employee, the dining services department, and the organization itself.
- The staff member who can identify with the organization and believe in it will be more willing to help the organization than will one motivated only by punishment and reward.

- Few people make an effort to analyze themselves objectively. The CDM, CFPP is challenged to recognize aspects of motivation that the employee may not be able to verbalize.
- Money is not a primary and important motivator for many employees. In fact, money is often a maintenance factor, not a motivation factor.
- Competition among employees or groups of staff members within the same organization generally does not motivate staff.

The CDM, CFPP should pay attention to what motivates different employees. By providing for basic needs and supporting the development and advancement of staff members, the manager can help employees want to perform on the job. For most employees, the desire to succeed and perform well is a more constructive and effective motivator than the fear or humiliation of losing the job.

Strong workplace motivators include a positive work climate, empowered employees, good teamwork, meaningful feedback, and consistent, honest recognition.

Work Climate

Work climate refers to how it feels to work in a given environment. It is the tone or attitude set by the CDM, CFPPs, and is often closely intertwined with the facility's philosophy. However, it is also greatly influenced by the attitudes and actions of all the staff.

A constructive work climate supports employee development and workplace participation. Essentially, work climate becomes the state of mind employees have on the job which, in turn, affects how they perform that job.

Clients are also affected by the work climate, as employees who feel positive about their jobs tend to treat them with more respect. Employees who are unhappy on the job may complain to clients, or perform their work grudgingly. All of this affects customer/client service and the image of the department.

Some of the factors that help promote a positive work climate include:
- A role model to respect and support.
- A belief in the value and talents of every individual in the organization.
- Support for employees' needs, especially training and development.
- Listening to others.
- Managerial attention to problems that create stress among employees.
- Encouragement of teamwork and enthusiasm.
- A sense of calm, even when there are deadlines and time pressures.
- Frequently expressed praise for the value of employees' accomplishments.
- An emphasis on teamwork whenever possible.

> **GLOSSARY**
>
> **Work Climate**
> Tone or attitude of how it feels to work in a given environment

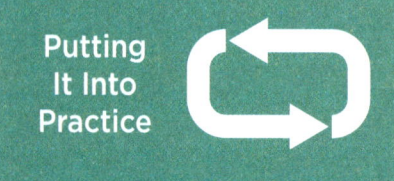

2. What are five practices you can implement at the workplace to move employees up Maslow's hierarchy?

Empowerment

Another idea that relates very closely to the work climate is **empowerment**. In contrast with old management theories that were highly autocratic, empowerment means that the CDM, CFPP encourages an employee to take action in situations. In doing so, an opportunity is given to the employee to achieve. As such, it is strongly motivating.

How does it work? Clearly, a manager cannot just say to employees, "Do whatever you want." A manager has to provide direction to this process. To empower employees, consider the following steps:

1. **Define objectives very clearly.** Let the employees know what the department is trying to achieve and keep these objectives in the forefront by discussing them often.
2. **Clarify policies so that employees have a solid framework for decisions they will make on their own.** For example, if you have a policy of always providing a substitution for a client who is unhappy with the food, make sure employees know this and follow the policy.
3. **Define the limits.** Tell employees what situations you support them in handling on their own, and what situations you wish to become involved. For example, employees might be empowered to accept a complaint, but are expected to involve management if a complaining client becomes abusive or violent.
4. **Communicate and coach.** As employees take power into their own hands, be accessible to coach them. Be willing to provide support at any time, and to discuss actions after to help an employee develop a greater range of skills. Ask to be informed, at least after the situation, about any information that is important to you as a manager.

> **GLOSSARY**
>
> **Empowerment**
> When management gives power to the employees to take action and resolve issues

Team Building

Another technique that is critical to the success of every dining services operation is team building. A team approach recognizes that each employee is not working alone. Instead, it means that all employees are working together to accomplish the defined objectives. The parallel to this teamwork is a sports team. For example, on a football team, the action of each player critically affects the bottom line—who wins the game. Players have to work together cohesively in order to win.

Actually, the same ideas hold true in a dining services department, as well as in a facility itself. The systems approach to management says that all the parts work together to accomplish the job. Serving a meal, for example, requires the coordinated efforts of people who purchase, receive, store, withdraw, prepare, and serve food. When the meal is successful, it is because everyone on the team performed well and worked together. Recognize that every position contributes to the success of the team: The cooks cannot prepare the meal if the pots have not been washed.

When a sense of teamwork does not exist, efforts can become disjointed and the work flow within systems can deteriorate. The result is poor performance and poor quality.

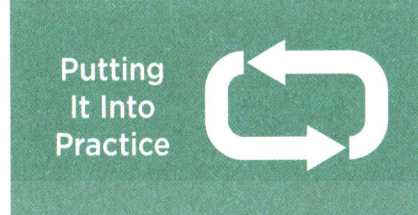

3. Write out an example where the employee is empowered at work to make decisions.

To encourage teamwork, you can take a number of actions, such as:

- **Communicate objectives.** Keep the objective in front of all staff members: "We are going to serve these clients the best food they have ever eaten!" or "We are going to re-define the meaning of excellent service." A common objective draws people together.
- **Believe in your team.** Your belief that the team can perform has a tremendous impact on what happens. Employees who are not sure what they can do will respond to your belief in their capabilities. Instilling confidence is a great motivator.
- **Use enthusiasm.** Enthusiasm is contagious and is a key factor in getting the team truly excited about meeting objectives. It also contributes to a very positive work climate.
- **Give team members roles and responsibilities.** Make the contribution of each team member clear.
- **Use informal leaders.** While a formal leader may have a position on the organization chart that defines authority over someone else, every business also has informal leaders. An informal leader is one who, through personality factors, tends to gain the cooperation of others. Informal leaders can help support the objectives of the team and help support each player.
- **Provide the resources needed.** The manager needs to equip the employee team with everything they need to do their work and meet their objectives.
- **Provide opportunities for fun.** Letting off steam from a tiring day, enjoying an appropriate joke, or attending a departmental picnic are all examples of how members of a team can have fun together. When work is finished and employees are relaxing, more team building takes place.
- **Resolve conflicts.** Conflicts naturally arise among employees from time to time. An effective manager recognizes conflict and works openly toward a resolution to keep the team together.
- **Celebrate successes.** Meeting a goal, completing a project, or earning recognition sometimes is by just getting through the meal.
- **Reward and recognize the team.** As the team meets objectives, this should become cause for cheering, celebration, and public recognition. These actions reinforce the efforts of the team and provide fulfillment to each team member.

Through effective teamwork, a CDM, CFPP can find that a group accomplishes more, employees gain satisfaction, and the systems function better. Thus a manager often needs to function as a coach and build each employee's identity as part of the team.

Tools for Meeting Goals and Objectives

To meet goals, motivation and tools are important. Several options to help meet these include: the organization chart, delegation, performance standards, policies and procedures, and communicating results.

Note the word "organization" in an organization chart. Remember, in the first part of this chapter on planning, you created a list of tasks that will be required to accomplish your goals. As you group these tasks and decide which staff members will be assigned to them, you are organizing. Use this chart to help with this. The organization chart illustrates the division of work, and can help determine to which employee the tasks should be delegated to.

Delegation is assigning tasks to the appropriate employee within the department. It is one way to develop the potential of employees. Remember that some employees may be motivated by the opportunity to take on added responsibility. Therefore, as you delegate, consider the following:

- Tasks must be communicated clearly and effectively.
- Employees must be empowered with the authority to accomplish these tasks.

It is not delegation if you assign the responsibility for a task but do not convey the authority to complete the task.

Goal Reporting

To monitor progress and ensure completion of the goal, many organizations utilize a quarterly or monthly reporting process. Typically the formal quarterly report sent to the administration is a follow-up to the Goal and Action Plan form in Figure 14.4. In addition, the manager is also frequently responsible with updating the department staff on **key performance indicators** (KPIs) for the facility and the department. KPIs are benchmark performance points tracked on a monthly basis and often relate to the department goals for improvement.

KPIs for foodservice management is an essential component to measure the current situation, as well as to measure progress over a period of time. It is one of the essential components to effectively review the objectives and strategies regularly. Foodservice KPIs are also linked to the overall goals of the organization.

For example, suitable key performance indicators in hospital food service would include KPIs on:

- Patient Satisfaction on Patient Food Services
- Number of Food-related Incidents and overall food safety
- Timely Patient Food Delivery
- Patient Plate Waste
- Number of Diets Served

See Figure 14.6 for a sample KPI report.

Summary

Policies and procedures, along with performance standards, help identify employees who are in the activities that have a direct effect on the goals. Who knows the current process better than those who currently do the tasks? The policies and performance standards define what is supposed to be done while the employees can clarify what is actually being done. Bridging the gap between what should be and what is will help you develop more realistic goals and action plans. With the input and buy-in of the staff, ownership of the outcomes is increased. Employees need motivation and team building at the workplace to achieve the goals and objectives for the organization.

> **GLOSSARY**
>
> **Delegation**
> Passing authority for tasks or assigning duties downward through the organization chart
>
> **Key Performance Indicators (KPIs)**
> Benchmark performance points tracked over time

Figure 14.6

Sample Key Performance Indicator Score Card for Dining Services

	ANNUAL	TARGET BUDGET	MET OR NOT MET TARGET	COMMENTS
Operational Efficiency Strategy				
Facility Finance-Reductions	$230,000	$525,000	↓	Our work needs to continue in reducing expenses to meet this budget.
Average Daily Census	106	116	↓	Continues to be below budget, it is better than last month.
Nutrition Care Expenses	$112,605	$114,436	↑	We are under budget year-to-date but need to continue looking for more reductions including: disposables, food and tube feeding,s and salaries.
Nutrition Care Revenue (Income)	$28,476	$26,528	↑	We are running 3.33% above our budget. These numbers are helping with offsetting our expenses—Good Job.
Number Meals Served	19,149	18,731	↑	Meals served increased by 418 from budget due to a small increase in the number of meals served per labor hour.
Employee Strategy				
Employee Engagement—First Choice—Department	3.89	4.08	↓	Work is being done on equipment needs and opinions count. **Are you using the suggestion box?** Exceeded 2019 goal of 3.66 work towards a goal of 4.08 for 2020.
Consumer Strategy				
Courtesy of Persons Serving Food	46%	50%	↓	March: Temp: 38%; Quality: 41%. Courtesy: 46%. Thanks for working so hard to please our patients. It's making a difference.
Special/Restricted Diet Explained	21%	100%	↓	Implement visit cards starting in June.
Food Temperature at Time of Meal Delivery	60%	90%	↓	Implementing new meals on-demand in TCU in July: 20% points YTD. Stay focused on prompt delivery of meals.

Chapter References

RESOURCES	
Employee Empowerment and Its Impact on Restaurant Business in Bangladesh	https://pdfs.semanticscholar.org/96c9/962dc04889e4488250157befbd6f4088d688.pdf
Hospital Food Service Key Performance Indicators	https://pdfs.semanticscholar.org/623e/2cb537d122d148c00d9286a7c7692d24471e.pdf
Maslow's Hierarchy of Needs	https://www.simplypsychology.org/maslow.html
S.M.A.R.T. Goals and Objectives	Smart-goals-guide.com

Communications and Managing Change

Overview and Objectives

Communication determines how effectively people work together in an organization. As a Certified Dietary Manager®, Certified Food Protection Professional® (CDM®, CFPP®) you are expected to be involved in interdepartmental teams, committees, and task forces; and apply good communication techniques in all your activities. After completing this chapter, you should be able to:

- Conduct effective department meetings
- Participate in meetings outside the department
- Participate in regulatory agency surveys
- Manage changes in the organization and assist employees in embracing the change
- Manage time and stress efficiently

Communication is simply the act of transferring information from one place, person, or group to another. Every communication involves at least one sender, a message, and a recipient. The transmission of the message from sender to recipient can be affected by a huge range of things. These include our emotions, the cultural situation, the medium used to communicate, and even our location.

In many respects, a CDM, CFPP functions as a communicator and facilitator. This role is especially true when representing the department at meetings. Understanding both the facility needs and expectations will help determine how the department team can carry them through. Ensuring that department activities are coordinated with those of the system would require cooperation and consistent ongoing communication at meetings.

Flow of Communciation in an Organization

In a facility, there is communication going in many directions. Some messages flow downwards, from superiors to managers, or from manager to the line staff. Others may flow upwards, from manager to supervisor, or from subordinates to manager. Some communication flows laterally, between and among peers.

In most organizations, **downward communication** is frequently used to convey policies, procedures, directives, objectives, and other information to subordinate personnel. It may be written or spoken. When a CDM, CFPP uses downward communication, it is often to give instructions, explain information or procedures, train employees, or communicate information that may have a bearing on employees' jobs.

Downward communication may be the only contact subordinates have with upper management. It usually follows the chain of command, meaning that you would receive the information from your supervisor who received it from his/her director or from the CEO. As a result, administration should:

- Be honest, accurate, and factual, whether the information is good or bad.
- Use words and phrases that subordinates can understand.
- Make the message specific; explain what effect it will have on the employee.

Your job, as the manager, is to continue communicating down the chain of command with accurate, reliable, and relevant information.

Employees also will communicate ideas, requests, and opinions to their supervisor. **Upward communication** is usually reporting and questioning. The CDM, CFPP is responsible for keeping a superior informed regarding the concerns and comments expressed by the staff.

In many facilities, upward communication is limited. Subordinates know the supervisor has the authority to fire, block promotions or salary increases, and give unpleasant assignments. So a reluctance to communicate upward is common. The supervisor must find ways to work with subordinates to maintain face-to-face communication that is free-flowing, open, honest, and respectful of differences in opinions.

Effective CDM, CFPPs help to invite this flow of communications by establishing an explicit open door policy. This policy states that: *My door is always open. Come talk to me any time about anything.* Stating this to employees helps to ease reluctance. This

---

GLOSSARY

Downward Communication
Used to convey policies, procedures, directives, objectives, and other information to subordinate personnel and follows the chain of command

Upward Communication
Used to communicate ideas, requests, and opinions to supervisors

policy can be challenging to honor, since a manager is busy. If you establish this policy and an employee asks to speak with you at an inopportune time, it is fair to say: *I really want to hear what you have to say. At the moment, there are some distractions. May we sit down together at 4:00 so that I can give you my full attention?*

If you have an open-door policy on communication, be sure to honor it. Nothing can be more disruptive to the department than to go back on your promise and violate trust.

Lateral communication among peers may involve discussions and meetings to solve problems and accomplish tasks that cross department or functional lines. This communication is critical in coordination, teamwork, and cooperation. Peers can be very effective at solving problems through discussion.

Informally, lateral communication can also involve the channel called the grapevine or the rumor mill. These exist in all organizations. The grapevine is a major communication tool in any organization, whether or not you recognize it. An effective manager keeps in touch with the grapevine, where the most uninhibited communications take place among employees. It is not realistic, or even wise, to attempt to close off the grapevine and prevent communications among employees. However, a manager should be aware that the grapevine can lead to distortion of messages, communication of rumors, and other problems.

How do you prevent problems on the grapevine? The best answer is to communicate openly with all employees. For example, if employees have reason to guess that a change is coming—such as a layoff or a major system overhaul—give them information. When you do not, they guess. Guesses become rumors. Then anxiety and ill feelings can escalate the problem. What if you don't have all the information yourself? Then, simply be honest. Tell employees what you know, what you don't know, and when you expect to know more.

Department Meetings

Having monthly department staff meetings is the norm in many facilities. The department manager holds meetings to update staff on facility and department activities, introduce new procedures, recognize the work of the department, clarify policies, gather feedback, and present ongoing training. Meetings help generate common understandings, stimulate creative problem-solving, and bring everyone onto the "same page" to promote teamwork.

Many CDM, CFPPs face time pressures in their work. It is, therefore, important to recognize that the time spent organizing, planning, and communicating in meetings can often improve productivity and effectiveness throughout the department.

When scheduling meetings, a manager may need to hold the same meeting, such as a training session, at several different times or days in order to reach all the employees. Also, staggering meetings or having them in small groups can be a good way to have a meeting without impacting all the departmental activities.

> **GLOSSARY**
>
> **Lateral Communication**
> Occurs among peers and may involve discussion and meetings to solve problems and/or accomplish tasks

Types of Meetings

The five basic types of meetings within the Dining Services department for which you may be responsible for are:

- Production meetings—daily and weekly
- Pre-meal line meetings
- Training meetings, such as an in-service
- Monthly department and goal progress meetings
- Teamwork meetings

Each of these meetings will have different guidelines, require different preparation, and will have a positive impact on the department. See Figure 15.1 for the details in conducting these meetings.

Figure 15.1
Types of Department Meetings

TYPE OF MEETING	PURPOSE	PREPARATION
Daily Production Meeting Weekly Production Meeting	• Review production, catering, and cafeteria needs	• Quick 15 minute stand-up meeting for updates • Held in kitchen • Review problems or concerns from day before • Plan for needs in coming days
Pre-Meal Line Meeting	• Review meal to be served, presentation of the meal, special needs	• Quick 15 minute stand-up meeting for updates • Held at the serving line • Discuss the display plate • Identify clients with concerns • Review problems or concerns from day/meal before
Training Meeting	• Conduct on-the-job training (OJT) and planned in-service meetings • Review sanitation and safety regulations	• 30-45 minute education meeting • Typically required attendance • May use outside trainer
Monthly Department and Goal Progress Meeting	• Review progress toward facility and department goals	• Formal 30-60 minute meeting • Review of department activities • Review of financial performance • Update on goals
Teamwork Meeting	• Develop department initiatives and performance goals • Work on interdepartmental goals	• Formal meeting • Team reports on task assignments • Progress reports • Action planning

Techniques for Effective Meetings

Planning is essential for effective meetings. The meeting leader should identify the specific purpose of the meeting, gather any necessary background information, and plan the agenda and time limit for the meeting.

When planning the meeting, determine who should attend, which specific objectives will be used, and the best approach to involve all the group members in discussion. You should:

- Select a time and day for the meeting that is most convenient for everyone.
- List the materials and equipment needed, such as audiovisuals, handouts, or equipment.
- Choose a place for the meeting that is quiet, comfortable, well lit, and big enough to accommodate all attendees.
- Notify all participants in advance.

Depending on the type of meeting, you should consult with key personnel prior to the meeting to include additional content and objectives. For instance, if the meeting is to review the progress of the department goals, you may want to meet with other interdisciplinary team leaders to collect information from them. Discuss with them how they present the organizational goals or obtain from them any training materials they use during the in-service training.

When appropriate, distribute an agenda for the meeting to each member in advance. An **agenda** is a planned outline or list and timetable for what will be discussed during a meeting. It should be reviewed verbally at the start of a meeting. A time limit should be established for each topic but this limit should not be so rigid that it cannot be adjusted. The agenda serves as an outline for the meeting and can help keep it on track. In planning an agenda, be sure to work with small, achievable objectives that can be accomplished within the established time-frame of the meeting.

If this is the first meeting of a new work group, introductions are very important. "Icebreaker" questions, such as, "What is your favorite home-cooked meal?" or "Where did you go for your last vacation?" can help introduce new members to the group. At the beginning of the meeting, clearly state the objective(s) and expected outcomes. Present all relevant information and encourage all attendees to participate actively. The leader should discuss the meeting's importance and encourage a friendly team spirit.

As the group leader, you have several responsibilities as the meeting evolves. On occasion, you can use a pre-meeting assignment to generate interest and discussion when the meeting convenes. Keep the group on track, the discussion moving forward, and include the unresponsive members of the group. You may have to actively ask for the opinions and experiences of all attendees, to ensure that one or a few of the group do not take over the discussion.

> **GLOSSARY**
>
> **Agenda**
> Planned objectives, outline, and timetable for a meeting

1. What are some techniques you would use to effectively hold a weekly production meeting?

If disagreement arises among group members, explore the reason for this and try to seek consensus from them. Clarify comments made by the attendees to ensure that their viewpoint is understood by everyone. Summarize progress and monitor that time is spent effectively and addresses the meeting objectives. If necessary, bring the group back by reviewing the problem, goals, and progress achieved.

As a group leader, you should watch the agenda as the meeting continues and take firm, polite action as required to conform to the timetable and objectives. Managing time during a meeting is easier if you state the time allotted for each part of the meeting at the beginning. For example, before discussing ideas for improving food temperatures on the trayline, you can say: *We have 10 minutes for discussion on this. What are your ideas?* About eight minutes into the discussion, you can say: *We have two more minutes for discussion about this. Is there anyone who hasn't spoken yet who would like to offer an idea?*

In a special procedure called **brainstorming**, participants are asked to list ideas for solving a problem. Explain that no idea is out of bounds, no idea is "good" or "bad," and discussion and judgment of ideas will be held until the brainstorming is completed. Even an idea that immediately proves ineffective can spark additional ideas.

During any meeting, each individual should be allowed to state his or her opinions. As a group leader, make sure that all the points made are considered fairly and openly. When establishing ground rules for a meeting, make it clear that all ideas will be respected and that each attendee should participate.

As a group leader, observe participants and look for feedback, including nonverbal communication. Identify and resolve any resistance or conflicts that may occur. If the discussion during a meeting brings out a conflict or a problem that is not part of the meeting's purpose, recognize it as important and set aside a separate time for it to be addressed. You may say: *Thank you for bringing this up. This sounds like an important issue for us to review. Since it is not related to our objectives at this meeting, we will need to set aside some time to focus on this separately. Would you please talk to me after the meeting and tell me more about it?*

Sometimes, members of a group need special attention as a meeting evolves. Figure 15.2 suggests some basic strategies that can be used in such situations.

At the end of the meeting, summarize the progress made. Identify the next actions to be taken, and see that everyone understands them. Review tasks assigned to individuals that may result from the meeting. When possible, identify the time and location of the next meeting.

Meeting Documentation

Documenting meetings is essential. The **meeting minutes**, a summary of what has been discussed and decided, provide a reference to everyone who has attended. Minutes can be used as a reference for the next meeting on an ongoing project. They should include a summary of the action plan, assignments, and deadlines, as applicable. If appropriate, a recorder should be appointed to document the meeting and include at least the following:

- Name of meeting
- Date
- Time the meeting started and ended

GLOSSARY

Brainstorming
Asking all participants to suggest ideas for solving a problem

Meeting Minutes
A summary of what was discussed and decided during a meeting

Figure 15.2
Strategies for Handling Group Problems

THE GROUP MEMBER WHO:	STRATEGY TO USE:
Wants to argue	Do not get involved. State/summarize the member's ideas and let the group decide upon their values.
Wants to help	Encourage the member to give ideas, especially when the discussion is veering off course.
Wants to discuss details	Acknowledge the member's points, but also remind the member of the meeting's objective and the time limit that has been set.
Will not stop talking	Interrupt the group member tactfully, then ask a question to bring the participant back to the topic.
Is afraid to speak	Ask the group member easy questions, recognize earlier contributions, and make the person feel important.
Wants to be recognized	Recognize the individual and ask the person for unique solutions to the problems at hand.
Is not interested	Ask the group member how the discussion will impact him/her.
Acts superior	Recognize this person's ability and ask this person the most difficult and challenging questions.
Wants to show cleverness	Identify any trick questions and give them to the group for response.

- Name of the leader and recorder
- Names of those present
- Key points and discussion topics (brief)
- Action to take
- Who is responsible to take the action and related deadlines

All participants should be provided with a copy of the minutes. Corrections, if needed, should occur at the next meeting.

In meetings conducted for training purposes, documentation is important to prove that employees have received training. This documentation may be requested by inspectors and surveyors to verify that established standards are being met. A training meeting typically includes an attendance roster and a summary of the presentation.

Effective Speaking

Each of us needs to learn more about speaking. In a business environment, we routinely speak with employees, supervisors, clients, team members, suppliers, and many others. Some spoken communications can be one-on-one and informal. Others are group presentations and may be very formal.

A number of basic tips can help with speaking, including:

- Know what you are going to say and develop a plan or outline, if needed.
- Identify the most important points of the message and organize what you are going to say around these points.
- Deliver your most important point(s) first. This is when the receiver's attention is likely to be at its peak. It also helps the receiver focus on the remainder of your message.
- Concentrate on the listener. Speak to listeners' perspectives, and notice feedback.
- Make eye contact.
- Share pride or compliments with employees when appropriate.

Figure 15.3 lists some of the traits and qualities that promote effective speaking.

In spoken communications, remember the value of silence and attention. Allow yourself to relax and listen to others. A manager who is a good listener can obtain work-related information, be more effective in interpersonal relationships, and generate information necessary to make good decisions. There are several basic principles helpful in effective listening. These are:

- Think about the central idea the speaker is trying to convey.
- Focus attention on what the speaker is saying rather than on distracting factors.
- Listen objectively to what is being said, without trying to make an immediate judgment.
- Listen for more than facts. There may be a hidden agenda or a subtle message the speaker is hesitant to convey.
- Understand the speaker's basic ideas before discussing or disagreeing.

What about situations in which spoken communication is a public presentation or a more formal event? Use presentations for a number of purposes, such as training or defending a budget or sharing information with colleagues, or asking for resources to implement a new idea.

Figure 15.3
Elements of Effective Speaking

- Confidence
- Knowledge
- Organization
- Pleasing Voice
- Concern
- Control of Emotion
- Language Command

- Friendliness
- Objectivity
- Empathy
- Open-Mindedness
- Trustworthiness
- Acceptable Appearance
- Honest

- Understanding
- Humility
- Concern for Listener
- Responsiveness
- Awareness of Situation
- Humor
- Forcefulness

- Sensitivity
- Charisma
- Concentration
- Spontaneity
- Tact
- Intelligence
- Enthusiasm

Formal Presentations

In presentations, a lecture alone can become boring. A wide variety of techniques will make them more effective. These include:

- **Demonstration.** In this mode, show people how to do something. For example, demonstrate methods for garnishing plates or taking an order for a meal.
- **Discussion.** This is a planned approach that uses group participation. For example, present basic information to a group and then permit the exchange of information through discussion.
- **Panel presentation.** With this method, the CDM, CFPP may serve as a member of a small group. Frequently, panel members make a presentation, share discussion with each other, and then open up the floor for questions and further discussion from the audience.
- **Role playing.** A technique in which participants assume the role of someone else in a defined situation and act it out. Role-playing is often effective in training because it gives participants a chance to try and practice new skills in a safe environment.
- **Case studies.** A description of a specific situation, either real or imaginary. Events are reported without explanation and attendees then use the experiences illustrated in the case as a basis for discussion.

When giving a presentation, it is natural to be nervous in front of a group. This feeling can be managed through practice and experience. Several tips are included in a Presentation Tips Page available online in the Supplemental Textbook Material.

View the Supplemental Material for this chapter to get Presentation Tips.

Meeting Follow-Up

If the meeting includes delegating staff members to accomplish a task after the meeting is over, it will be important to follow up with them before the next meeting. Depending on the task, it may be helpful to work with the staff members to develop a timeline to complete their tasks. Then, check with them to make sure they are following their timeline. The manager's role is to check progress and ensure that tasks are being completed.

Meeting follow-up also includes publishing meeting minutes. Some recommend that minutes should be distributed within 24 hours of the meeting. Correct any errors in a timely manner rather than waiting weeks to review the proceedings.

E-Mail Etiquette

Much of today's business communication occurs through email. Consider these simple rules if you communicate through email.

- It is no different than writing a letter so use a greeting, a closing, and a signature line with contact information.
- Always reread the email before you send it to make sure there are no errors and the tone of the email is friendly and professional.

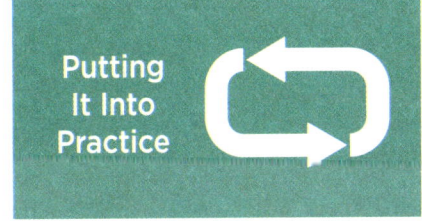

2. During your monthly in-service trainings, two employees keep interrupting and the group loses focus. How would you best handle the problem using effective strategies and verbal communication?

- Do not use emoticons and refrain from using "texting" abbreviations.
- Refrain from sending an email if you are angry; communicate in person.
- Respond in a timely manner or at least let the person know when you can respond. Timely is generally within 24 hours.

Writing a Memo

A memo is a specific type of written business communication that is used frequently. A memo is a brief document that provides a message about new information, such as a new procedure, or requests a reader to take an action, such as approving a plan or attending a meeting. To make a memo effective, direct it specifically to the reader(s), and spell out the action being requested.

A memo has five parts: a heading, an opening, a background, a brief discussion, and a summary. The heading includes these components: to, from, date, and subject. The opening should state the purpose of the memo. The background gives the context of the information or request. A simple discussion section provides more detail about the plan or request. The summary is a short statement that ties in with the opening, reminding the reader what should happen next.

External Meetings

There are at least two categories of external meetings where the manager needs to represent the department: interdepartmental meetings and professional association meetings. On an interdepartmental basis, the manager may need to hold or participate in meetings that can help ensure organization-wide problem-solving, quality management, and/or systems revision.

Interdepartmental Meetings

Interdisciplinary Care Team

In healthcare facilities, there is usually a team approach in the care of clients. The team may be composed of a Certified Dietary Manager, Certified Food Protection Professional, a Registered Dietitian Nutritionist, a Dietetic Technician, a Nurse, a Physical Therapist, an Occupational Therapist, a Speech Therapist, a Social Worker, a Clinical Pharmacist, a Physician, and/or many others. How a team is structured and the roles of each team member are governed by healthcare standards as well as the policies and practices of each facility. The role of the CDM, CFPP in Care Team Meetings is discussed in Chapter 14 of the *Nutrition Fundamentals and Medical Nutrition Therapy* textbook.

Task Forces and Committees

As a CDM, CFPP, you may be asked to represent the foodservice department on a number of facility committees and task forces led by an appointed chairperson. Meetings are regularly scheduled. In meetings such as these, attendance and minutes typically are recorded and distributed to all members. Committees and task forces are established to:

- Coordinate activities within the organization.
- Solve problems.
- Evaluate or revise systems.
- Devise plans for meeting objectives.

As a CDM, CFPP, you may be asked to serve on facility-wide committees, such as:

- **Infection Control.** This committee's usual purpose is to develop policies and procedures for sanitation techniques, isolation procedures, reporting of infectious diseases, and educating and training all personnel.
- **Safety Committee.** A typical purpose of this committee is to review all unsafe acts within the facility both for clients and others. Establishing fire safety and disaster preparedness, the implementation, Occupational Safety and Health Administration (OSHA) and other regulatory standards are also the concern of a safety committee, along with providing education and training materials to all personnel.
- **Cost Control.** The purpose of this committee may be to provide, develop, and implement cost-effectiveness procedures and plans.
- **Quality Assessment and Improvement.** The purpose of this committee is to monitor, evaluate, and document actions for the provision of quality service and products for all clients.
- **Customer/Client Service.** A committee such as this may focus on ways to improve customer/client service and satisfaction in all areas.
- **Marketing Committee.** Be involved, particularly if the facility is expanding services related to dining services.

There may be other committees to which the manager belongs. The number and types of committees vary from one facility to the next. In a committee, a group of persons work together to address and solve problems as well as perform assigned administrative activities. Committees may be temporary or permanent. They are usually appointed for ongoing activities, and may be mandated by regulatory agencies.

Task forces are usually appointed to deal with specific problems. Members of a task force analyze a problem, complete research, and make recommendations for action. Once the problem is solved, the task force is usually disbanded.

Survey and Agency Meetings

As the author and/or reviewer of the Policy and Procedure Manual, Standard Operating Procedures (SOPs), and personnel documentation, the manager has the most direct knowledge of the department. The manager is the primary contact for the accreditation surveyors, healthcare inspectors, unemployment officers, lawyers, risk management coordinators, as well as other official boards of inquiry.

The best preparation for any governmental or legal meeting is the knowledge of your own documents. When the written department guidelines comply with the regulations, or consistently document personnel actions (both positive and negative), then responding to a surveyor's question can be complete and professional.

Clinical Care Meetings

Participation in the clinical activities that many CDM, CFPPs are responsible for is addressed in Chapter 14 of the *Nutrition Fundamentals and Medical Nutrition Therapy* textbook.

Change Management

Change is anything that requires revisions in the roles and routines of a workforce. Sometimes a change is made voluntarily, as when employee groups generate ideas about performing work more effectively. At other times, change may be forced upon the department from the higher administrative levels in the facility or from external agencies, such as Centers for Medicare & Medicaid Services (CMS), or The Joint Commission (TJC), or the local health department.

Change is a continuing process and not an activity with a distinct start and finish. The facility in general and the dining services department specifically are evolving at all times. In fact, experts in organizational behavior agree that change is a sign of a healthy, successful organization. An organization that is not able to change also is not able to adapt and excel. Change can generate excitement, commitment, and pride, but it should be managed in a way that can help employees feel positively about it.

All elements in the dining services department and within the organization itself are closely related. Therefore, a change made in one area is likely to have an impact on other areas as well.

For any change to be effective, the CDM, CFPP should first show the employees the reason for the change. It is important to be honest and provide the needed facts. And whenever possible, the employees should be involved in the earliest planning phases of the change.

While dining services employees may not have the option of rejecting change, they should have the option of participating in decisions on how to implement a change. CDM, CFPPs can use participative management approaches to involve employees in planning. As employees are trained, coached, and counseled about the changes being proposed, their involvement will, ideally, reduce their resistance to the change. Typically, employee ownership and commitment will grow in direct relation to the amount of input they have into the entire process.

Examples of impending change include: mergers, new software, new dining services equipment, remodeling, menu revisions, new regulations, budget cuts, census variations, new administrative staff and/or philosophies, and evolution of professional practice.

Resistance to Change

It is human nature to be anxious and hesitant about the uncertainty of a change. The employees' resistance to change, therefore, makes it difficult for the CDM, CFPPs to implement change. The reasons for resisting change can include the following:

- **Economic concerns.** Sometimes change has a negative economic impact upon employees.
- **Inconvenience.** Some changes will require employees to learn new operating procedures or become responsible for extra duties.
- **Anxiety.** Fear of the unknown makes people feel threatened or insecure about their own work situations.
- **Changing relationships.** Some new work assignments and reporting structures can alter working relationships.
- **Increased control by others.** Some changes take away employees' independence. For example, increased supervision may be part of implementing a new procedure.

- **Low trust.** A sense of mistrust or fear of what will happen next can make change difficult, including concern that the company, supervisors, or fellow workers cannot competently manage the change.
- **Concerns about performance.** Some changes generate fear that one is no longer doing a good job. A dedicated employee may be troubled by a change and worry about his/her ability to perform the new tasks, new procedures, or work with new tools.

An organizational change, such as a move to a better office, can be well accepted simply because of its obvious advantages. But not all changes fit into this category. Where changes create ambiguity and uncertainty, then resistance to change is likely to emerge.

Changes are inevitable in every organization. Sometimes the change is a carefully planned transition from one process to another. In health care, a change is often the result of evolving regulations or decreasing reimbursements. All too often, the change is the result of a crisis or unexpected event.

If you can accept that change is a normal part of the workplace, then planning for and implementing change becomes a way of doing your job. It becomes part of the culture. Successful implementation of change leads to a willingness to try more.

Involvement of all levels of the staff early on helps develop a better plan. Too often, the changes are planned with little input by the frontline staff. Yet, they are the ones who know more about how the job is done, and how it could be done faster. Thus, you should begin with involving them in planning goals, objectives, and action plans. Early participation of frontline staff in the planning and evaluation stages of implementing change will also increase their appreciation for and acceptance of the new processes, location, or structure.

Your credibility as a manager, and in turn, your ability to implement major changes, is established through a history of open communication, honesty, and a concern for the welfare of the staff. Frequent communication of the plan, progress, and outcomes is invaluable. Also, note that fear of hidden agendas and unknown goals increases the staff's resistance to change.

Managing change along with the day-to-day workload can be challenging. As a CDM, CFPP, it is important to manage time and stress.

Time Management

CDM, CFPPs use various tools to assist with time management. A simple calendar, whether on paper or electronic, can help organize and track to-do items. When making to-do lists, the CDM, CFPPs set priorities for each item to help stay focused as interruptions or surprises occur throughout the day. As a CDM, CFPP, if you cannot accomplish everything on the list, at least focus on the most important tasks in order.

Today, access to a wide variety of computer-based tools helps with time management. Some CDM, CFPPs use email to manage a calendar, track recurring events, and manage to-do and tickler lists. To track commitments further in the future and follow up on action items, and/or the time-related responsibilities of others who report to you, also use a tickler list. A tickler list is designed to "jog" your memory about selected items or tasks. Figure 15.4 illustrates a tickler list. Smartphones provide excellent tools with the additional advantage of portability. Setting reminders and repetitions on your mobile calendar or desktop calendar also helps you stay organized and ensures completion of tasks.

The calendar may also issue an audible alarm or reminder for an upcoming deadline or appointment. In some facilities, a project management software application is used throughout the facility to help track and coordinate work. Through email and voice mail, messages and instructions can be quickly passed and acknowledged.

Stress Management

Stress is a condition that arises from physical or mental strain, anxiety, and overwork. It is familiar not only to CDM, CFPPs, but to most employees in the workplace. The demands and schedules of the job can be strenuous. Client interactions can be satisfying but draining. Along with work-related stress, you may experience stress from factors outside the workplace. Stress is a natural experience and it is not unique to CDM, CFPPs. A few ideas can help manage stress in the everyday work life:

- Take breaks. Physical breaks, emotional breaks, and mental breaks are all important. Examples include: talking a walk, stopping to enjoy a joke, or switching tasks for a while. Each of these helps to restore energy.
- Accept what you cannot change. It takes a lot of emotional energy to worry about things you cannot control, or feeling angry about something you cannot influence.
- Use relaxation exercises. Physical and mental relaxation exercises can help loosen tense muscles or release negative thoughts.

Focus on one task at a time to concentrate your energy. Thinking about other tasks at the same time only creates more stress.

- Focus on the positive results of your efforts. In addition to hard work and job-related pressure, you can usually see results and satisfaction in the outcomes. Good food and satisfied clients help balance out the stress.
- Be realistic. Setting goals and expectations that are out of reach is very stressful. Refer to S.M.A.R.T. goals discussed in Chapter 14.
- Keep a positive outlook. A healthy perspective is one in which you remember the big picture and focus on the things that can be accomplished. Keep the details in mind but do not get caught in the fine print.
- Seek help when needed. Request assistance and tap into available resources when the tasks call for it. If stress is taking a greater toll, do not hesitate to seek professional help.

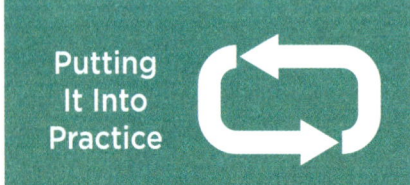

3. Your hospital is being bought by a big consortium of hospitals. This may lead to changes in the department. How would you communicate this to your staff?

Figure 15.4
Tickler List

March 1	• Quality Improvement Plan due
	• Employee Recognition Dinner
April 10	• Quarterly QA Reports due
	• Annual P&P Updates due
April 20	• Quarter 1 Financial Variance Report due

Summary

Effective communication is invaluable in the workplace. It is best to use the tools of communication, participation, and negotiation to help employees accept change. If necessary, a manager may use his or her authority as a tool in implementing change. It is helpful to involve both formal and informal employee groups and their leaders in the change process. Training programs are often necessary as changes are implemented. To help overcome resistance, employees need an opportunity to learn new procedures and gain confidence.

Commitment of senior leadership, visible support by administration, and celebration of successes all start at the top. Senior leadership can encourage the cooperation of multiple departments to ensure participation, which in turn, will improve the likelihood of success.

After change has been implemented, it must be evaluated. It is important to see whether the change has been beneficial and whether any additional changes are needed to further improve the effectiveness of the dining services department. The CDM, CFPP should also assess whether there has been any unexpected spin-off effects of the change.

Chapter References

RESOURCES	
Effective Communication in the Workplace	https://www.tdcj.texas.gov/divisions/cjad/presentations/Effective_Communication_in_the_Workplace.pdf
Gregoire, Mary (2013). Foodservice Organizations, A managerial and systems approach, 8th ed. Upper Saddle River, NJ: Pearson Prentice Hall	
International Association of Business Communication	https://www.iabc.com/
How to Run Effective Business Meetings	https://www.thebalancecareers.com/effective-meetings-produce-results-before-the-meeting-1918729
Ventura, Steve and Templin, Michelle (2005). Five Star Teamwork-How to Achieve Success Together	

Professional Development and Ethics

Overview and Objectives

As a professional, the manager has many responsibilities. One of these is managing professional development and growth through self-assessment and lifelong learning. Another is the responsibility to act ethically. After completing this chapter, you should be able to:

- Understand the importance of continued competence for professional development
- Discover resources for lifelong learning
- Learn the importance of professional ethics for a Certified Dietary Manager®, Certified Food Protection Professional® (CDM®, CFPP®)

Professional Development

A CDM, CFPP is a professional. A CDM, CFPP has passed a nationally-recognized exam and is recognized as having the training and experience to perform the responsibilities outlined in the CDM, CFPP Scope of Practice. See the Supplemental Material for the CDM, CFPP Scope of Practice. Continuing education (CE) is required to maintain credentialed status. Completion of continuing education helps a CDM, CFPP stay at the forefront of evolving changes in the nutrition and foodservice industries.

Generally, continuing education is required to some degree, especially in health care. However, there is a growing shift from continuing education to continued competence. **Continued competence** embraces a more comprehensive view that each individual is responsible for their own professional development and demonstrates application of knowledge and skill. This view creates a need for a CDM, CFPP to self-reflect on their professional development needs and choose education to meet those needs.

Completing a gap analysis is a great tool to assess yourself. ANFP has created a tool based on the CDM, CFPP competencies. For further details on how this tool can be used, see the Supplemental Material for this chapter.

Lifelong Learning

It is not uncommon for a CDM, CFPP to pursue additional training at some point during a career to develop new skills. The following could be considered:

- One may choose to go to culinary school.
- Another may choose to obtain an associate's or bachelor's degree.
- Another may pursue a degree in business management.
- Yet another may seek additional credentials.

When planning your own development, give some thought to both short-term and long-range goals. In the short term, learn more about standards, or labor unions, or another specific topic. Use results-oriented objectives for something you need to do or will need to do soon, and work backward to identify resources for training or acquiring training.

Resources for development may come from a professional association, in-house training department, community resources, local schools, business seminars, the Internet, and self-study courses. An online or advanced study course is one way a CDM, CFPP can pursue additional education while still holding down a full-time job with variable hours. Along with formal classroom training, develop knowledge through getting industry updates online, food books, trade magazines, and websites.

Professional Association Meetings

What could be next for the CDM, CFPP? Consider joining one or more professional associations of like professionals. This will allow growth, both professionally and personally. The following are some examples of the benefits of membership:

- **Networking opportunities.** Networking, or interacting with others in the profession, can be an excellent source of support, resources, ideas, and friendship. By networking with others, you usually discover that management challenges are not unique and that colleagues can help each other advance the practice of foodservice management. Some professional associations, such as Association of Nutrition & Foodservice Professionals (ANFP), offer web-based discussion areas or chat rooms,

---

GLOSSARY

Continued Competence
Embraces a more comprehensive view that each individual is responsible for their own professional development and demonstrates application of knowledge and skill

Professional Ethics
Professionally accepted standards of personal and business behavior, values, and guiding principles

View the Supplemental Material for this chapter to see the CDM, CFPP Scope of Practice and the CBDM Gap Analysis Tool.

where members can meet with others from diverse locations to discuss professional issues. These associations may also offer local meetings to become involved in.

- **Educational opportunities.** Professional associations are one of the best resources for educational sessions, meetings, and materials that help develop skills and continue professional growth.
- **Research.** A professional association typically conducts research on matters of interest to its members, such as salaries, benchmarking, professional practices, and other issues. This research is shared with members.
- **Publications.** A professional association issues publications that address the unique needs and interests of its members.
- **Employment services.** Many professional associations operate job boards on the Internet. Here, find information about employment opportunities that relate to your qualifications.
- **Contact with suppliers.** Through trade events and vendor relationships, professional associations become a conduit for information about suppliers and vendors.
- **Legislative activity.** A professional association may lobby for the interests of its members in state and regional governments, supporting legislation that supports the interests of the profession and the industry.

Professional Ethics

The CDM, CFPP is often challenged ethically working in an institutional environment. The concept of ethics refers to views, attitudes, and practices about what is right or wrong. It describes moral standards. **Professional ethics** take into account many basic values such as integrity, honesty, fairness, responsibility, and trust. The foodservice operation traditionally maintains high standards that are reflected in current policies and procedures. These policies help maintain the integrity of the operation and its customers. A healthcare facility presents an even greater challenge in the area of ethics because it is a highly regulated environment that puts patient safety, care, and privacy above everything. Violating HIPAA regulations, for example, would put patient privacy at risk which can be costly not only to the organization, but can also lead to job loss and possibly professional consequences that could follow a manager for years to come.

View the Supplemental Material for this chapter to see articles on professional ethics from Nutrition & Foodservice Edge magazine.

The Certifying Board for Dietary Managers® (CBDM®) which is the credentialing agency for the Association of Nutrition & Foodservice Professionals (ANFP), has a formal policy: the CDM, CFPP Code of Ethics. It is important for the CDM, CFPP to understand and comply with the 18 principles listed in Figure 16.1, which outlines the Code of Ethics. This is a serious matter as any misconduct that clearly indicates incompetence, unethical behavior, and physical or mental impairment affecting the performance of the CDM, CFPP may result in disciplinary action, up to and including revocation of certification.

1. You are required to manage petty cash in your department. You need money for personal use one day, so you decide to take from the petty cash with the intent of paying it back shortly. Is this ethical? Discuss your answer.

Figure 16.1
Principles Guiding the Code of Ethics for the CDM, CFPP

1. The Certified Dietary Manager, Certified Food Protection Professional provides professional services with objectivity and with respect for the unique needs and values of individuals.
2. The Certified Dietary Manager, Certified Food Protection Professional avoids discrimination against other individuals on the basis of race, creed, religion, sex, age, national origin, and complies with EEOC & ADA requirements and the Rehabilitation Act of 1973.
3. The Certified Dietary Manager, Certified Food Protection Professional fulfills professional commitments in good faith.
4. The Certified Dietary Manager, Certified Food Protection Professional conducts himself/herself with honesty, integrity, and fairness.
5. The Certified Dietary Manager, Certified Food Protection Professional endeavors to act impartially in all decisions while fulfilling professional duties and agrees to disclose any existing or potential conflicts of interest.
6. The Certified Dietary Manager, Certified Food Protection Professional practices dietary management based on professional principles.
7. The Certified Dietary Manager, Certified Food Protection Professional assumes responsibility and accountability for personal and professional competence in practice.
8. The Certified Dietary Manager, Certified Food Protection Professional maintains confidentiality of all protected information and adheres to privacy and security rules of the Health Insurance Portability and Accountability Act of 1996 (HIPAA) and all other federal, state, and local requirements.
9. The Certified Dietary Manager, Certified Food Protection Professional exercises professional judgment within the limits of his/her qualifications and seeks counsel or makes referrals as appropriate.
10. The Certified Dietary Manager, Certified Food Protection Professional provides sufficient information to enable clients to make their own informed decisions.
11. The Certified Dietary Manager, Certified Food Protection Professional promotes or endorses products in a manner that is neither false nor misleading.
12. The Certified Dietary Manager, Certified Food Protection Professional permits use of his/her name for the purpose of certifying that dietary services have been rendered only if he/she has provided or supervised the provision of those services.
13. The Certified Dietary Manager, Certified Food Protection Professional accurately presents professional qualifications and credentials.
    a. The Certified Dietary Manager, Certified Food Protection Professional uses "CDM and CFPP" or Certified Dietary Manager and Certified Food Protection Professional only when certification is current and authorized by the Certifying Board for Dietary Managers.
    b. The Certified Dietary Manager, Certified Food Protection Professional complies with all requirements of the Certifying Board's certification program in which he/she is seeking initial or continued credentials from the Certifying Board for Dietary Managers.
    c. The Certified Dietary Manager, Certified Food Protection Professional is subject to disciplinary action for aiding another person in violating any Certifying Board certification requirements or aiding another person in representing himself/herself as a Certified Dietary Manager when he/she is not.
14. The Certified Dietary Manager, Certified Food Protection Professional presents substantiated information and interprets controversial information without personal bias, recognizing that legitimate differences of opinion exist.
15. The Certified Dietary Manager, Certified Food Protection Professional provides objective evaluation of candidates for professional association memberships, awards, scholarships, or job advancement.
16. The Certified Dietary Manager, Certified Food Protection Professional voluntarily withdraws from the professional practice if personal circumstances could negatively affect or harm the client or organization that serves the client.
17. The Certified Dietary Manager, Certified Food Protection Professional complies with all applicable laws and regulations concerning the profession. The Certified Dietary Manager, Certified Food Protection Professional is subject to disciplinary action under the following circumstances:
    a. The Certified Dietary Manager, Certified Food Protection Professional has been disciplined by a state chapter and at least one of the grounds for discipline is the same or substantially equivalent to these principles contained herein.
    b. The Certified Dietary Manager, Certified Food Protection Professional has committed an act of misfeasance or malfeasance which is directly related to the practice of the profession as determined by a court of competent jurisdiction, a licensing board, or any agency or a governmental body.
18. The Certified Dietary Manager, Certified Food Protection Professional accepts the obligation to protect society and the profession by upholding the Code of Ethics for the profession of Dietary Management and by reporting alleged violations of the Code through the review of the Certifying Board for Dietary Managers.

Source: The Certifying Board for Dietary Managers (CBDM)

Before understanding the principles guiding the Code of Ethics, it is important to know why a Code of Ethics is important for the CDM, CFPP. The Certifying Board for Dietary Managers believes it is in the best interests of the profession and the public it serves that a Code of Ethics provide guidance to CDM, CFPPs in their professional practice and conduct. This code reflects the ethical principles guiding the CDM, CFPP and outlines commitments and obligations of the manager to self, client, public, and the profession. It assists in the effective management of foodservice operations, safety and welfare of the public by establishing and enforcing qualifications for Dietary Manager certification and for issuing voluntary credentials to individuals who have attained those qualifications. The Certifying Board has adopted this Code to apply to individuals who hold these credentials.

Living in a diverse environment, every foodservice employee should operate without any bias or prejudice. The first two principles ensure that the CDM, CFPP is engaged in the task of providing services for every customer in the organization, regardless of their ethnicity, race, age, or gender. Additionally, a typical CDM, CFPP is responsible for financial management including cash and inventory. Ethics here would imply honesty in daily transactions and cash handling. Additional obligations include working effectively with vendors, patients/residents, and employees who all have protected rights. Many of the decisions a leader faces come down to doing the right thing.

Some ethical issues are straightforward, but from time to time ethical choices as a professional may be less clear. For example, ethical practices in purchasing usually prohibit accepting gifts from a supplier or potential supplier. Now, what happens when you attend a food show and are invited to register for a free drawing? Are you accepting a gift? Are you violating sound ethical practices?

Another example is a policy about client confidentiality that specifies you should not disclose information about clients to others (family, friends, co-workers, etc.) who are not directly involved in their clinical care. A diet aide delivers a tray to the room of a beloved resident. The resident shares some personal information about herself. The diet aide is concerned and addresses the issue in the elevator to the CDM, CFPP while there are other people in the elevator, thus compromising HIPAA or patient confidentiality. So, while intentions may be good, it is important to realize that the principle precedes the intent.

When faced with an ethical dilemma, what should you do? A few steps can help reach a resolution. First, check the codes of ethics for the professional association(s) and the facility. Next, talk the situation over with peers and colleagues. Ask whether they have faced a similar dilemma. If so, ask how they considered the issue and what resolution they reached. Of course, think about the situation from your own perspective. What feels right—and why?

Figure 16.2 shows an ethical decision-making model. This model can be used to examine the ethical issue to aid in the decision-making. Also discuss a job-related ethical dilemma with your supervisor. When making a difficult decision, your supervisor may draw from additional experiences and be able to assist you. In addition, they should be alerted to the issues and concerns, so there will be no surprises or questions down the line. Enlisting approval and support ahead of time protects you, your supervisor, and the facility.

Figure 16.2
Visual of the Ethical Decision Making Model

- Identify the Ethical Problem
- Collect Information
- State the Options
- Apply Ethical Principles to the Options
- Make the Decision
- Implement the Decision

Summary

As a CDM, CFPP, remember you are a professional. It is important to reflect on your professional needs and growth throughout your career.

Acting ethically is an integral part of having the CDM, CFPP credential behind your name. Understanding the CDM, CFPP Code of Ethics and knowing steps to make ethical decisions will help guide you through ethical issues you may face.

Chapter References

RESOURCES	
Academy of Nutrition and Dietetics Code of Ethics	eatrightpro.org/resources/career/code-of-ethics
The Certifying Board for Dietary Managers (CBDM) Code of Ethics	https://www.cbdmonline.org/docs/default-source/legacy-docs/docs/codeethics.pdf

Safe Food Handling: Personnel

Overview and Objectives

Ensuring safety in a foodservice operation is the responsibility of the manager of that operation. This includes the safety of employees and clients of that operation and the safety of the food served. In this chapter, we examine the role of the Certified Dietary Manager®, Certified Food Protection Professional® (CDM®, CFPP®) in risk management, thus ensuring safety in the use of equipment and work flow. After completing this chapter, you should be able to:

- Instruct employees in safety and sanitation
- Enforce employee compliance with safety and sanitation regulations
- Understand the Food Code and federal safety laws/regulations
- Write cleaning procedures for utensils, equipment, and work areas
- Evaluate equipment in terms of maintenance needs and costs
- Interpret safety data sheets
- Inspect all areas of department for sanitary conditions

The Food Code

The U.S. Food and Drug Administration (FDA) publishes the Food Code, a model that assists with food safety at all levels of government. It provides a scientifically sound technical and legal basis for regulating the retail and foodservice segment of the industry such as restaurants, and grocery stores, and institutions such as nursing homes. Local, state, and federal regulators use the FDA Food Code as a model to develop or update their own food safety rules and to be consistent with national food regulatory policy.

Chapter 2 of the 2017 Food Code focuses on employee health and safety. It defines a **permit holder** in an operation and the responsibilities of a **person in charge** who should demonstrate to the regulatory authority during inspection, knowledge of foodborne disease prevention, application of HACCP principles, and the requirements of the Food Code. Additionally, the person in charge must also demonstrate knowledge in:

- Personal Hygiene and its impact on food safety
- Symptoms of foodborne illness
- Time/Temperature Control for Safety (TCS) Food, formerly known as Potentially Hazardous Foods (PHF)
- The hazards of consuming undercooked meat, poultry, eggs, and fish
- Temperatures for hot holding, storing, cooling, and reheating TCS food
- Prevention of cross-contamination
- Standards for avoiding bare hand contact with food
- Adequate and effective handwashing
- Cleaning and sanitation
- Food-safe equipment
- Safe water
- Safe use of chemicals
- Employee health restrictions/exclusions
- Food allergy awareness
- Proper training of employees in food safety, including food allergy awareness.

The designated person in charge works with the staff and administration to develop policies and procedures for carrying out these duties.

Personal Hygiene for All Employees

All foodservice employees must observe personal hygiene practices to reduce the likelihood of contaminating the food. They must also observe safe work practices. It is the responsibility of the CDM, CFPP to develop and implement policies on hygiene and the responsibility of every foodservice employee to observe the standards of personal hygiene to ensure food safety.

Personal hygiene and handwashing are critical controls for food safety. Many foodborne illnesses travel from people to food and then to clients, who may then become ill. Employees should observe the following standards for personal hygiene:

- Bathe daily.
- Cover mouth when coughing or sneezing; wash hands after.

GLOSSARY

Permit Holder
The entity that is legally responsible for the operation of the food facility such as the hospital, nursing facility, school district, or restaurant owner

Person in Charge
The manager of the dining services operation who is responsible for developing, carrying out, and enforcing procedures aimed at preventing foodborne illness

- Do not eat, drink, or use tobacco or chew gum while preparing food. Do these only on breaks and wash hands after.
- Restrain and cover hair.
- Frequently wash hands following established procedures.

Handwashing and Hand Care

Preparing and serving foods with hands is a common way of transferring pathogens and other food hazards from people to food. Handwashing, therefore, is the most important step that all dining services employees can take to protect food. All employees should be trained in proper handwashing procedures. To reinforce this important practice, post reminder signs at every handwashing sink employees use. The most effective way to determine the employee compliance with handwashing standards is to observe their on-the-job practices. Hands must be kept clean before, during, and after preparing foods. According to the Food and Drug Administration (FDA) Food Code, hands should be washed:

- After touching bare human body parts.
- After using the restroom.
- After coughing, sneezing, using a tissue, using tobacco, eating, or drinking.
- After handling soiled equipment or utensils.
- Before food preparation.
- During food preparation, as often as necessary to remove soil and avoid cross-contamination.
- When switching between raw foods and ready-to-eat foods.
- After engaging in any activity that might contaminate hands.

Dining services personnel must clean their hands, wrists, forearms, and other exposed parts of their body with a cleaning compound (antibacterial soap is recommended).

As shown in Figure 17.1, proper handwashing requires the application of the cleaning compound and then vigorously rubbing the hands for at least 10-15 seconds, followed by a rinse with potable water.

Ensuring the cleanliness of areas underneath the fingernails and in between fingers is particularly important. A nail brush may be used to clean under fingernails, particularly after handling raw food, parts of which may be trapped under the fingernails, or after using the restroom. Recommendations about whether to use nail brushes vary. If used, they must be sanitized on a regular basis.

Dining services staff must keep their fingernails trimmed, filed, and maintained so the edges and surfaces are smooth and cleanable. Fingernail polish or artificial nails are not allowed for employees working with food unless the nails are covered by a sanitary, disposable glove in good condition.

Personnel must be provided with a sink specifically intended for washing hands. It is not acceptable for the staff to wash their hands in sinks intended for food preparation or for them to complete the food preparation activities in hand sinks. At least one sink must be designated for handwashing and more may be required to ensure their convenient use by employees. These handwashing sinks should be easily accessible to employees. They should be available in food preparation, dining services, and warewashing areas, as well as in restrooms. A handwashing sink in the lavatory must provide water at a temperature of at least 100°F through a mixing valve or faucet. Some models of hand sinks are equipped with infrared sensors or flow control devices, eliminating the need for the staff to touch the sink faucets The lavatory must be supplied with a hand cleanser and materials for hand drying such as individual, disposable towels, a heated-air drying device, or a non-heated pressurized air device. When food exposure is limited and handwashing lavatories are not conveniently available—such as in some mobile or temporary food operations or at some vending machine locations—employees may use chemically treated towelettes for handwashing. Remember, though, that towelettes are not as effective as handwashing and are not accepted by all local food codes.

Hand antiseptics (previously called hand sanitizers) are permitted for use at the food and dining services, according to the FDA Food Code. A hand antiseptic solution should be either approved by the FDA or contain antimicrobial ingredients listed by the FDA. A hand antiseptic may be used only after an employee has washed his or her hands, following established procedure. In other words, *using a hand antiseptic is not a substitute for washing hands*. It is only a supplementary option.

Jewelry

Dining services staff should limit hand and arm jewelry to one single band ring since these can trap the microorganisms, making it difficult to keep clean.

The Food Code clarifies the use of medical alert jewelry, such as a band indicating a drug allergy or medical condition. Medical information jewelry is not an exception to the "no-jewelry" guideline. It is not permitted on hands or arms. The Food Code guidance explains that an employee can wear an alert bracelet as a necklace or on the ankle.

Disposable Glove Usage

The use of disposable gloves/single-use gloves in dining services operations is increasingly common. It is important to note that wearing gloves is not a substitute for appropriate, effective, thorough and frequent handwashing. Single-use gloves should be stored and dispensed in a manner that prevents contamination. Gloves should be intact and free of tears or other imperfections. Before putting on a pair of gloves, wash

Figure 17.1
Handwashing Procedures

1. Rinse under clean, running warm water.
2. Apply an amount of cleaning compound recommended by the cleaning compound manufacturer.
3. Rub together vigorously for at least 10-15 seconds while:
    a. Paying particular attention to removing soil from underneath the fingernails during the cleaning procedure.
    b. Creating friction on the surfaces of the hands and arms or surrogate prosthetic devices for hands and arms, fingertips, and areas between the fingers.
4. If using antimicrobial soap, 15 seconds of vigorous washing is required.
5. Thoroughly rinse under clean, running warm water.

NOTE: To avoid recontaminating their hands, food employees may use disposable clean towels or similar clean barriers when touching surfaces such as manually operated handles or restroom door handles.

Adapted from 2017 FDA Food Code, sections 2-301.12 to 2-301.16 your hands, following the established procedure. Replace gloves at least hourly when changing food preparation tasks; after sneezing, coughing; or touching hair, face, or non-disinfected surfaces. Skin lesions, cuts on the hands, wrists, or exposed portions of the arm must be covered with an impermeable cover such as a finger cot or stall. If the lesions are on the hands or wrists, a disposable glove should be worn over the impermeable cover.

Clothing

Dining services employees should always wear clean clothing to prevent contamination of food, equipment, utensils, and linens. If employees are expected to change into a uniform after reporting to work, you need to provide a suitable changing area separate from food preparation and storage areas. Employees should not bring personal items such as coats, hats, and purses into food preparation areas.

To further minimize the risk of foodborne illness transmission from employees or employee work habits, protective clothing should be worn to keep the body parts from being in contact with the exposed foods. Hair restraints and beard restraints should be worn to reduce contact with human hair. Aprons and disposable gloves are also used to reduce the transfer of microorganisms to an exposed food. Aprons and disposable gloves should be changed frequently.

Avoid Hand Contact With Food

In addition to handwashing, the risk of foodborne illness can be reduced by eliminating direct contact of hands with ready-to-eat food. Except when washing fruits and vegetables, dining services employees should not touch exposed, ready-to-eat food with their bare hands. Instead, they should use suitable utensils such as deli tissue, spatulas, tongs, single-use gloves, or dispensing equipment. Dining services personnel should also minimize bare hand and arm contact with exposed food that is not in a ready-to-eat form.

Tasting Food

Dining services personnel should be trained in proper tasting techniques. To prevent contamination, employees should not taste food while standing over it. A dining services employee may not use a utensil more than once to taste food that is to be sold or served. A utensil used to taste food cannot be returned to the pot. It is a good idea to have a container of tasting spoons/forks close to the food preparation area to avoid using the preparation utensil for tasting.

Handling Sanitary Surfaces

Employees should avoid touching the eating ends of the utensils, the tops or insides of drinking glasses, the surfaces of plates, or any other utensil or serviceware in a manner that might allow their hands to contaminate the item.

1. The employee on the trayline has come to work with a long gold necklace and hoop earrings. You notice that she goes to the bathroom with her gloves on and comes out with them still on her hands. Is this a safety concern? How would you resolve these issues?

Employee Health

Proper management of a food establishment operation begins with employing healthy people and instituting a system of identifying employees who present a risk of transmitting foodborne pathogens to food or to other employees. The person in charge is responsible for ensuring all food employees and conditional employees are knowledgeable and understand their responsibility to report listed symptoms, diagnosis with an illness from a listed pathogen, or exposure to a listed pathogen to the person in charge. The person in charge is also responsible for reporting to the regulatory official if a food employee reports a diagnosis with a listed pathogen. This reporting requirement is an important component of any food safety program. A food employee who suffers from any of the illnesses or medical symptoms or has a history of exposure to a listed pathogen in this Code may transmit disease through the food being prepared. The person in charge must first be aware that a food employee or conditional employee is suffering from a disease or symptom listed in the Code before steps can be taken to reduce the chance of foodborne illness. See Figure 17.2 for a decision tree of when to restrict an employee who reports a listed exposure under the Food Code.

A conditional employee is a potential food employee to whom a job offer has been made, conditional on responses to subsequent medical questions or examinations. The questions or examinations are designed to identify potential food employees who may be suffering from a disease that can be transmitted through food and done in compliance with Title 1 of the Americans with Disabilities Act of 1990. A conditional employee becomes a food employee as soon as the employee begins working, even if only on a restricted basis. When a conditional employee reports a listed diagnosis or symptom, the person in charge is responsible for ensuring that the conditional employee is prohibited from becoming a food employee until the criteria for reinstatement of an exclusion are met (as specified under section 2-201.13 of the Food Code). When a symptomatic or diagnosed conditional employee has met the same criteria for reinstatement that apply to an excluded symptomatic or diagnosed food employee (as specified under section 2-201.13 of the Food Code), the conditional employee may then begin working as a food employee.

Reportable Health Information

The Food Code lists a number of health conditions that food employees must report to the person in charge. Each employee has the responsibility for reporting any information that may have an impact on food safety. The FDA Food Code draws special attention to six pathogens that may be transmitted by dining services employees: Norovirus, Shigella, hepatitis A, Salmonella Typhi, nontyphoidal Salmonella, and Shiga toxin-producing E. coli (STEC). An employee diagnosed with any of these illnesses must report this to the person in charge who is responsible for taking action to prevent any disease transmission.

In addition, the Food Code indicates that even if employees have only symptoms—such as diarrhea, fever, vomiting, jaundice (yellowing of the skin, which can be a symptom of hepatitis), sore throat with fever, or an infected wound that is open, draining, and/or contains pus—this is cause for action. Each of these may potentially indicate that a foodborne pathogen is present. Thus, each of these must be reported to the person in charge. **Exclude** simply means to prohibit employees from coming to work. A medical clearance is required for the employee to return to work. Also, note that if an employee is actually diagnosed with a foodborne illness, he or she should be excluded from work and the health department must be notified. Guidelines offered

---

GLOSSARY

Exclude
Prohibit employees from coming to work

Figure 17.2
When to Restrict a Food Employee Who Reports a Listed Exposure Under the Food Code

KEY
STEC = Shiga toxin-producing Escherichia coli
HSP = Highly Susceptible Population
NTS = Nontyphoidal Salmonella

Source: 2017 FDA Food Code

by the Food Code may be considered minimum standards, based on commonly-cited culprits in actual foodborne illness outbreaks. Local authorities and/or the facility's health policy may dictate further restrictions.

If the employee has an infected wound, the employee can come to work but must cover the wound with an impermeable cover.

Guidelines for responding to symptoms or illness are more liberal if serving a general, healthy population. Rather than exclude employees, restrict employees who have Norovirus with no symptoms, Shiga toxin-producing Escherichia coli (STEC) with no symptoms, or sore throat with fever, for example. **Restrict** means to limit an employee's activities, so that there is no risk of transmitting any foodborne illness. For example, a restricted employee should not work with food or clean equipment, dishes, utensils, or linens. An infected cut or wound must be bandaged and covered with an impermeable

GLOSSARY

Restrict
To limit an employee's activities so there is no risk of transmitting foodborne illness (such as reassign the employee to a non-food related position)

cover. If the wound is on the hand or wrist, this must also be covered with a clean, disposable glove.

The Food Code also addresses the question of an employee who suffers sneezing, coughing, or a runny nose. Any employee who has a discharge from eyes, nose, or mouth should not work with exposed food, clean equipment, utensils, or linens; they also should not unwrap single serve items. This means that if an employee has a common cold, the manager may need to restrict the employee from work.

In addition to employee wellness and contact with food products is the management of the work environment. Maintaining a safe workplace and equipment as well as managing risk is a daily activity.

The Food Code requires that both conditional and regular food employees acknowledge, in writing, their responsibility for reporting certain symptoms, diagnoses, and health conditions to the CDM, CFPP. Employees must also acknowledge their responsibility to comply with restriction or exclusion, when applicable. At the same time, the person in charge must acknowledge in writing, the responsibilities outlined in the Food Code for managing employee health. This means, that when the facility offers a dining services job to someone, they should ask that person to sign a reporting agreement. The FDA provides a sample form (see Figure 17.3). In addition, the Food Code stipulates that a dining services operation must have a written employee health policy. The policy must address, at a minimum, how the operation complies with the rules for reporting illness/symptoms and managing restrictions or exclusion.

Risk Management

In a food production and dining services environment, risks confront both management and employees. Managing them can lead to lower employee injury rates and higher productivity. **Risks** are the possibility of injury. **Risk management**, therefore, is the practice of managing the possibility of injury to employees and clients or harm to the organization.

A food production department presents many risks. There are open flames, steam-releasing machines, sharp knives, hot liquids, wet or slippery floors, and heavy objects. Employees often move fairly quickly in an effort to meet deadlines. An accident, then, can result in harm to an employee or client. It can damage morale and image. It can also generate lost work days, and other costs to a facility. The U.S. Bureau of Labor Statistics reports that industries with high rates of employee injuries are food service, hospitals, and nursing homes.

What causes accidents? Initially, there is the presence of a risk, or situation that is potentially dangerous. Accidents happen when someone is not paying attention. Examples of safety risks appear in Figure 17.6. As you can see from these examples, a risk sets the stage for an accident to occur. For example, a sharp knife sitting in a sink full of soapy water is an invitation for an employee to reach his or her hand in and get

GLOSSARY

Risk
The likelihood of a potential dangerous situation

Risk Management
Managing the possibility of dangerous situations to employees, clients, or the organization

---

Putting It Into Practice

2. An employee has diarrhea as a result of Crohn's disease which cannot be transmitted. Would you put any exclusions to work? What would you emphasize? Review Table 17.3. What questions would you ask and what would you avoid asking?

Figure 17.3
Table 4 Summary of Requirements for Symptomatic Food Employees

SYMPTOM	EXCLUSION OR RESTRICTION		Removing Symptomatic Food Employees from Exclusion or Restriction	RA Approval Needed to Return to Work?
	Facilities Serving an HSP	Facilities Not Serving an HSP		
Vomiting	EXCLUDE 2-201.12(A)(1)	EXCLUDE 2-201.12(A)(1)	When the excluded food employee has been asymptomatic for at least 24 hours or provides medical documentation 2-201.13(A)(1). *Exceptions:* If diagnosed with Norovirus, Shigella spp., E. coli O157:H7 or other EHEC/STEC, HAV, or typhoid fever (S. Typhi) (see Tables 1b & 2).	No, if not diagnosed
Diarrhea	EXCLUDE 2-201.12(A)(1)	EXCLUDE 2-201.12(A)(1)	When the excluded food employee has been asymptomatic for at least 24 hours or provides medical documentation 2-201.13(A). *Exceptions:* If Diagnosed with Norovirus, E. coli O157:H7 or other EHEC/STEC, HAV, or S. Typhi (see Tables 1b & 2).	No, if not diagnosed
Jaundice	EXCLUDE 2-201.12(B)(1) if the onset occurred within the last 7 days	EXCLUDE 2-201.12(B)(1) if the onset occurred within the last 7 days	When approval is obtained from the RA 2-201.13 (B), and: • Food employee has been jaundiced for more than 7 calendar days 2-201.13(B)(1), OR • Food employee provides medical documentation 2-201.13(B)(3).	Yes
Sore Throat with Fever	EXCLUDE 2-201.12(G)(1)	RESTRICT 2-201.12(G)(2)	When food employee provides written medical documentation 201.13(G) (1)-(3).	No
Infected Wound or Pustular Boil	RESTRICT 2-201.12(H)	RESTRICT 2-201.12(H)	When the infected wound or boil is properly covered 2-201.13(H)(1)-(3).	No

NOTES:
- Food employees and conditional employees shall report symptoms immediately to the person in charge.
- The person in charge shall prohibit a conditional employee who reports a listed symptom from becoming a food employee until meeting the criteria listed in section 2-201.13 of the Food Code, for reinstatement of a symptomatic food employee.

Key for Tables 1, 2, 3, and 4:

RA = Regulatory Authority

EHEC/STEC = Enterohemorrhagic, or Shiga toxin-producing Escherichia coli

HAV = Hepatitis A virus

HSP = Highly Susceptible Population

Source: FDA 2017 Food Code 2-201.12 Table 4: History of Exposure, and Absent Symptoms or Diagnosis Page 442

cut. Water accumulating on the floor raises the likelihood that someone walking there will fall.

Safety and Safety Inspections

Risks are situations a CDM, CFPP can identify and correct through routine inspection. The most important thing to do is simply note the risk and then take action. A tool for accomplishing this is a safety inspection checklist. Figure 17.5 shows an example of a safety inspection checklist, which can help organize the foodservice operation when examining it for risks. A structured inspection process is one that has

Figure 17.4
ADA and Employee Health

The Americans With Disabilities Act (ADA) regulations protect persons with disabilities. They prohibit discrimination in employment decisions. They also stipulate that an employer must make reasonable accommodations for an employee with a disability. As defined by the law, a disability is a medical condition or disorder that substantially limits a person in doing basic life activities. According to the Equal Employment Opportunity Commission (EEOC) guidance, an employee who has the key symptoms that could indicate foodborne illness is NOT disabled. Because a foodborne illness is generally a short-term condition, the ADA regulations do not apply. In other words, a manager can restrict or exclude an employee, following Food Code guidelines.

However, a foodborne illness occasionally leads to long-term disability, such as chronic liver failure following a Hepatitis A disease. If this occurs, the ADA regulations do apply. In this case, you must follow the steps outlined by the ADA. You must first determine if there is a reasonable way to eliminate the risk of the employee transmitting the illness. If not, or if the adjustment would create undue hardship on the department, you should next check on reassigning the employee to a non food-handling position. According to the EEOC guidance, even when Food Code indicates that you should exclude the employee, you still have an obligation to follow a thinking process and plan of action outlined by the ADA. Furthermore, you must handle all health issues carefully when making hiring decisions. Here are some disability-related questions from the EEOC that should and should not be asked of a (potential) employee:

1. **Disability-Related Questions & Medical Exams During Employment Application & Interview Stage**

   The law places strict limits on employers when it comes to asking any job applicants to answer disability-related questions, take a medical exam, or identify a disability. For example, an employer may not ask a job applicant to answer disability-related questions or take a medical exam before extending a job offer. An employer also may not ask job applicants if they have a disability (or about the nature of an obvious disability). An employer may ask job applicants whether they can perform the job and how they would perform the job, with or without a reasonable accommodation.

2. **Disability-Related Questions & Medical Exams After a Job Offer for Employment**

   After a job is offered to an applicant, the law allows an employer to condition the job offer on the applicant answering certain disability-related questions or successfully passing a medical exam, but only if all new employees in the same type of job have to answer the questions or take the exam.

3. **Disability-Related Questions & Medical Exams for Persons Who Have Started Working as Employees**

   Once any employee is hired and has started work, an employer generally can only ask disability-related questions or require a medical exam if the employer needs medical documentation to support an employee's request for an accommodation or if the employer believes that an employee is not able to perform a job successfully or safely because of a medical condition. The law also requires that employers keep all medical records and information confidential and in separate medical files.

Source: Ref: Disability Discrimination | U.S. Equal Employment Opportunity Commission
https://www.eeoc.gov/laws/guidance/job-applicants-and-ada

Figure 17.6
Safety Risk Examples

- A pile of boxes obstructs a hallway where many employees need to walk or in aisle of storeroom or freezer.
- A ladder has a broken rung.
- A slicer has a frayed power cord.
- A puddle of water is accumulating on the floor.
- A pot has a loose handle.
- The hot water temperature is set too high.
- A loose tile sits awkwardly on the floor.
- A sharp knife is sitting in a sink full of soapy water.
- Knives in the kitchen have become dull, requiring an employee to use more pressure when using them.
- A cart used for transporting coffee has a loose wheel.
- The safety guard for a slicer or mixer is missing.
- An urn of hot coffee is balanced precariously on several trays on the counter.
- The safety valve on a steam-jacketed kettle is clogged.
- Broken mugs appear on the floor in the dishroom.
- Hallways or stairways are poorly lit.
- Heavy boxes are placed on higher shelving.

an established plan, time, forms, and evaluation, and is essential to help monitor safety needs on a routine basis.

Who should perform a safety inspection? Conducting a safety audit may be rotated among small teams or work groups. Ideally, a CDM, CFPP delegates the responsibility of safety inspections to groups of employees while retaining final responsibility and accountability. Involving all employees in safety audits builds awareness and commitment.

The frequency of a safety inspection may vary from one facility to the next but should follow an established schedule. Some perform weekly inspections and others do it bi-weekly. Regardless of the frequency, build a state of daily watchfulness for any safety risk among all employees.

View the Supplemental Material for this chapter to see Figure 17.5, Food Service Manager Self-Inspection Checklist.

There may be a facility-wide safety team that visits each area of the workplace. This is a valuable resource where a new set of eyes are reviewing the environment. If the facility is being inspected by a team, welcome the opportunity and learn all you can from it.

Likewise, if someone in your department is invited to join a safety team, recognize this as an excellent learning experience.

Any identified significant risk should be corrected on the spot or if it is due to a piece of equipment, it should be taken out of service. When a safety inspection has been completed, carefully review the results. Some CDM, CFPPs use a column on the inspection form itself to note corrections made with a date and time.

Some of the ongoing risk prevention activities in a food production dining services department involve equipment maintenance. When a steam release valve is clogged or an electrical cord is frayed, the CDM, CFPP should identify this and take quick action to place any dangerous equipment or location "off limits" to all and arrange for repairs. For more detailed risks common in a foodservice operation and their possible interventions, refer to Figure 17.7. Note that this is an excellent list of rules for any type of facility.

Employee Practices

Beyond risks, employee practices have great influences on safety. Even in a safe environment an employee can make an error that results in an injury. In fact, a majority of food production accidents occur when an employee simply is not paying attention or thinking about his or her action.

Here are some examples:

- A cook is feeling rushed to get the hot entrée out to the dining room. She grabs a pan without using a pot holder.
- A cafeteria server uses a wet rag to wipe the counter, and then to handle a pan for the steam table.
- A pantry employee microwaves a covered tray of food, and then carelessly removes the cover with steam venting towards his hand.
- A cook decides to grab another box of cake mix from the top shelf of the storeroom. He stacks a couple of boxes and climbs up.
- A trayline employee had punched in late and begins running to the trayline.
- A supervisor rushes through the door to the cafeteria without checking to see if the doorway is clear.
- An employee in the dishroom tries to carry too many soiled dishes at a time.

Each of these—and many more—constitutes a situation in which human action is likely to cause an accident. An accident can affect the careless employee, co-workers, or clients, so each employee has a responsibility to everyone in the vicinity to work safely. Common accidents in food production and dining services operations include slips and falls, cuts, burns, and muscle strains. To manage the human factor, a CDM, CFPP can take the following actions:

Build awareness. While the manager is aware of the risk of accidents in the operation, not everyone walking through the doors will automatically have the same awareness. In orientation for new employees and in ongoing training sessions, explain to the employees that the food production operation does indeed have hazards, and that each person has a role in ensuring safety. Make sure that part-time employees also receive this training.

Define expectations. Let every employee know that safety is a priority and ask them to make safety their priority, too. When possible, share the facility's safety statistics with the work team on an ongoing basis. If they are not optimal, ask the team for a commitment to improve them. Build a goal with objectives and action plans to focus on workplace safety.

Build safety into procedures. As employees are trained to accomplish certain tasks and procedures are written, incorporate specific safety requirements. Explain what tools are required for safe work performance, such as a ladder for reaching high places, a dry pot holder for handling hot pots and pans, a blade guard for the slicer, and so forth. Include actions the employees must take during this procedure to provide protection. For example, a procedure for cleaning electrical equipment includes the basic step of unplugging the equipment first.

Make inspection everyone's job. Whether or not each employee is involved in formal safety inspections, tell the employees what hazards to watch for. Ask them to identify and help correct (or report) safety risks.

Figure 17.7
Food and Employee Safety Checklist—School Foodservice Department

PERSONAL SAFETY

- Hands washed frequently and correctly (A handwashing sign is posted).
- Fingernails well trimmed and clean. No nail polish/artificial nails. Inappropriate jewelry or watches not worn during production and service.
- Hand sinks used for washing hands only. Pot sinks are not used for washing hands.
- Gloves worn when handling ready-to-eat foods without utensils.
- Gloves are changed when task is interrupted and possible contamination can occur. (Example: While making sandwiches, more meat is needed. Employee touches box containing meat and then goes back to making sandwiches).
- Employees trained on lifting heavy objects.
- Employees are in clean and proper uniform, including proper shoes.
- Effective hair restraints are used properly.
- Employee sick reporting log posted.

EQUIPMENT-FOOD SAFETY

- Floors are clean and dry to prevent falls.
- Thermometers calibrated weekly and documented.
- Temperatures of received items documented properly on receiving log.
- Refrigeration equipment maintained at 41°F or below.
- NSF approved cutting boards in good condition and stored vertically for proper draining and quick drying.
- Knives are sharp and stored properly to prevent unnecessary cuts.
- All towels in use are stored in properly concentrated sanitizing solutions. Solution is changed as it becomes dirty.
- Equipment is clean and in good repair: Hot holding equipment, coolers/freezers, can openers (including blade), drawers and racks, exhaust hood and filters.
- Gas equipment is working properly and gas lines are checked regularly for proper operation.
- Can openers are clean and in good working order to prevent employee cuts.
- Steam equipment is in good working order and operated correctly to prevent employee injury.
- Proper handling of hot pans (pot holders) is available to prevent burns.
- Kitchen garbage containers are clean and not overflowing.
- There is good lighting in the department work areas.
- If used: Dishmachine is working properly, temperatures are within range and documented. minimum temperatures for heat sanitizing compartments is 180°F (165°F for stationary racks).
- If used: three-compartment sink is properly set up for warewashing; sanitizing sink is free of suds and temperature is a minimum of 171°F and documented.
- There are proper fire extinguishers available and all staff knows how to use them.

FOOD SAFETY

- FIFO (First In, First Out) method of inventory management.
- Documentation of 'keep' or 'discard' on every food item before meal starts.
- Initial and batch temperatures documents.
- Holding temperatures documented every two hours for 'keep' items.
- Documentation of cooling temperatures on all leftover 'keep' items, (At least two temperatures are taken).
- Food reheated to 165°F or above and documented on production sheet.
- Documentation is complete on production guide for items prepped, items sold, and items left. Numbers match and if not, reasoning is documented.
- All foods are properly wrapped/contained, labeled and dated. **No expired foods**.
- Food is stored a minimum of 6" off floor.
- Unwashed produce stored below ready-to-eat items (Example: Raw broccoli below lunch meat)
- No outside food stored in coolers or freezers.

Continued

Figure 17.7
Food and Employee Safety Checklist—School Foodservice Department *(Continued)*

- Chemicals clearly identified.
- Chemicals are stored away from food and food-related supplies.
- Safety Sheets are available for all chemicals in the event of an unplanned exposure.
- Sanitizing solutions prepared in correct concentrations and documented.

Source: Adapted from the MN School District 196 Food Safety Checklist, used with permission.

Ask for caution. Remind employees to be alert, to focus on what they are doing, and to exercise care. Do not allow rough-and-tumble activities or other situations that could cause a safety hazard. Ask the employees not to distract one another when they are involved in dangerous tasks. Ask them to watch out for each other, and alert others when they see a dangerous or careless action in progress.

Offer ongoing reinforcement. As you walk through food production areas from day to day, observe what employees are doing. If you see an unsafe practice tell the employee on the spot. If you see a safe practice praise the employee. Safety, like sanitation, is a way of life. If the CDM, CFPP makes that an expectation, the employee will remember its importance.

Fire Safety

The potential for fire exists in all food production and dining services operations. Possible causes of fire include: unemptied grease traps, grease build-up on exhaust vents, equipment malfunction, faulty or frayed electrical cords, improper storage of flammable items, ignition of trash because of cigarettes being improperly discarded, or food left unattended during preparation. Employees must be familiar with all possible sources and kinds of fire, the locations of fire suppression equipment, and the actions to

Figure 17.8
Fire Extinguishers

CLASS	TYPE OF FIRE	RECOMMENDED EXTINGUISHER	COMMENTS
Class A	Normal combustible materials	Foam, soda acid, pump tank (plain water), gas cartridge, multipurpose dry chemical	
Class B	Grease and oil	Foam, carbon dioxide, multipurpose dry chemical, ordinary dry chemical	Never use plain water or a water extinguisher. This spreads the fire.
Class C	Electrical	Carbon dioxide, multipurpose dry chemical, ordinary dry chemical	Never use plain water or a water extinguisher. This can cause electrical shock.

Putting It Into Practice

3. The chef smells gas from the gas oven range. What is the first step you should take for his safety?

take in the event of a fire. As with all safety issues, a self-audit is a strong preventative tool. A sample fire safety audit appears in Figure 17.9, found in the Supplemental Material for this textbook.

When responding to a fire, the first few minutes or even seconds are the most important. A fire requires three conditions: fuel, oxygen, and a heat source. The goal in extinguishing a fire is to remove one or more of the required elements. Fires are classified according to the material combusting, as shown in Figure 17.8. Extinguishing a Class A fire may require removing the heat or the fuel source, while Class B and Class C fires generally require the removal of oxygen. Fire extinguishers have an identification system that indicates which type of fire they will extinguish.

View the Supplemental Material for this chapter to see Figure 17.9, Fire Safety Audit.

The best all-purpose fire extinguisher for a food production operation is the multipurpose dry chemical type. Extinguishers should be inspected regularly to ensure that they are still properly charged.

Employees should receive annual training about fire safety. Training should include the emergency response procedures. Topics to address include:

- Fire prevention plan and responsibilities.
- Location, purpose, and use of devices in the department, such as heat detectors, smoke detectors, fire alarm box, and fire extinguishers.
- How to respond to a fire.
- Sounding the alarm.
- How to use a fire extinguisher.
- How to protect yourself if clothing catches fire.
- Evacuation plan and exit routes.
- Procedures for protecting/evacuating clients in case of an emergency.

During training, employees should walk through the facility and locate the signaling devices. They should also walk through the evacuation routes (not just view them on a map). It is also a good idea for employees to practice using a fire extinguisher in a controlled environment. In some facilities, a fire safety officer or team will conduct fire safety training.

A common failing in a fire response is waiting to see whether the fire will become serious before calling for help. In fact, some employees may hesitate, trying to extinguish a fire on their own. It is always safer to call for help, even if it may not be needed. A CDM, CFPP should specifically direct employees to sound the alarm, even if the fire seems small. Training aids that can help employees remember some basic response techniques are described in Figure 17.10.

Heat Exhaustion

Another safety concern in a food production environment is heat stress. This can happen any time the employees find themselves in a hot, humid environment. Everyone should be alert to symptoms of heat stress. Timely intervention can prevent serious problems. When a person becomes overheated, symptoms such as profuse sweating, muscle cramps, and skin rash may occur. These are early signs of heat exhaustion, a medical condition in which the body cannot cool itself quickly enough.

Figure 17.10
Training Aids for Fire Response

RACE	PASS	STOP, DROP, AND ROLL
Steps for responding to a fire: 1. **Remove** everyone from danger. 2. Turn on the **Alarm.** 3. **Confine** the fire. 4. **Extinguish** fire, if it can be done safely.	Steps for using a fire extinguisher: 1. **Pull** the pin. 2. **Aim** at the base of the fire. 3. **Squeeze** trigger and keep extinguisher in an upright position. 4. **Sweep** across the base of the fire.	**Stop, Drop, and Roll** if your clothes catch on fire.

If left untreated, heat exhaustion can progress to symptoms of pale/clammy skin, weak and/or rapid pulse, low blood pressure, headache, intense thirst, weakness, dizziness, nausea, and vomiting. Intervention is important to prevent heat exhaustion from leading to heat stroke. In a heat stroke, a person may develop a high fever (>102°F), experience seizures, or become unconscious. This is a medical emergency. Interventions are described in Figure 17.11.

A CDM, CFPP should be aware of heat-related risks and prevent problems by using air conditioning and fans, encouraging employees to wear lightweight, loose-fitting clothing that conforms with the dress code, encouraging employees to take breaks if they are working in heat, and most importantly—encouraging employees to drink plenty of fluids when working in heat, even if they don't feel particularly thirsty. (Note: The FDA Food Code requires that employee beverages must be in a closed container.)

Figure 17.11
Interventions for Heat Exhaustion

FIRST AID	DO NOT...	CALL 911 IF
• Have the person lie down in a cool place. Elevate the person's feet about 12 inches. • Apply cool, wet cloths (or cool water directly) to the person's skin and use a fan to lower body temperature. Place cold compresses on the person's neck, groin, and armpits. • If alert, give the person beverages to sip (such as Gatorade), or make a salted drink by adding a teaspoon of salt per quart of water. Give a half cup every 15 minutes. Cool water will do if salt beverages are not available. • For muscle cramps, give beverages as above and massage affected muscles gently, but firmly, until they relax.	• **DO NOT...** underestimate the seriousness of heat illness. • **DO NOT...** give the person medications that are used to treat fever (such as aspirin or acetaminophen). They will not help; and they may be harmful. • **DO NOT...** give the person salt tablets. • **DO NOT...** give the person liquids that contain caffeine. • **DO NOT...** use alcohol rubs on the person's skin. • **DO NOT...** give the person anything by mouth (not even salted drinks) if the person is vomiting or unconscious.	Call immediately for emergency medical assistance (911) if: • The person loses consciousness or experiences a change in alertness (e.g., confusion or seizures). • The person has a fever over 102°F. • Other symptoms of heat stroke are present (like rapid pulse or rapid breathing). • The person's condition does not improve, or worsens despite treatment.

Source: U.S. National Library of Medicine

Government Regulations—OSHA

The Occupational Safety and Health Act (OSH Act) of 1970 was passed to "assure safe and healthful working conditions" for today's employees. It mandates that employers provide a safe work environment for employees. In 1971, the Occupational Safety and Health Administration (OSHA) enforced this regulation. In some cases, OSHA enforcement is handled by state agencies.

OSHA is involved in all aspects of employee safety on the job. It provides standards to ensure a safe work environment. It requires the maintenance of safety records, the filing of safety reports, and strict adherence to good safety practices. Employers are required to maintain records of employee accidents and to report serious accidents and fatalities to OSHA.

OSHA periodically inspects businesses to monitor the level of compliance. If a business is found to be in violation of a health and safety regulation OSHA may issue a citation, fine the employer, or in some cases, order the employer to close the business until compliance is attained.

OSHA also provides training information for employers, employees, compliance tools, and references on its Web site at www.osha.gov. Specifically, OSHA standards relate to safe equipment, electrical safety, machine usage, fire safety, accident prevention, and sound ergonomic practices. Guidelines listed in the Safety Inspection and Fire Safety Audits provided in this chapter reflect many of the OSHA standards.

To comply with OSHA standards, a CDM, CFPP should review standards, monitor and correct hazards, report and document injuries, and provide ongoing training for employees. Employers are required to display a poster prepared by the Department of Labor summarizing the major provisions of the Occupational Safety and Health Act and telling employees how to file a complaint. The poster must be posted in a conspicuous place where employees and applicants for employment can see it.

Accident Investigation and Reporting

If an accident or injury occurs in the operation, it is the manager's responsibility, by law, to report it. It is likely that the facility has an accident or incident reporting form that must be completed. See Figure 17.12 in Supplemental Material for an OSHA sample reporting form. OSHA advises completing a reporting form within seven days of an incident and keeping it on file for five years after the incident.

The form is a tool to help gather all relevant information to support systematic information review. The manager and other reviewers should look for the causes and identify the ways to prevent this type of accident from recurring. The employer (the facility) must maintain record-keeping for OSHA. It is important to know that the form contains confidential employee information. Therefore, always handle the form in a confidential manner, sharing it only with those in the facility who need to review it in order to help manage safety concerns.

View the Supplemental Material for this chapter to see Figure 17.12, Injury and Illness Incident Report.

Putting It Into Practice

4. Fill out an injury report for an employee who has just cut their hand while using the deli slicer.

> **GLOSSARY**
>
> **Work-Related Injury**
> Injury that occurs at work that results in days away from work, restricted work activity, medical treatment, loss of consciousness, or death
>
> **Ergonomics**
> The science of fitting the work environment to the employee
>
> **Musculoskeletal Disorders (MSDs)**
> Disorders affecting any part of the systems of skeleton, muscles, and tendons

OSHA defines a **work-related injury** or illness as one that results in days away from work, restricted work activity or job transfer, medical treatment (beyond first aid)—or in the most extreme case—loss of consciousness or death. In addition, a needlestick, hearing loss, or tuberculosis infection may require reporting under certain circumstances.

As a critical personnel policy, all employees should report any accident or injury to a supervisor. If an accident occurs, the steps are to first take care of the employee, obtaining first aid or medical help as needed. Second, complete the accident reporting form. During this process, include questions about how the accident occurred and how the accident could have been prevented. If the employee is in a condition to discuss this, ask the employee to make suggestions. Finally, follow internal procedures for handling the emergency and completing the form.

As accidents are tabulated and analyzed in the facility (such as by a safety committee or safety officer), review the accident statistics and trends. Target areas that need improvement and use the steps outlined above to improve the safety record. Accident review should become an integral part of quality assurance activities.

Ergonomics in Food service

Another area of increasing concern today is the ergonomics of foodservice work. **Ergonomics** is the science of fitting the work environment to the employee. A key objective of ergonomic analysis and intervention is to prevent injury related to repetitive motions and related work factors.

Repetitive motion injuries are common in many industries including food production and dining services. Unlike an accident or sudden event, a repetitive motion injury occurs gradually, over time. It comes from the motions an employee makes, over and over.

Examples of repetitive motion include:
- Using a scoop over and over to portion applesauce into bowls.
- Bending down to lift boxes and placing them on a shelf over and over again.
- Reaching for a plate cover and turning to place it on a tray moving along the trayline over and over.
- Racking plates for the dishmachine again and again.

Examples of injuries that can result from repetitive motions include:
- Carpal tunnel syndrome. This is an inflammation of tendons in the wrist, causing numbness or tingling.
- Tendonitis. This is inflammation of a tendon, anywhere in the body. A tendon is connective tissue that attaches muscles to bones.

More broadly, experts are also looking at other factors that cause injury to muscles, nerves, tendons, ligaments, and joints. In addition to repetitive motion, factors such as awkward posture, force, and vibration can bring on injury. A broader term for injury related to work environment and tasks is **musculoskeletal disorders (MSDs)**. These are disorders affecting any part of the systems of skeleton, muscles, and tendons.

Today, safety experts in all industries focus a great deal on how the work environment can be designed to help prevent these injuries. First, ask employees to report and investigate symptoms that may indicate development of an MSD. These include:

- Painful joints
- Pain in wrists, shoulders, forearms, knees
- Pain, tingling, or numbness in hands or feet
- Fingers or toes turning white
- Shooting or stabbing pains in arms or legs
- Back or neck pain
- Swelling or inflammation
- Stiffness
- Burning sensation

In addition, review any information that becomes available in the workplace that can help pinpoint MSDs that are occurring. Look carefully at workstations, at the posture of employees, and at movements. Look for opportunities to improve the work environment to minimize injury. Train employees how to use good body mechanics. Figure 17.13 lists ergonomic hazards in food service, along with solutions.

Figure 17.14 lists examples of training points and interventions in the food production and dining services workplace for preventing MSDs.

Safety Data Sheets

Every department is required to maintain a notebook of **Safety Data Sheets (SDS)** for each "hazardous" chemical or product used within the food production or dining services areas. Until recently, manufacturers and vendors provided printed material that included information such as health risks, handling instructions, first aid, and safe disposal of the products. While some manufacturers still provide a SDS printed sheet, most have gone to an online availability of the information to be downloaded and printed by the department for access by employees in the event of an accident or spill.

Putting it Into Action

Training, policies and procedure, audits, and inspections are all important pieces of the safe workplace. Ensuring access to appropriate and well-maintained equipment helps protect staff from injuries. However, the most important component of safety on the job is the employee. The role of the manager is to develop a culture of safety, and when observing unsafe practices or equipment misuse address the issue. The entire department staff and clients benefit when you hold employees accountable for their compliance to safety regulations.

GLOSSARY

Safety Data Sheet (SDS)
A printed information sheet for each "hazardous" chemical or product used within the department

Figure 17.13
Ergonomic Hazards and Solutions

Dietary employees must perform many lifting, reaching, and repetitive tasks as part of their job duties. Employee activities in this area, if occuring with sufficient duration, magnitude, and/or frequency, may create a musculoskeletal disorder (MSD).

POTENTIAL HAZARD: REACHING/LIFTING

Frequent elevated extended reaches for supplies or heavy containers can cause back and shoulder injury resulting in muscle strain, bursitis, tendonitis, and rotator cuff injuries.

Possible Solutions

Assess worksites for ergonomic stressors and identify and address ways to decrease them such as:

- Provide height-adjustable workspaces appropriate for the task being performed, so that workers can keep elbows close to the body. For example, lower countertops, or use height adjustable countertops or stands, or provide work stands for employees.
- Redesign or reposition tasks to allow elbows to remain close to the body (e.g., turn boxes over on side to allow easier access).
- Avoid awkward postures (e.g., reposition work in front of worker so that he does not have to reach above or behind to get supplies).
- Use mechanical aids to reduce the need to lift. Use a spring device to automatically lift a load (e.g., use automatic plate and cup riser dispensers).
- Lighten a load that needs to be lifted or get help when lifting.
- Train workers to use proper lifting techniques.

POTENTIAL HAZARD: REPETITIVE MOTIONS

Rapid hand and wrist movements from frequent cutting, chopping, or scooping may lead to hand disorders such as tendonitis or carpal tunnel syndrome. Example: A kitchen worker scoops ingredients with a flexed wrist.

Possible Solutions

Assess worksites for ergonomic stressors and identify and address ways to decrease them such as:

- Rotate workers through repetitive tasks.
- Use mechanical aids for chopping, dicing, or mixing foods (e.g., food processors, mixers).
- Select and use properly designed tools. For example, kitchen scoops or kitchen knives that allow the wrist to remain straight.
- Maintain a neutral (handshake) wrist position.
- Restructure jobs to reduce repeated motions, forceful hand exertions, and prolonged bending.

Source: http://www.osha.gov/SLTC/etools/hospital/dietary/dietary.html

Figure 17.14
Musculoskeletal Disorders (MSDs): Training Points

- Use proper lifting techniques.
- Lighten the load; do not try to lift too much at once.
- Provide mechanical aids for lifting as warranted.
- Avoid reaching or working above shoulder height.
- Seek to avoid motions that require bending the wrists. Instead, try to keep wrists comfortably straight as much as possible.
- Teach safe postures: As often as possible, elbows should be at 90° angles; shoulders should be relaxed and low; and arms should be close to the body.
- Be sure standing workers are working at comfortable counter heights that do not require them to bend excessively.
- Avoid repeated twisting and arrange the work area to support this.
- For workers involved in prolonged repetitive movements, provide frequent breaks from the task.
- Rotate workers through jobs to reduce the repetition of movements on any one worker.
- As possible, minimize the amount of force or pressure a worker must use to accomplish a task.
- Look for utensils with ergonomically designed grips, especially for utensils that are used repeatedly. These are thicker than ordinary handles and may minimize strain.
- Ask a qualified expert, such as an occupational health nurse, to train employees to stretch safely to avoid injury.
- Talk with workers and ask them what steps they believe could make their jobs more comfortable.

Figure 17.15
Ergonomically Sound Techniques

Lifting

1. Get close to the load. Bend at the hips and knees. Firmly grasp the load.
2. Keep head and shoulders erect. Lift, using legs for power.
3. Maintain a wide base.
4. To transfer the load, turn with your feet. Do not twist at the wrist.
5. Lower the load by bending at the hips and knees.

Straight Wrists

Avoid the situations illustrated below. Instead, keep wrists as straight as possible.

Holding a Can

Avoid picking up a large can with one hand.

Instead, pick up a large can with two hands on the sides.

Source: The Grossbauer Group. Used with permission.

Chapter References

RESOURCES	
Americans with Disabilities Act Rights of Employees	ada.gov
Disability Discrimination | U.S. Equal Employment Opportunity Commission	https://www.eeoc.gov/laws/guidance/job-applicants-and-ada
FDA Food Code	fda.gov
OSHA Ergonomic Hazards and Solutions	https://www.osha.gov/SLTC/etools/hospital/dietary/dietary.html
OSHA Occupational Safety and Health Administration	osha.gov
OSHA Occupational Safety and Health Administration, Dietary	osha.gov/SLTC/etools/hospital/dietary/dietary.html
OSHA Safety Data Sheets	https://www.oshalgov/Publications/OSHA3514.html
U.S. Equal Employment Opportunity Commission (EEOC)	eeoc.gov
UC San Diego, Food Safety for Food Service Employees	https://blink.ucsd.edu/safety/resources/training/food.html

Safe Food Handling: Purchasing, Receiving, and Storage

Overview and Objectives

Ensuring food safety depends on selecting a safe food vendor, obtaining food from approved sources, and carefully controlling the receiving, storage, and distribution practices. After completing this chapter, you should be able to:

- Identify appropriate grades and inspections for food
- Procure food and water from approved sources
- Verify the quality and quantity of food supplies and equipment received
- Check supplier invoices against facility purchasing order
- Recognize the hazards associated with types of food packaging
- Recognize the signs of contamination upon receipt and in storage
- Process rejections for unacceptable products
- Label, date, and monitor food to ensure rotation
- Prevent environmental contamination of food
- Establish and maintain security procedures

GLOSSARY

Approved Source
A source that is inspected based on federal, state, or local laws and has appropriate HACCP procedures in place

Inspection
A mandatory process that addresses wholesomeness and safety of fresh meats, dairy, and produce

Shellfish Identification Tags
Special labels that can be used to trace a product such as oysters, mussels, or clams back to the source in the event that illness occurs

Grading
A voluntary process providing a descriptive term or number to designate quality

Purchasing

For a food production operation, purchasing is the first step in the flow of food. Food and water must be purchased from **approved sources**. An approved source is one that is inspected based on federal, state, or local laws and has the appropriate Hazard Analysis and Critical Control Points (HACCP) procedures in place. The Centers for Medicare & Medicaid Services (CMS) guidelines F812 and F813 specify that food must be procured "from sources approved or considered satisfactory by Federal, State or local authorities."

Vendor specifications should include:

- Quality standards such as grading and HACCP verification
- Wholesomeness indicators such as inspection

In addition, delivery times and intervals may also be included in the vendor specifications. The manager needs to exercise careful planning when purchasing food. Purchasing excessive quantities of food can result in spoilage, increased costs, and greater likelihood of foodborne illness. Perishable products—such as produce, seafood, meats, eggs, and dairy products—should be purchased in a quantity that will be used within a short time period. Non-perishable foods such as canned and frozen foods can be purchased in quantities that allow for longer storage times, if desirable.

Inspection

All food shipped in interstate commerce (from one state to another) must meet the requirements of one or more federal laws. The U.S. Department of Agriculture (USDA) has established uniform standards for state and federally inspected meats, poultry, and eggs. **Inspection** is a mandatory process that addresses wholesomeness and safety of fresh meats, dairy products, and produce. Some products that are not shipped across state lines may have to be inspected by state programs with their own standards—some higher than those of federal programs. Food production operations may only purchase meat, poultry, and eggs that have been inspected by the USDA or by a state department of health or agriculture. Inspected food is considered to be safe for consumption. However, inspection does not imply any quality standard.

Seafood and fish must be purchased from approved suppliers. This is especially important for molluscan shellfish such as oysters, scallops, mollusks, and clams because they may be consumed raw or undercooked. To ensure safety when received, these foods must be accompanied by a certification that documents where and when they were harvested (**Shellfish Identification Tags**). This certification must be kept for 90 days to allow time for evidence of a hepatitis A virus infection. The Public Health Service maintains the lists of Certified Shellfish Shippers. Suppliers should be selected from this list or from state-approved lists.

Grading

Grades are classifications of foods by a descriptive term or number to ensure uniform quality and give an indication of desirability. **Grading** is a voluntary process. Most grades are assigned by government agencies and follow strict guidelines. Grades refer to attributes such as visual appearance, color, size, marbling, and uniformity.

Canned vegetables and fruits are usually graded and each vendor has its own terminology. Beef, veal, pork, and lamb are graded by the U.S. Department of Agriculture (USDA). For beef, the USDA grades are: prime, choice, select, standard, commercial, utility, cutter, and canner. The last three grades are not used in food production operations. Examples of inspection stamps and grade shields appear in Figure 18.1.

Figure 18.1
USDA Inspection Stamps and Grade Shields

Vendor Selection

Selecting a vendor is an important part of the purchasing process. The Certified Dietary Manager®, Certified Food Protection Professional® (CDM®, CFPP®) should consider the extent to which the potential vendor will be able to meet the quality, service, and cost expectations of the food production operation. The relationship between the manager and the vendor should be based on mutual understanding, cooperation, and trust.

Selection of a vendor is a business decision. Although a personal history with a sales representative is a valuable asset, the final decision should be based on the needs of the organization. Visits to the vendor's distribution center and inspections of delivery vehicles are advisable in the process of selecting a vendor. (Note that food prepared in the home cannot be served in quantity foodservice operations.)

As the CDM, CFPP, determine if the facility has a purchasing agreement and if you are required to purchase exclusively with a vendor. Many managers spend time on weekly meetings with a number of sales representatives from multiple vendors. While access to a local market or vendor can be helpful for the occasional missing item, professional organizations purchase the majority of their inventory from a limited number of prime vendors.

In today's marketplace, most healthcare and school operations participate in a **Group Purchasing Organization (GPO)**. The GPO functions as a contract buying program that negotiates favorable pricing for items most frequently used by their members. Not all items, nor all brands, purchased are covered by the GPO pricing program, however.

> **GLOSSARY**
>
> **Group Purchasing Organization (GPO)**
> A contract buying program that negotiates favorable pricing for its members

Putting It Into Practice

1. When receiving a shipment of frozen meats, fish, shellfish, and poultry, how would you best inspect the products?

Even items not on the GPO contracted price are usually less expensive through the prime vendor than through the local or back-up vendors. If the facility does have a GPO program available, it is generally to the manager's benefit to access the purchasing agreement. Another advantage of the GPO is they typically pre-approve the vendors for safety, sanitation, and delivery services.

Some of the considerations leading to selection of a safe food vendor include:

- Is the vendor inspected by an independent source to ensure food safety?
- Can the supplier provide you with written proof of government inspection for meats?
- Does the vendor have a Hazard Analysis Critical Control Point (HACCP) system in place?
- Are the vendor's delivery vehicles clean and well maintained?
- Are the delivery trucks for refrigerated foods adequately refrigerated?
- If purchasing frozen foods: do delivery trucks have freezer sections?
- Can the vendor provide business references?
- Can the vendor meet the delivery needs (daily, weekly, monthly) of the facility to ensure a safe flow of food?
- Does the vendor have a reputation for providing quality products?
- Will the vendor allow staff to inspect products upon receipt?
- Is the vendor cooperative if you refuse products because of food safety concerns?
- Where is the vendor located relative to the foodservice operation?

Once a reputable vendor is found, it is important to monitor quality continuously to ensure that the vendor has a long-term commitment to providing safe, quality food.

Receiving

Receiving is an important phase in the flow of food through a food production operation. Food items should be carefully inspected before being placed into storage. The person receiving must be knowledgeable in food safety, quality standards, and purchasing specifications. It is essential that food is inspected immediately upon delivery. Product not meeting the facility's quality and safety standards should be refused and returned to the vendor.

If possible, schedule deliveries at times convenient for the receiver to inspect food carefully or change the scheduled work time of receiving staff to be available at the time of planned deliveries. Even government inspected foods must be examined since federal inspection programs do not inspect food at every step in the flow of food from producer to vendor to foodservice operation. Storage areas should be prepared to accept new deliveries and the staff should also be available to compare the invoice to the order and store the food immediately.

Of special concern today is fish, such as large tuna or farm-raised (aquaculture) fish that might be consumed raw or undercooked, as in sushi. If you purchase frozen fish for this purpose, it must contain a label indicating that is was properly frozen. (Otherwise, these fish may contain a parasitic worm that can infect your clients.)

Purchased juice products, as well as pureed fruits and vegetables that are served to highly susceptible populations, such as the sick and the elderly, must contain a label stating that the products have been pasteurized.

Potentially hazardous foods must be received at a temperature of 41°F or below. A frozen food must be received in a frozen state and at 0°F or below, in most cases. You need to carefully inspect all refrigerated and frozen foods for any sign of temperature abuse during transportation and delivery. For instance, large ice crystals are evidence that frozen food was thawed and refrozen—and should be rejected on delivery. A receiving checklist in the Supplemental Materials (Figure 18.2) can help employees check and document the condition of foods.

When receiving food:
- Reject food in damaged packaging.
- Check for inspection stamps, date codes, labels/tags for fish or juice.
- Check the temperature of frozen and refrigerated foods, including milk.
- Verify freshness by color, odor, touch, and package condition.
- Look for signs of pest infestation and/or spoilage.

View the Supplemental Material for this chapter to see Figure 18.2, Receiving Checklist.

Figure 18.3 shows how to check temperature of foods, and Figure 18.4 shows quality and safety indicators to check for many common foods.

Food Packaging

Technologies for packaging food to promote safety are constantly evolving. Some of the technologies used are presented below.

Modified Atmosphere Packaging (MAP). Most spoilage microorganisms are **aerobic**, meaning they need oxygen to grow. In modified atmosphere packaging, oxygen is commonly replaced with a mixture of ozone, carbon dioxide, or nitrogen. This type of packaging can extend freshness of the product by maintaining a reduced-oxygen environment. Many food products are now packaged this way including vegetables, salad greens, fresh pasta, meat, fruit, cheese, seafood, and pre-prepared foods such as sandwiches and bakery products.

GLOSSARY

Modified Atmosphere Packaging (MAP)
A type of packaging that extends the life of the product by maintaining a reduced oxygen environment

Aerobic
Requires oxygen to survive—many microorganisms are aerobic

Figure 18.3
Verifying Food Temperature During Receiving

Image courtesy of Cooper-Atkins

Figure 18.4
Quality Indicators for Receiving Safe Food

FOOD ITEM	ACCEPT	REJECT
Fresh Beef	• Light pink to bright red color (aged beef may be darker) • Firm and elastic	• Dark brown or greenish color, sour or rancid smell
Fresh Poultry	• Slightly yellow appearance • Firm flesh • Not sticky to touch • Received at or below 41°F	• Dark appearance under wings • Sticky to touch
Marine Foods	• Gills of fresh fish are pink • No iridescence (shimmering) • Eyes clear, not sunken	• Excessive fish or ammonia smell
Milk and Dairy Products	• Intact packaging • Clean containers • Butter with firm texture • Cheese free of mold • Received at or below 41°F	• Damaged or leaking containers • Expired dates
Egg and Egg Products	• Clean eggs, uncracked shells • Received at or below 45°F	• Cracked or dirty eggs
Fresh Produce	• Bright color, no mold or wilt	• Signs of insect damage or plant disease • Bruises or soft produce
Canned Foods	• No dents • All foods labeled	• Dented or rusted cans
Dry Goods	• Intact packaging	• Ripped or torn packaging
Frozen Fish	• Labeled that it was properly frozen	• If label is missing • If large ice crystals are present
Molluscan Fish	• Contains a shellfish ID tag	• If tag is missing
Juice or Pureed Fruits/Vegetables	• Is labeled "pasteurized"	• If not pasteurized

Putting It Into Practice

2. While receiving an order for frozen beef, you notice ice crystals on the outside of a carton. What does that mean and what would you do?

Although the packaging can extend shelf life, it will not always prevent microbial growth. For example, an **anaerobic** pathogen such as Clostridium botulinum may thrive in this low-oxygen environment. Another concern with Modified Atmosphere Packaging (MAP) foods is that they may not "look" or "smell" spoiled when, in fact, they may have become unsafe for consumption. It is up to the manufacturers to protect the clients from illness by providing instructions on how to store and handle the product safely and marking dates. It is up to the operator to make sure that these products are received and stored properly. Thus when receiving and storing MAP foods, you should:

- Read the label. Note that recommended handling practices vary from product to product.
- Check for a **time/temperature indicator (TTI) strip**. This strip changes color if the product is outdated or has been temperature abused.
- Check for an expiration date or use-by date on the package. Do not use packages past recommended dates.
- Check for air bubbles. Vacuum packaged foods should be free of air bubbles.
- Maintain MAP packaging under refrigeration.
- Keep MAP packaging sealed until ready to use them. Once a MAP package has been opened, the advantages of a low-oxygen environment disappear. Pathogens can now grow more rapidly.

Modified Atmosphere Packaging (MAP) techniques are very safe and provide advantages. However, a CDM, CFPP must, nevertheless, recognize and control hazards, as with any food product.

Ultra High Temperature Processing (UHT). UHT products are treated by flash sterilization and then packed into sterilized, airtight containers. Milk that is processed using the UHT (shelf-stable milk) can be stored at room temperature for the time period indicated on the label. The most common UHT products are dairy products but the use is expanding to fruit juices, wine, soups, and stews. After opening, the product must be refrigerated and used within the time listed on the product label. For instance, a milk-based soup that was processed with UHT has the following directions on the label: "After opening, keep refrigerated and use within 7-10 days."

Storage

Proper storage is an important aspect of food protection. Storage is more complex than simply having adequate space. Storage involves the variables of light, temperature, ventilation, and air circulation. Food must be stored 6" above the floor, on clean, slatted racks or shelves, and in a manner that prevents environmental or cross-contamination. Slatted shelving allows for proper air circulation around food and should not be covered with foil or other material. Food must also be stored away from walls and ceilings. Food not intended for further preparation before serving must be stored in a way that prevents contamination from food requiring preparation.

For instance, raw foods, such as meat, should never be stored above ready-to-eat foods like fresh fruit, salads, or desserts. The raw food may splash or drip onto the ready-to-eat food and result in cross-contamination. Food may not be stored in locker rooms, toilet areas, dressing rooms, in garbage rooms, mechanical rooms, under sewer lines that are not adequately shielded, under open stairwells, under a water leak, or near any other potential source of contamination. Chemicals must never be stored near food.

> **GLOSSARY**
>
> **Anaerobic**
> A pathogen such as Clostridium botulinum that can thrive in this low-oxygen environment—without air
>
> **Time/Temperature Indicator (TTI) Strip**
> Strip that changes color if the product is outdated or has been temperature abused
>
> **Ultra High Temperature Processing (UHT)**
> UHT products are treated by flash sterilization and then packed into sterilized, airtight containers

Figure 18.5
Storage Temperatures

Dry storage	50°F–70°F
Refrigerated storage	41°F or below
Deep chilling storage	26°F–32°F
Freezer storage	0°F or below

Every food has a shelf life, which is the amount of time the product can be expected to remain reasonably safe, if properly stored. The foodservice staff must monitor the dates on the foods to ensure that they are used before their expiration. New deliveries should be stored behind previous deliveries to ensure that the oldest product is used first. This method of stock rotation is called **First In, First Out (FIFO)**.

Certain foods may be difficult to identify after they are removed from their original packaging. Foods such as salt and sugar look the same, but if they are mixed up for clients on special diets it can be disastrous. Some oils or granulated foods may look like cleaning compounds. Packaged food labels contain nutrition information as well as valuable ingredient information that may be needed for consulting with clients with allergies. For those reasons, containers holding food or food ingredients that are removed from original packaging for use in the foodservice operation should be labeled with the common name of the food and the date the package was opened.

When storing raw meats, fish and pork should be kept separated from poultry because of the possible higher bacterial count in the poultry. As mentioned, meats should be stored below ready-to-eat foods to avoid dripping during thawing.

Dry storage area temperatures should be maintained between 50°F–70°F. For short-term holding of perishable foods, maintain refrigerators between 34°F–41°F. Sometimes a food is not quite as cold as the temperature around it. Maintaining refrigeration temperatures below 38°F will help ensure that actual food temperatures remain out of the hazard zone. The Food Code suggests placing a thermometer in the warmest part of the refrigerator. New technology allows employees to measure a simulated product temperature for better accuracy.

Ideally, meats, poultry, and fish should be stored in a deep chilling unit. Very low temperatures may damage food and affect quality for some items such as produce and dairy products. Often separate coolers are used for the produce and dairy with slightly higher thermostat settings.

Detailed information on food safety and foodborne illness is covered through the food handler certification programs. Check with state and local regulations for specific requirements regarding food handler certification or food handler cards. Figure 18.7 provides a summary of guidelines for purchasing, receiving, and storing food.

GLOSSARY

First In, First Out (FIFO)
A storage practice to ensure that older products are used first

View the Supplemental Material for this chapter to see Figure 18.6, Storage Temperature Log.

Putting It Into Practice

3. You received 5 gallons of milk on the first of the month and used 3 of them. Another 5 gallons have been purchased for use for the following week. What would you do with the 2 gallons from the previous purchase?

Product Recalls

Periodically, manufacturers identify quality issues that affect the safety or integrity of their product in the marketplace. Issuing a product recall is a major process for the manufacturer and distributor to coordinate. If a product has been designated for recall, typically the distributor contacts all customers who have purchased the specific lot numbers of the item and advises the customer on the appropriate steps for disposal. Normally, the vendor does not want to "pick up" the product from a facility. Many of the major vendors also list complete details of product recalls on their website.

Summary

Ensuring the safety of the food served to clientele starts with the vendor and their acquisition of food from approved growers. The purchase, delivery, and storage within the department is designed to maintain the quality and safety of the food until the time of preparation. In the next chapter, food safety shifts to the actual preparation and presentation of meals for the clients.

Figure 18.7
Guidelines for Purchasing, Receiving, and Storing Food

ITEM	PURCHASE	RECEIVE	STORE	SHELF LIFE
Meat	• USDA or state inspected	• Receive frozen at 0°F • Receive refrigerated at 41°F or below	• Store frozen at 0°F or below • Store refrigerated at 41°F or below, separate from poultry	• Fresh beef: 6-12 months in freezer; 3-6 days in refrigerator • Ground beef: 3-4 months in freezer; 1-2 days in refrigerator
Poultry	• USDA or state inspected	• Receive frozen at 0°F • Receive refrigerated at 41°F or below	• Store frozen at 0°F or below • Store refrigerated at 41°F or below	• 6 months in freezer; 1-2 days in refrigerator
Fish and Shellfish	• From an approved supplier • Shellfish must have shellfish identification tag	• Receive frozen at 0°F • Receive refrigerated at 41°F or below	• Store frozen at 0°F or below • Store refrigerated at 41°F or below, separate from poultry	• All: 2-4 months in freezer • 1-2 days in refrigerator
Milk and Dairy Products	• Pasteurized milk and milk products	• Receive frozen (ice cream) at 6°F to 10°F • Receive refrigerated at 41°F	• Store frozen at 0°F or below • Store refrigerated at 41°F or below • Unopened UHT package may be stored at room temperature	• Milk: Use by expiration date on carton • Ice cream: 6 months in freezer

Chapter References

RESOURCES	
Clemson Food Systems and Safety	clemson.edu/extension/food
F Tag Food Safety Requirements	https://www.licamedman.com/ftag/746/f812-food-procurement-store-prepare-serve-sanitary
Group Purchasing Organizations (GPOs)	en.wikipedia.org/wiki/Group_purchasing_organization
U.S. Department of Agriculture (USDA) *Grading Standards*	ams.usda.gov/grades-standards
U.S. Department of Agriculture (USDA) *Inspection Standards*	fsis.usda.gov/wps/portal/fsis/topics/food-safety-education/get-answers/food-safety-fact-sheets/production-and-inspection

Safe Food Handling: Food Preparation

Overview and Objectives

Did you ever consider how many processes food goes through before we actually consume it? Safe purchasing, receiving, and storage procedures are just the beginning of what are needed to keep our food safe. In this chapter, we will evaluate foodborne diseases and their causes, explain all phases in the flow of food, and review the HACCP guidelines. After completing this chapter, you should be able to:

- Identify potentially hazardous foods and susceptible populations
- Recognize the causes, symptoms, and types of foodborne illnesses
- Monitor the time and temperature to limit growth of or destroy microorganisms
- Prevent cross-contamination of food
- Identify appropriate techniques for temperature retention
- Ensure the safe cooling of food
- Understand HACCP and develop procedures to identify and monitor the critical control points (CCP)
- Devise effective recordkeeping systems that document HACCP
- Anticipate emergency preparedness procedures necessary to assure a safe food supply
- Develop a crisis management plan to address an outbreak of foodborne illness

Foodborne Illness: Causes & Preparation

A foodborne illness is a major public concern. In 2011, the Food Safety Modernization Act (FSMA) was implemented to expand and improve the security and safety of our nation's food supply. This was historic legislation designed to build a new system of food safety oversight. Why is this important legislation needed? According to the Centers for Disease Control and Prevention (CDC), "each year, foodborne illness strikes 48 million Americans, hospitalizing a hundred thousand and killing over three thousand."

Although many people experience foodborne illnesses, they do not report them, brushing off the symptoms as "the flu." A **foodborne illness** is a disease that is transmitted by food. The most frequent cause is harmful microorganisms—or poisons produced by the harmful microorganisms. Symptoms of a foodborne illness vary according to the cause of the illness and the person who is afflicted. However, the common symptoms may include vomiting, diarrhea, fever, and headache. In some cases, death is a very real risk.

Some individuals are more susceptible to foodborne illness than others. Their symptoms may be more severe, and their risk of death may be higher. Preschool age children, the elderly, pregnant women, and persons with weakened immune systems are among the high-risk groups. They are also called **highly susceptible populations (HSP)**. Serving these HSP groups requires special awareness of their increased vulnerability—and sometimes special precautions in ingredient selection and meal preparation are warranted.

Often, when there is a reported case of a foodborne illness in one food, expect more of the same foodborne illness in the same food. A **foodborne illness outbreak** occurs when two or more persons become ill after ingesting the same food and a laboratory analysis confirms that the food was the source of the illness. Also, a foodborne illness caused by a chemical is also considered an outbreak even though only one person is affected.

The annual cost of foodborne illness is estimated to be $152 billion. According to the Centers for Disease Control and Prevention (CDC), there are more than 250 different types of diseases caused by contaminated food or beverages. And there are also new strains of harmful foodborne microorganisms constantly evolving.

Food Hazards

A food can become unsafe in a number of ways. Also, there are many **hazards** in the environment that can affect the safety and quality of food served to people. Hazards are present in food, air, and water, on work surfaces, and on the hands as well as the dining services employees themselves. Food-related hazards fall into three major categories: biological, chemical, and physical, as shown in Figure 19.1. The presence of substances in food that can cause harm is called **contamination**.

Biological Hazards

Biological hazards include bacteria, viruses, parasites, and fungi. Viruses and bacteria threats to the safety of the food supply are also commonly cited in foodborne illness outbreaks. There are many bacteria in the environment and in our bodies. While some serve useful purposes, others cause serious foodborne illnesses. These microorganisms that cause foodborne illness are called **pathogens**.

GLOSSARY

Foodborne Illness
A disease that is transmitted by food

Highly Susceptible Populations (HSP)
Persons who are more likely to experience foodborne disease because they are immunocompromised, preschool age children, pregnant women, or older adults

Foodborne Illness Outbreak
Time when two or more cases of a similar illness result from eating a common food

Hazards
Biological, chemical, or physical property that may cause an unacceptable consumer health risk that must be controlled

Contamination
The presence of biological, physical, or chemical substances in food that could cause harm

Pathogens
Microorganisms that cause foodborne illness

Figure 19.1
Food Hazards

BIOLOGICAL	CHEMICAL	PHYSICAL
• Bacteria • Parasites • Viruses • Fungi • Natural Toxins • Prions	• Pesticides • Toxic Metals • Cleaning Chemicals	• Dirt • Hair • Broken Glass • Metal Shavings

Pathogens may already be in the food supply or may be introduced at any time from the point of harvest to the processor, manufacturer, distributor, or at the food production operation.

Pathogens can be categorized as bacteria, viruses, parasites, fungi, and natural toxins. Some species are valuable and useful in preserving food or producing alcohol if they are specially cultured and used under controlled conditions. Improper operating procedures and food preparation practices allow improper microbial activity which can be a primary cause of foodborne illness or intoxication (see Figure 19.2).

Bacteria

There are many types of bacteria, with differences in their growth habits and requirements. **Anaerobic** bacteria grow in an environment with little or no oxygen. These bacteria might contaminate canned foods or Modified Atmosphere Packaged (MAP) products. They may also grow in the center of large quantities of food. Then there are the **aerobic** bacteria which require oxygen to grow.

Types of Illness

Exactly how pathogens cause illnesses varies. Some microorganisms enter the body in an active state and continue to grow. The type of illness that results is called a **foodborne infection**, because the person who eats the food is literally infected with the pathogens. For example, Salmonella bacteria enter the body in a live state and grow in the body, causing fever, nausea, diarrhea, and other symptoms. This illness is called salmonellosis.

Other microorganisms produce a poison or toxin that is not destroyed in cooking. The bacteria may not be alive anymore, but their toxins are still present and cause illness. This illness is called **foodborne intoxication**. For example, Clostridium botulinum bacteria produce a toxin. Botulism is the illness that results from eating the affected food.

> **GLOSSARY**
>
> **Foodborne Infection**
> Condition when pathogens enter the body in an active state and continue to grow (e.g., Salmonella)
>
> **Foodborne Intoxication**
> An illness that occurs from the toxin or poison left from bacteria that are no longer alive (e.g., Clostridium botulinum)

Figure 19.2
Causes of Foodborne Illness

| Pathogens are naturally present in the food supply. | Contamination or mishandling occurs during processing, transport, storage, preparation, and/or service. | Pathogens may grow. New pathogens may be introduced. Other biological, chemical, and physical contaminants may also enter food. | Food is consumed and foodborne illness results. |

> **GLOSSARY**
>
> **Toxin-Mediated Infection**
> A condition when live bacteria enter the body and produce a dangerous toxin (e.g., E. coli bacteria)
>
> **FOTTWA**
> Acronym for the conditions needed for bacterial growth: Food, Oxygen, Temperature, Time, Water, Acidity

Finally, some microorganisms enter the body in a live and growing state, producing toxins. The resulting illness is a **toxin-mediated infection**. Shiga toxin-producing E. coli bacteria (STEC), for example, cause an illness that involves severe diarrhea and vomiting.

Types of Pathogens

Due to environmental and growth conditions, most pathogens favor certain foods. For example, Listeria bacteria are often associated with unpasteurized cheese and processed meats, Salmonella with eggs, Shiga toxin-producing E. coli with ground beef, and Norovirus with shellfish.

The Certified Dietary Manager®, Certified Food Protection Professional® (CDM®, CFPP®) should be able to recognize symptoms that could signal foodborne illness and warrant medical evaluation. However, it is important to note that control mechanisms for foodborne illness are fairly universal. A comprehensive set of food protection practices can prevent illness from a wide range of pathogens. The CDC lists the top five pathogens causing illness, hospitalization, and death: These are: Norovirus (a virus, formerly called Norwalk virus), Salmonella (bacteria), Clostridium Perfringens (bacteria), Campylobacter (bacteria), and Staphylococcus aureus (bacteria). These top five pathogens are highlighted on the following pages (Figure 19.3).

Conditions for Bacterial Growth and Toxin Formation

To protect clients from foodborne illness, first consider the conditions that allow bacteria to grow or toxins to develop. The conditions are similar to what humans need: air, food, moisture, and warmth. Bacteria require food, too. Often, they favor food high in protein, such as meat. But at times, they will settle for vegetables, fruits, and other plant foods. In addition to food, bacteria grow most rapidly in an environment which also provides moisture, warmth, neutral or slightly acidic pH, oxygen at a level favored by the bacteria, and time. Moisture is measured as available water (a_w) in a food. Examples of food with a high a_w content include meat, cheese, and produce. Meats, fresh fruits, and fresh vegetables, for example, have an a_w of close to 1.0, while crackers have an a_w of 0.1.

The term pH describes the level of acidity or alkalinity. Optimal conditions for microorganisms are typically neutral or slightly acidic. Generally, as foods become more acidic, they are less likely to support bacterial growth. Meats, fish, and vegetables tend to be slightly acidic and support bacterial growth. Foods that are very acidic, with a pH below about 4.2, do not favor bacterial growth. Based on a_w and level of acidity, you can see why traditional methods of food preservation use techniques like dehydrating food products (to *reduce a_w*) and pickling or adding vinegar (to reduce pH to extremes where bacteria cannot thrive).

Time and temperature are critically interrelated in controlling bacterial growth and the formation of toxins. When all other conditions are suitable for microorganisms, a key question is: How much time does the microorganism have in which to flourish? For example, in one environment bacterial growth may be controlled if the temperature and time are managed. However, if the temperature is the same, but the bacteria have twice as much time to grow, there may be increased (a hundred times more) bacteria present. The more time a microorganism has under favorable conditions, the more it will multiply or produce toxins. This is one reason that holding time, cooling (for hot foods), reheating time (for leftovers), storage time, and other time-related factors are important for ensuring safe food. Conditions that help bacteria grow can be summarized by the acronym **FOTTWA**: Food, Oxygen, Temperature, Time, Water, Acidity, shown in Figure 19.4.

Figure 19.3
Common Foodborne Pathogens

TYPE	SOURCE	SYMPTOMS AND COMPLICATIONS	PREVENTION
Bacillus cereus Bacteria	Milk, cereals, rice, and starchy foodstuffs	Diarrhea, fever, chills, and dehydration. Onset is usually within 12-50 hours.	Keep food out of the hazard zone. Keep dry products away from moisture.
Campylobacter jejuni Bacteria	Raw meat, poultry and shellfish, contaminated water and unpasteurized milk	Muscle pain, headache and fever followed by diarrhea, abdominal pain and nausea. Onset is usually 2-5 days.	Thoroughly cook meat and poultry. Use pasteurized milk and products. Control time/temperature. Use clean utensils. Use chlorinated drinking water.
Clostridium botulinum Bacteria	Grows in anaerobic environment—canned and reduced oxygen packaged foods or soups and sauces that have been improperly cooled. Also found in honey. Produces a toxin.	Double vision and difficulties in speaking, swallowing and breathing. May result in nerve damage and life-threatening illness. Illness is called botulism. Onset is usually 12-48 hours.	Dispose of canned foods that are leaking or bulging, or are dented or damaged. Inspect vacuum-packaged foods for tears and time/temperature abuse.
Clostridium perfringens Bacteria	Naturally present in the soil. Any raw food may contain the spore or bacteria. Called the "cafeteria germ" because many outbreaks result from large quantities of food being held at room temperature or cooked too slowly.	Abdominal pain and diarrhea. Onset is usually 8-22 hours.	Thoroughly cook foods containing meat or poultry. Maintain food at safe temperatures. Cool foods quickly by dividing into small, shallow containers. Use ice as an ingredient, use an ice bath, or use a blast chiller. Reheat refrigerated foods adequately.
Listeria monocytogenes Bacteria	Commonly found in the intestines of animals and humans, in milk, soil, and leafy vegetables. Also found in unpasteurized dairy products and processed meals.	In adults: sudden onset of fever, chills, headache, backache, abdominal pain, and diarrhea. In newborns: may cause respiratory distress, refusal to drink, and vomiting. Can cause miscarriage or stillbirth in pregnant women. Onset 3-70 days.	Avoid unpasteurized milk and dairy products. Cook ground meats thoroughly. Maintain food temperature out of the hazard zone. Bacteria may grow at refrigerated temperatures, so follow use-by and sell-by dates on processed foods.
Salmonella enteritidis Bacteria	Often found in meat and poultry products. Can survive in frozen food and grow with or without oxygen. Common cause is poor personal hygiene or cross-contamination.	Nausea, vomiting, cramps, and fever. Onset is within 12-36 hours. Can be fatal to high-risk groups, such as the elderly.	Avoid serving raw eggs or undercooked poultry. Never pool eggs. Use pasteurized egg products. Sanitize work surfaces and utensils. Cook food thoroughly.
Shiga toxin-producing *Escherichia coli* (STEC) Bacteria	Ground beef has been implicated in several severe outbreaks. Beef was often contaminated during processing and then mishandled during preparation. Also found in raw seed sprouts, lettuce, unpasteurized milk.	Produces a toxin which causes hemorrhagic colitis. Symptoms include abdominal cramps, watery diarrhea, nausea, vomiting, and low-grade fever. Acute kidney failure is a possible complication. Onset is usually 3-8 days.	Cook ground beef to 155°F for 15 seconds or more. Reheat properly. Use good sanitation and hygiene practices. Store and hold foods properly.

Continued

Figure 19.3
Common Foodborne Pathogens *(Continued...)*

TYPE	SOURCE	SYMPTOMS AND COMPLICATIONS	PREVENTION
Shigella Bacteria	An infected foodservice employee (carrier) or contaminated water supply are frequently cited sources. Prepared salads, gravies, and milk have been implicated.	Symptoms include diarrhea, fever, chills, and dehydration. Onset is usually within 12-50 hours.	Ensure a safe source of water. Restrict foodservice employees with infectious disease from the foodservice operation. Ensure good personal hygiene.
Staphylococcus aureus Bacteria	Illness is caused by a toxin. Improperly sanitized equipment and poor handwashing practices are culprits. Ham, cold meats, custards, cream-filled desserts are implicated foods.	Nausea, vomiting, and abdominal cramps. Can be fatal to elderly, infants, and other high-risk populations. Onset 1-6 hours.	Keep food out of the hazard zone by storing and cooking properly. Ensure good personal hygiene. Do not allow employees with infected cuts to handle food.
Yersinia enterocolitica Bacteria	Found in meats, oysters, fish, and raw milk. Poor sanitation and food preparation practices contribute to outbreaks.	Fever, headache, nausea, abdominal pain, and diarrhea. Onset 24-48 hours.	Heat food thoroughly to destroy the bacteria. Practice effective handwashing.
Giardia Bacteria	Found in contaminated water, infected food handlers, possibly fresh produce.	Diarrhea, abdominal cramps, bloating, weight loss, or malabsorption. Typical onset is 1-2 weeks after contact; may last 6 weeks or much longer. Person may have no symptoms.	Practice proper handwashing and good personal hygiene. Use approved water sources.
Anisakis Parasite	Roundworm found in fish, transmitted through ingestion of raw or partially cooked marine foods.	Can be painful and is often misdiagnosed as appendicitis, Crohn's disease or gastric ulcer. Can require surgery to remove the parasite.	Cook marine foods thoroughly to destroy the parasite.
Trichinella spiralis Parasite	Roundworm found in pork and wild game. Illness caused by consuming pork that was not thoroughly cooked.	Muscle pain and fever.	Thoroughly cook pork to destroy parasites.
Hepatitis A Virus	Virus is transmitted from one person to another through food. Water, shellfish and salads are frequently implicated foods.	Fever, abdominal pain, loss of appetite and jaundice. Typical incubation time is 10-15 days, but can be up to 50 days.	Practice proper handwashing and good personal hygiene. Restrict infected persons from foodservice operation.
Norovirus Virus	Contaminated shellfish or foods washed in contaminated water. Employees infected with the virus.	Nausea, vomiting, diarrhea and abdominal pain.	Avoid serving raw shellfish. Observe good personal hygiene and cooking practices.
Vibrio vulnificus Bacteria	Contaminated shellfish, especially from warm seawater.	Fever, skin lesions, collapse, cystic shock.	Avoid serving raw shellfish.

Figure 19.4
Conditions for Bacterial Growth: Food, Oxygen, Temperature, Time, Water, Acidity (FOTTWA)

Food	Food must contain appropriate nutrients for growth. Bacteria generally require protein and carbohydrates.
Oxygen	Some bacteria require oxygen (aerobic). Some bacteria cannot tolerate oxygen (anaerobic). Others grow with or without oxygen (facultative).
Temperature	Temperature is probably the most critical factor in the growth of bacteria. The hazard zone of 41°F-135°F is the range in which microorganisms grow and produce toxins most rapidly.
Time	A single bacterial cell can multiply into 1 million cells in 5 hours under ideal conditions. A general rule is that food in the hazard zone for 4 or more hours may be unsafe.
Water	Moisture is measured based on water activity (available water or a_w). Pathogens generally grow in foods with an a_w value greater than 0.85.
Acidity	Many pathogens tend to prefer conditions that are near a pH of 4.3-7.5, which is neutral or slightly acid.

Time and temperature control for safety (TCS) is needed to prevent the growth of pathogens or the formation of toxins in foods. Some examples of these TCS foods include meat, poultry, eggs, fish, seafood, cut melons, raw seed sprouts, garlic/oil mixtures, baked potatoes, cooked plant foods such as beans or rice, and some fresh vegetables (e.g., lettuce, tomatoes). These foods typically contain the nutrients, available water, and acidity levels that bacteria require for growth. Many plant foods are TCS. In fact, foodborne illness outbreaks over recent years have been traced to plant foods such as chopped parsley, lettuce, spinach, fresh berries, green onions, tomatoes, fruit juices, and other products.

> Shell eggs that have been treated to destroy possible Salmonella bacteria are omitted from the list of TCS. These are often called pasteurized shell eggs.

The 2017 FDA Food Code definition of TCS emphasizes the fact that TCS requires control of both time and temperature to control hazards. The old definition targeted foods that might support "rapid and progressive growth" of pathogens. Today, however, "rapid" is not as meaningful. Pathogens do not need to grow rapidly to create illness. Prolonged, progressive growth, such as that of Listeria bacteria in lunch meats or hot dogs held under refrigeration for extended periods of time, is enough to cause illness.

Danger Zone

An awareness of Food, Oxygen, Temperature, Time, Water, Acidity (FOTTWA) is the first step towards understanding how to prevent the growth of harmful bacteria. Many food protection practices involve controlling temperatures. The temperature range in which most bacteria grow rapidly is 41°F-140°F, called the **danger zone**.

The CDM, CFPP can help minimize bacterial growth during preparation and service by controlling the time food is in a temperature range favorable to bacterial growth. In general, temperature control means keeping cold food cold and hot food hot, while

GLOSSARY

Danger Zone
The temperature range in which most bacteria grow rapidly (41°F - 135°F)

minimizing the time the food is in the hazard zone. In fact, a potentially hazardous food that is allowed to remain in the hazard zone for a cumulative time of four hours or more during all phases of receiving, storage, preparation, and service is considered unsafe to eat.

Virus

A **virus** is the smallest and simplest known form of life. Viruses can be transmitted from a dining service employee to a foodservice client. They do not grow or multiply in food. Viruses need a living host such as a human, an animal, or a fish in which to grow. Shellfish can also be sources of foodborne viruses. Preventing viral foodborne illness requires the health screening of employees, the removal of employees with viral illnesses from the work schedule, sound personal hygiene habits, and careful selection of marine foods.

Parasite

A **parasite** is a small or microscopic organism that lives within another organism called a host. The parasite can be transmitted from animals to humans when the food is not cooked thoroughly. For example, Trichinella is a parasite found in pork (rarely seen in commercially grown pork in the United States and Europe), and wild game. The parasite is actually a roundworm that causes an infection (trichinosis) in the person who consumes it. Cooking pork to the proper temperature and holding that temperature for a recommended minimum time destroys the parasite.

Fungi

Molds and yeasts are types of **fungi**. Some play a role in food processing. For example, yeasts are used in the production of bread while molds are used in the processing of cheese. However, molds and yeasts can also be a threat to food safety. Molds grow well on most types of food and appear as brightly colored, fuzzy growth. Certain molds produce a toxin which can result in a foodborne illness. Toxins produced by fungi, called mycotoxins, may be found in dry and/or acidic foods. Guidelines for handling food that has mold appear in Figure 19.5.

Yeasts

Yeasts are not a significant cause of foodborne illness but they can still contaminate food and cause it to spoil. Yeasts prefer sweet, liquid foods and are well known for fermenting cider and fruit juices. An indication of yeast spoilage is a fermenting, alcoholic smell, and discoloration.

Natural Toxins

Toxins can occur naturally in foods such as fish, shellfish, mushrooms, and certain plants. A foodborne illness called ciguatera (pronounced "sig-wah-terrra") is caused by consuming fish that has, in turn, ingested toxins present in algae. Shellfish can also be toxic if they consumed poisoned algae. An example of shellfish-related illness

---

GLOSSARY

Virus
Source of foodborne illness that does not grow in food but is transmitted from people, animals, or fish/shellfish

Parasite
A small organism, such as Trichinella, that lives within another living organism, such as in pork or wild game

Fungi
Molds or yeast that can cause an illness or produce a toxin that causes the illness

---

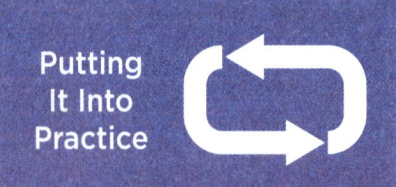

1. At a picnic, the potato salad was served for lunch at 11 am. The leftovers were then kept on the picnic table until it was time to go home around 4 pm. The potato salad was then put in the refrigerator so it could be eaten the next day. Should it be served or thrown away? Why?

Figure 19.5
Guidelines for Handling Foods Containing Mold

Some foods that develop mold must be discarded. Other foods can be used, but if so, the mold must first be cut out and then at least an inch of the food under and around it.

DISCARD	CUT AND USE
• Cucumbers • Tomatoes • Spinach, Lettuce, Leafy Greens • Bananas, Peaches, Melons • Berries • Breads, Cakes, Rolls, Flour • Soft Cheeses like Brie or Mozzarella • Lunch Meat and Cheese (slices) • Yogurt, Tub Spreads, Cream Cheese • Canned Foods • Peanut Butter • Juices • Cooked Leftovers	• Bell Peppers • Broccoli, Cauliflower • Cabbage • Garlic, Onions • Potatoes • Turnips • Zucchini, Winter Squash • Apples, Pears • Hard Cheeses like Cheddar or Swiss

is paralytic shellfish poisoning. Scombroid poisoning is the result of eating certain varieties of fish that release a toxin called histamine when they begin to spoil. Mushroom poisoning can result from eating certain varieties of mushrooms. Generally these toxins are not destroyed by cooking. So the best protection is prevention: purchase seafood and mushrooms only from approved sources.

Chemical Hazards

Chemical hazards include pesticides that are sprayed on food, preservatives used to maintain food, toxic metals in cooking equipment and utensils, and chemical cleaning materials used in the foodservice operation.

Preservatives and Food Additives

Some chemicals are added to food to help preserve the quality. Sulfites are one example that is used for fresh fruits and vegetables, shrimp, lobster, and wine. Sulfites may cause an allergic reaction in some people so sulfiting agents added to a product in the processing plant must be declared on labeling. Do not use a sulfiting agent on raw produce.

Other chemicals added to enhance food quality that may cause allergic reactions are nitrites/nitrates in meats and monosodium glutamate (MSG) used in Asian or Latin American foods.

Allergens

Food allergies are a separate, but classified as chemical, type of food-related illness warranting the attention of CDM, CFPPs. The FDA Food Code has added an emphasis on food allergies: "Food allergy is an increasing food safety and public health issue affecting approximately 4% of the U.S. population or twelve million Americans."

The 2017 FDA Food Code lists the following topics that managers need to know regarding food allergies:

- The eight major food allergens
- Food allergen ingredient identities and labeling
- How to avoid cross-contamination during food preparation and service

A food allergy is an adverse reaction to food that involves the immune system. An allergic reaction depends on the allergen, a specific protein in the food that triggers an immune system response. For example, the protein in peanuts or eggs may function as an allergen for sensitive individuals. Figure 19.6 shows the foods associated with the most common food allergies. The best control measure to use in the foodservice department is to prevent cross-contamination between allergenic and non-allergenic ingredients.

Figure 19.6
The Most Common Food Allergens

- Milk
- Eggs
- Fish
- Shellfish (e.g., crab, lobster, shrimp)
- Tree Nuts (e.g., almonds, pecans, walnuts)
- Wheat
- Peanuts
- Soybeans
- A food ingredient derived from one of these: peanut oil, baked goods containing eggs, sauces containing wheat flours, etc.

Pesticides

Chemicals used to keep produce grown in the United States free from plant diseases and insect infestations are regulated by the government and should not cause foodborne illness when applied at recommended levels. But some foods originating from international sources with less government regulation and monitoring should be checked. Remember to wash all fresh fruits and vegetables to remove chemical residues before serving.

Toxic Metals

Metals that can cause foodborne illness include cadmium, antimony, lead, zinc, and copper. Antimony, zinc, and copper may cause contamination after prolonged contact with acid foods. Carefully select foodservice equipment to control this hazard.

2. Raw meat has been placed on the refrigerator shelf above the raw vegetables. What type of contamination would this be?

Cleaning Supplies

Cleaning products may also cause contamination when improperly used or stored. Cleaning supplies and other toxic materials must be stored separately from the food preparation and service areas. Never use a food container to store chemicals, and never use chemical containers to store food. Containers used for cleaning—such as buckets and pails—should be clearly marked and dedicated for use in cleaning only.

Physical Hazards

Physical hazards are foreign materials that enter the food accidentally. Some examples are glass fragments, pieces of bone, metal shavings, staples from produce crates, and other objects that fall into food and cause serious physical harm or injury. Methods or techniques to prevent contamination of food from physical hazards include: visually inspecting food during preparation, maintaining equipment in good repair, keeping food covered to prevent fragments from falling into it, and discarding food that has been exposed to broken dishware.

Foodborne Illness Prevention

Foodborne illness is a real and present danger. This places a great responsibility on every CDM, CFPP and food production and dining services staff member to protect clients. It is essential to take steps to protect food and control hazards. The steps follow the movement of food throughout your operation—from purchasing ingredients to receiving and storing; to preparing and serving food; to managing leftovers.

United States government research indicates that the five top causes of foodborne illness outbreak are:

- Improper holding temperatures
- Contaminated equipment
- Poor personal hygiene
- Inadequate cooking
- Food from unsafe sources

A CDM, CFPP must ensure safe practices in all phases of foodservice management. To know what a safe practice can include, use the Food and Drug Administration (FDA) set of food protection standards, called the FDA Food Code, which provides the basis for this chapter.

Anyone managing a food production operation must be aware of the constant hazards that can result in foodborne illness. In the U.S. today, foodborne illness is a serious public health concern. In some cases, failure to observe food safety practices can result in illness, hospitalization, or even the death of a client. While the responsibility is grave, we fortunately have the knowledge of the factors causing foodborne illness and the means to control them. This is the charge of every CDM, CFPP.

The movement of food through the various stages of purchasing, receiving, storage, preparation, transport, holding, service, cooling, and reheating is called the **flow of food**. Each step in this flow presents hazards and challenges for food protection. In this section, we will focus on the latter segment of this flow, beginning with food preparation.

> **GLOSSARY**
>
> **Physical Hazards**
> Foreign materials that enter food accidentally
>
> **Flow of Food**
> Movement of food through a food production facility including purchasing, receiving, storage, preparation, transport, holding, service, cooling, and reheating

Preparing Safe Food

Temperature is a critical variable and must be monitored at each step in the flow of food. To ensure safe handling, keep temperature logs in all storage, preparation, and service areas. Involve all staff members in monitoring temperatures and be sure that all staff are trained in the proper procedures for recording food temperatures.

Time is also an important control for food protection. Label all food items with the latest time for use when moving it from storage to preparation areas. Once food has been removed from a monitored, temperature-controlled environment, serve or dispose of it within four hours. For instance, if meals are served through room service and the lunch entrée was prepared at 10:00 a.m. for a room service request, it must be served or refrigerated properly before 2:00 p.m.

Dispose of the food if it is in unmarked containers or if the expiration date has since passed. Communicate food labeling and monitoring practices to all members of the food production and dining services team.

Cross-Contamination

Cross-contamination is the transfer of pathogens from any item to food. The source of contamination may be a non-food item, such as a work surface, another food, or the hands of a foodservice employee. Food production and dining services professionals must take steps to prevent cross-contamination during all phases of food preparation and service. Figure 19.7 identifies examples of how cross-contamination can occur. To prevent cross-contamination:

- Follow proper procedures for cleaning and sanitizing equipment and utensils.
- Observe handwashing practices and standards for glove use.
- As much as possible, isolate raw foods from ready-to-eat or prepared foods in all phases of the flow of food.

Raw fruits and vegetables must be thoroughly washed in water to remove soil and other contaminants. They should be washed before being cut, combined with other ingredients, cooked, served, or offered for service in a ready-to-eat form.

Pathogens like Salmonella or chemicals such as pesticides may be present on the outside surface of fruits and vegetables. The FDA Food Code states that "All fresh produce, except commercially washed, pre-cut, or bagged produce, must be thoroughly washed under running, potable water before eating, cutting, or cooking." This is required even if you plan to peel the produce prior to eating. If using pre-washed, bagged produce in an opened bag, it must be considered a potentially hazardous food.

GLOSSARY

Cross-Contamination
The transfer of pathogens from any item or human to food

Figure 19.7
Examples of How Cross-Contamination May Occur

- A foodservice staff member prepares tuna salad while wearing gloves and then puts a pan of macaroni and cheese into the warmer without changing gloves and washing hands.
- A cook dices beef for stew on a cutting board and then chops onions on the same board without cleaning and sanitizing the surface between jobs.
- A cook uses the same spatula to put raw burgers on the grill and to remove cooked burgers from the grill.
- A foodservice staff member allows raw egg mixture to splash over prepared foods near the steam table.
- An employee picks up trash from the floor and then enters the walk-in refrigerator without first washing hands.

Ice that is used for displaying fresh produce or cooked shellfish cannot be used further for cooking or service.

Thawing

Foods must be thawed in a manner that would avoid placing the food in the hazard zone for an excessive amount of time. Frozen food should never be thawed at room temperature. The following are four options for thawing food safely:

- Thaw gradually under refrigeration that maintains the food temperature at 41°F or less.
- Thaw completely submerged under cold, potable, running water (70°F or less), with water pressure sufficient to continuously agitate any food particles off the surface. With this method, thawing time should be less than two hours, or until food reaches 41°F. (This method may not be effective for thawing large pieces of meat.)
- Thaw during the cooking process by cooking frozen food in the oven in a continuous process.
- Thaw and cook single-service items completely in the microwave from a frozen state and then cook immediately.

Food that is removed from the freezer to thaw gradually under refrigeration should be marked to indicate the date it was removed from the freezer. The food should be consumed seven days or less after that date (when the food was removed from the freezer) and held at 41°F or below.

Slacking

Slacking is the process of moderating the temperature of frozen foods before preparation (such as in deep-fat frying). For example, when deep-fat frying chicken nuggets that are at -10°F, bring their temperature up to 25°F first. Regulations about slacking TCS foods vary from one jurisdiction to another.

The FDA Food Code says that if slacking is used you should:

- Maintain the temperature of the food being slacked under refrigeration at or below 41°F.
- Maintain the product at any temperature, as long as it remains frozen.

Cooking

Cooking is a very important step in the flow of food. Failure to cook TCS food thoroughly can cause foodborne illness. Cooking food thoroughly destroys most (but not all) biological hazards.

For TCS foods, the FDA Food Code suggests cooking standards that combine time and temperature. An **endpoint temperature** is the temperature a food reaches at the end of cooking.

Endpoint temperature should be measured with a calibrated measuring device such as a thermometer or thermocouple. Measure in the part of the food that is heated last—usually the center or thickest part of the food. See Figure 19.8 for more tips on measuring temperatures.

After using a thermometer probe, always clean and sanitize it with an isopropyl alcohol wipe. The Food Code stipulates that a thermometer is like a utensil because it contacts food and therefore requires sanitization.

> **GLOSSARY**
>
> **Endpoint Temperature**
> The temperature a food reaches at the end of cooking

Figure 19.8
Measuring a Food Temperature

Food Item
- Insert the thermometer into geometric center or into thickest portion.
- Insert away from the bone, fat, or gristle on a food product.
- Insert sideways into small items.

Food Packaging
- Fold bag over the thermometer or probe for bulk milk or liquids.
- Place between frozen packages of food.

General Guidelines
- Wait 5-10 seconds for an accurate reading.
- Sanitize thermometer after each use.
- Submerge until at least two inches deep in milk and other liquids.

Reaching a specified temperature alone is not adequate for ensuring descruction of pathogens. Cooks should be instructed to hold the endpoint temperature for a specified length of time, as shown in Figure 19.9. For mixed foods, such as casseroles and soups, find the ingredient with the most stringent time and temperature standard, and apply that standard.

Cooks should monitor and record cooking times and temperatures in a log, as shown in Figure 19.10, found in the Supplemental Material.

Some TCS foods pose special concerns. In cooking pork and game animals it is imperative to destroy the possible parasites. Ground meats and seafood have an increased surface area resulting from grinding. This creates more opportunity for pathogens to flourish. Stuffed foods, such as ravioli or stuffed turkey, also provide a favorable breeding ground for foodborne pathogens. The FDA time and temperature standards reflect these concerns.

Highly Susceptible Populations

If serving a highly susceptible population, be aware that both eggs and juices receive special attention in the Food Code. Generally, you should avoid using fresh, shell eggs for food preparation. Instead, use pasteurized egg products for quantity cooking. Pasteurized in-shell eggs are fine for both single-service and quantity production. (The use of shell eggs, pasteurized shell eggs, and liquid eggs was discussed in Chapter 4.)

For highly susceptible populations, the Food Code cites the FDA and CDC health advisories to avoid eating fresh seed sprouts, such as mung bean or alfalfa sprouts. It also stipulates that raw or undercooked meats, such as raw, marinated fish, soft-cooked eggs, or rare meat may not be served. (In foodservice operations serving a general population, this may be permitted as long as the operation provides a consumer advisory about the associated risks.)

Due to the incident and impact of E. coli on young children, a children's menu may not list undercooked hamburger or other ground meat.

Figure 19.9
Minimum Food Temperatures and Holding Times Required for Reheating Foods for Hot Holding

FOOD ITEM	MINIMUM TEMPERATURE	MINIMUM HOLDING TIME at the Specified Temperature	MAXIMUM TIME to Reach Minimum Temperature
¶ 3-403.11(A) and (D) Food that is cooked, cooled, and reheated	74°C (165°F)	15 seconds	2 hours
¶ 3-403.11(B) and (D) Food that is reheated in a microwave oven	74°C (165°F)	and hold for 2 minutes after reheating	2 hours
¶ 3-403.11(C) and (D) Food that is taken from a commercially processed, hermetically sealed container or intact package	57°C (135°F)	No time specified	2 hours
Roasts: Option A ¶ 3-403.11(E) Unsliced portions of meat roasts cooked as specified under ¶ 3-401.11(B)	Same oven parameters and minimum time and temperature conditions as specified under ¶ 3-401.11(B)	Same oven parameters and minimum time and temperature conditions as specified under ¶ 3-401.11(B)	Not applicable
Roasts: Option B ¶ 3-403.11(E) Unsliced portions of meat roasts cooked as specified under ¶ 3-403.11(A)	74°C (165°F)	15 seconds	2 hours

Source: 2017 Food Code pg. 751

Microwave Cooking

When preparing food in a microwave:

- Rotate or stir the food item throughout or at the midpoint of cooking to distribute the heat evenly.
- Cover to retain surface moisture.
- Cook to a temperature of at least 165°F in all parts of the food item.
- Allow to stand covered for two minutes before serving to obtain temperature equilibrium.

Serving Safe Food

During service, a combination of time and temperature is used to prevent or slow down the microbial growth. TCS foods must be held out of the hazard zone as much as possible, as shown in Figure 19.11. Figure 19.12 illustrates examples of monitoring temperature during preparation and service.

View the Supplemental Material for this chapter for Figure 19.10, Endpoint Temperature Log.

Putting It Into Practice

3. The cook is preparing whole chickens for dinner. How does he ensure that the chickens are cooked and safe to eat? What tools can he use to document time and temperature?

Figure 19.11
Safe Food Handling: Food Preparation

Figure 19.12
Monitoring Temperatures During Preparation and Service

Image courtesy of Cooper-Atkins

View the Supplemental Material for this chapter for Figure 19.13, Holding Temperature Log.

Figure 19.3 in the Supplemental Materials features a log which can help employees monitor and document holding temperatures, which should be measured at least every two hours.

Hot Holding

Hot foods must be held at 135°F or above, with the exception of roasts cooked to a time and temperature as shown in Figure 19.9. Stir foods during holding to redistribute heat throughout the food. Keep food containers covered to retain heat and to prevent environmental contaminants from entering the food.

Steam tables and food warmers are examples of equipment that may be used to retain heat and control food temperatures. Steam tables are not meant to cook foods—only to hold them after cooking. Food warmers (also called "hot-boxes") are usually equipped with an ambient thermometer. Steam tables usually have a temperature control knob but generally do not measure the actual food temperature. When holding hot foods for service, measure the food temperature at least every two hours. If the food temperature falls into an unsafe range, immediately follow the procedures for reheating previously cooked food. When restocking hot food products, finish one pan completely before bringing in a refill; do not pour new product on top of older product.

Cold Holding

To slow down the growth of bacteria, cold food must be held below 41°F. Special considerations are required for using ice as a coolant. Packaged food should not be stored in direct contact with ice or water if the entry of water is possible due to the packaging or its location in the ice or water. Ice that has been used as a coolant may not be used as food or food ingredient. Unpackaged food may not be stored in direct contact with undrained ice. Exceptions to this include:

- Whole, raw fruits or vegetables—such as celery or carrot sticks or whole potatoes—may be immersed in ice or water.
- Raw chicken and raw fish that are received immersed in ice in shipping containers may remain in that condition while in storage awaiting preparation or service.

During holding and service, utensils should be kept in the food. Utensil handles should be kept above the top of the food and the container. Between uses, a utensil can be stored in water that is at least 135°F. During service, food on display must be protected from contamination. During transport, the food must be covered and kept out of the hazard zone.

Self-Service Food Bars

Self-service food bars, such as buffets and salad bars, present special food protection risks. Client actions and habits create the potential for contamination. You need to label all the food items in self-service areas to discourage the clients from sampling food items. Sneeze guards must be used on service lines, salad bars, and display cases. Also, self-service food bars should be monitored by the dining services employees trained in food protection practices. Each client is required to use a clean plate for each food item from a food bar to prevent contamination from soiled dishes and utensils.

Ready-to-Eat Foods

The FDA Food Code has specific guidelines for serving ready-to-eat food without additional preparation to achieve food safety such as bakery items (breads, rolls, cakes, pies), fruits and vegetables that are served raw, or dried meat products such as jerky or beef sticks. Self-service of these foods must include utensils or effective dispensing methods that protect the food from contamination.

Cooling

Large food items such as roasts, turkeys, and large containers of rice, refried beans, or soup/stews take longer to cool because of the bulk of the food. According to the FDA Food Code, TCS food should be cooled from 140°F to 41°F within a total maximum time of six hours. The first step of this process is to bring the food temperature down to 70°F within the first two hours.

If the food, such as tuna from a can, is at room temperature, you need to cool it down to 41°F within four hours. Figure 19.14 identifies methods for rushing the cooling process. Once cooled, the food should be covered, dated, and labeled according to the date marking standards.

Figure 19.14
Proper Cooling Methods

- Place food in a shallow container (2" deep) to increase the surface area and reduce the cooling time.
- Divide a large food mass into several smaller masses (e.g., a 20 lb. roast divided into five 4 lb. masses).
- Stir the food in a container which is placed in an ice water bath.
- Use rapid cooling equipment such as a blast chiller.
- Add ice as an ingredient.

Date Marking

TCS food prepared in the food production operation and held at or below 41°F should be labeled at the time of preparation with the date by which the food should be consumed. Prepared foods should be used within seven days or less of preparation if held at 41°F or below.

The practice of date marking is detailed in the FDA Food Code. When a date is marked on a food product, it means that the food must be used or discarded by that date. A key objective of this practice is to address the time element of bacterial growth. The longer a TCS food remains in storage, the more chance that the Listeria bacteria will grow—and they can do so even at or below 41°F.

Date marking applies not only to leftovers. Generally, after opening a package of TCS food it must be marked with the date. The food should be used or discarded within seven days, starting with the day the package was opened as Day 1.

Certain products, such as hard cheeses or cheeses that contain up to 50% moisture (e.g., cheddar, Parmesan, gorgonzola, jack), yogurt, sour cream, buttermilk, and certain shelf-stable processed meat products are exempt from the date-marking procedures. Date-marking guidelines also do not apply to deli salads obtained from a food processing plant, because they already apply the processes to prevent bacterial growth. Instead, refer to the manufacturer's use-by date. Remember that if a TCS food in storage is not maintained at or below 41°F, it should be discarded.

Reheating

Frozen, ready-to-eat food taken from commercially prepared, intact packages must be heated to at least 135°F for hot holding. Reheating for hot holding should be done as rapidly as possible.

A previously cooked food (a food that was prepared, cooked, and cooled in the food production operation) must be reheated to an internal temperature of 165°F for a minimum of 15 seconds. This process must be completed within two hours.

Reserving of food is also governed by the FDA Food Code. Food that is unused or returned by the client may not be offered to others. If the food is individually packaged, such as crackers, salt, pepper, or sugar packets, it may be served again if the packaging is in good condition. No food, including secure packets, may be served again if it is returned from clients in medical isolation or quarantine.

HACCP Basics

Hazard Analysis Critical Control Point (HACCP) is important in food protection. The HACCP system is a preventative food safety program that greatly reduces the likelihood of foodborne illness. HACCP (pronounced has-sip) was developed years ago to ensure a safe food supply for astronauts. It is now being implemented throughout the food processing and service industries.

HACCP uses a systematic approach to identify, evaluate, and control the food safety hazards. It focuses on the flow of food rather than on individual procedures. A CDM, CFPP who uses HACCP principles in combination with basic sanitation and a solid employee training program can prevent, eliminate or reduce the occurrence of foodborne illness in his/her facility.

HACCP builds on essential food safety practices that should already be in place. These are called standard operating procedures (SOPs). They include the sanitation guidelines outlined in the FDA Food Code and discussed in other chapters of this book—such as the practices for:

- Purchasing, receiving, and storing food
- Personal hygiene policies
- Thawing, cooking, holding, and cooling food
- Cleaning and sanitizing

They are prerequisites for implementing an effective plan. Without them, any HACCP plan could fail.

Although using HACCP is not directly a part of the Food Code, the FDA recommends implementing it throughout the food industry. HACCP plans may be required in food production operations, processing juice in-house, preparing pureed food, or operating a cook-chill system. Furthermore, school foodservice operations participating in the National School Lunch Program (NSLP) are required to have the HACCP plans in place. The local health department may also require implementation of a HACCP system.

The success of HACCP is dependent on a number of variables. CDM, CFPPs learn the principles and concepts of the HACCP system and can demonstrate to effectively use it by applying their knowledge. In turn, it is essential that the managers educate and train all members of their food production and dining services team on the principles of HACCP and their role in its implementation.

4. While making meat sauce for the spaghetti, what are the steps that are taken to thaw the ground beef and hot hold the meat sauce at the right temperature after cooking? How would the meat sauce be best reheated for use the next day?

Implementing a HACCP System

A HACCP system revolves around seven principles, summarized in Figure 19.15.

1. Analyze Hazards

Identify the hazards associated with foods in recipes and on menus. These items could be hazardous due to the ingredients, the processes involved in preparation, the holding and handling during service, or their ultimate use. Hazards may vary from one food production operation to another—even with the production of the same menu item. Differences include:

- Ingredient sources
- Product formulations
- Processing or packaging techniques
- Preparation methods and equipment
- Storage and service plans
- Who will be consuming the food
- Employees' understanding of safe food practices

While HACCP is concerned with the safety of all food, particular attention should be given to TCS foods which can support progressive bacterial growth or the development of toxins. It's also important to examine the flow of food through the food production system. As you track each TCS food, find out where the hazards are. Check what

Figure 19.15
Seven Principles of HACCP

#	Principle
1	Analyze hazards.
2	Identify critical control points (CCPs).
3	Establish critical limits for critical control points (CCPs).
4	Establish procedures for monitoring critical control points (CCPs).
5	Establish corrective actions.
6	Establish procedures to verify that the system is working.
7	Establish a record-keeping system.

Putting It Into Practice

5. What would be the CCPs in a beef lasagna recipe?

dangerous microorganisms have the opportunity to grow. Developing a flow chart or diagram of food movement can help identify hazards and control points.

2. Identify Critical Control Points

The parts in the flow of food at which a potential hazard can be controlled or eliminated are called **control points**. These occur throughout the flow of food, such as during receiving, storage, thawing, cooking, holding, and chilling, and are generally addressed through standard operating procedures. For each control point, find out if the loss of control can lead to an unacceptable health risk. This is called a **critical control point (CCP)**. To determine whether a step is a CCP, refer to the CCP Decision Tree (Figure 19.17). Critical control points vary depending on the food item being prepared and the preparation techniques being used. Often, cooking to the recommended time and temperature standard becomes a CCP. However, in a cook-chill operation, blast chilling food to a recommended temperature within a specified time is also a CCP.

Following the CCP Decision Tree, there is generally only one CCP for any food or menu item. However, advice varies: some HACCP examples include only one step in the flow of food and designated as a CCP while in other models there are several. Whether one or several, either are acceptable because you are implementing critical control. However, beware of designating too many steps as CCPs. This can make the system too complex for employees to carry out. Instead, review the standard operating procedures and use them as control points (not CCPs with documentation requirements) as appropriate.

3. Establish Critical Limits for Critical Control Points

There must be a **critical limit** for each CCP identified. A critical limit defines the limits of certain properties that are accepted for a given product at a given stage in the flow of food. It is observable and measurable. For a cooked food, a critical limit might specify minimum internal temperature for the endpoint of cooking, along with the minimum time that temperature must be held. The standards used for critical limits should come from the local food code, the FDA Food Code, or a similar guideline.

4. Establish Procedures for Monitoring Critical Control Points

Determine how and by whom CCPs will be monitored. Monitoring procedures may be included in standardized recipes. Observe and measure to determine whether critical limits are met. Critical limits may also be included in recipes, and food production personnel should be required to measure all CCPs and document them in HACCP logs.

5. Establish Corrective Actions

When monitoring shows that a critical limit has not been met, there must be an established procedure to follow. These procedures, called **corrective actions**, are specific to each food production operation. Corrective actions should be clearly written and understood by food production personnel. For example, when baking meatloaf

> **GLOSSARY**
>
> **Control Point**
> Point in the flow of food where a hazard can be controlled: a step can be taken to minimize the risk of foodborne illness
>
> **Critical Control Point (CCP)**
> Step in the flow of food which, if not controlled, could lead to an unacceptable health risk for consumers of the food
>
> **Critical Limit**
> Specified limits or characteristics of a physical, chemical, or biological nature that help you measure whether you have adequately controlled a hazard at a CCP
>
> **Corrective Actions**
> The procedure to follow when monitoring shows that a critical limit has not been met

6. You are monitoring the HACCP plan for your facility. What would some time and temperature records include that need to be maintained?

Figure 19.16
Analyzing Hazards: Questions to Ask

- Does the food contain any sensitive ingredients that may present known hazards (e.g., Salmonella, Staphylococcus, aflatoxin)?
- What are the sources (e.g., geographical region, specific supplier)?
- Does the process include a controllable processing step that destroys pathogens? If so, which pathogens?
- Does the microbial population change during the normal time the food is stored prior to consumption?
- Does the layout of the facility provide an adequate separation of raw materials from ready-to-eat (RTE) foods if this is important to food safety? If not, what hazards should be considered as possible contaminants of the RTE products?
- Will the equipment provide the time-temperature control that is necessary for safe food?
- Is the equipment properly sized for the volume of food that will be processed?
- Can the equipment be sufficiently controlled so that the variation in performance will be within the tolerances required to produce a safe food?
- Is the equipment reliable or is it prone to frequent breakdowns?
- Is the equipment designed so that it can be easily cleaned and sanitized?
- To what degree will normal equipment wear affect the likely occurrence of physical hazard (e.g., metal) in the product?
- Is the package clearly labeled "Keep Refrigerated" if this is required for safety? Does the package include instructions for the safe handling and preparation of the food by the end user?
- Is each package and case legibly and accurately coded? Does each package contain the proper label?
- Can employee health or personal hygiene practices impact the safety of the food being processed?
- Do the employees understand the process and the factors they must control to assure the preparation of safe foods?
- Will the employees inform management of a problem which could impact safety of food?
- What is the likelihood that the food will be improperly stored at the wrong temperature?
- Would an error in improper storage lead to a microbiologically unsafe food?
- Will the food be heated by the consumer?
- Will there likely be leftovers?
- Is the food intended for the general public?
- Is the food intended for consumption by a population with increased susceptibility to illness (e.g., infants, the aged, or immunocompromised individuals)?

Source: FDA

(a CCP), the critical limit is to reach 155°F for a minimum of 17 seconds. You check the temperature in the deepest part of the meatloaf at the end of cooking and it's only 140°F. A corrective action might be to return the meatloaf to the oven immediately and continue cooking to reach 155°F for 17 seconds. Other examples of corrective actions might be: contacting the CDM, CFPP for direction, reheating immediately to a specific temperature, or disposing of food that was improperly cooked.

GLOSSARY

Verification
The use of equipment to determine that the HACCP system is in place and achieving the desired objectives

6. Establish Procedures to Verify the System Is Working

Calibration of temperature monitoring devices and review of HACCP logs for accuracy and completeness will help to verify the system is fulfilling its mission to improve food safety. Review HACCP logs, records of monitoring CCPs, and corrective actions taken by staff members. Conduct random checks to ensure that CCPs are being monitored appropriately by staff and that temperature monitoring equipment is working properly. Figure 19.18 lists some activities a manager may use in the **verification** process.

Figure 19.17
Critical Control Point (CCP) Decision Tree

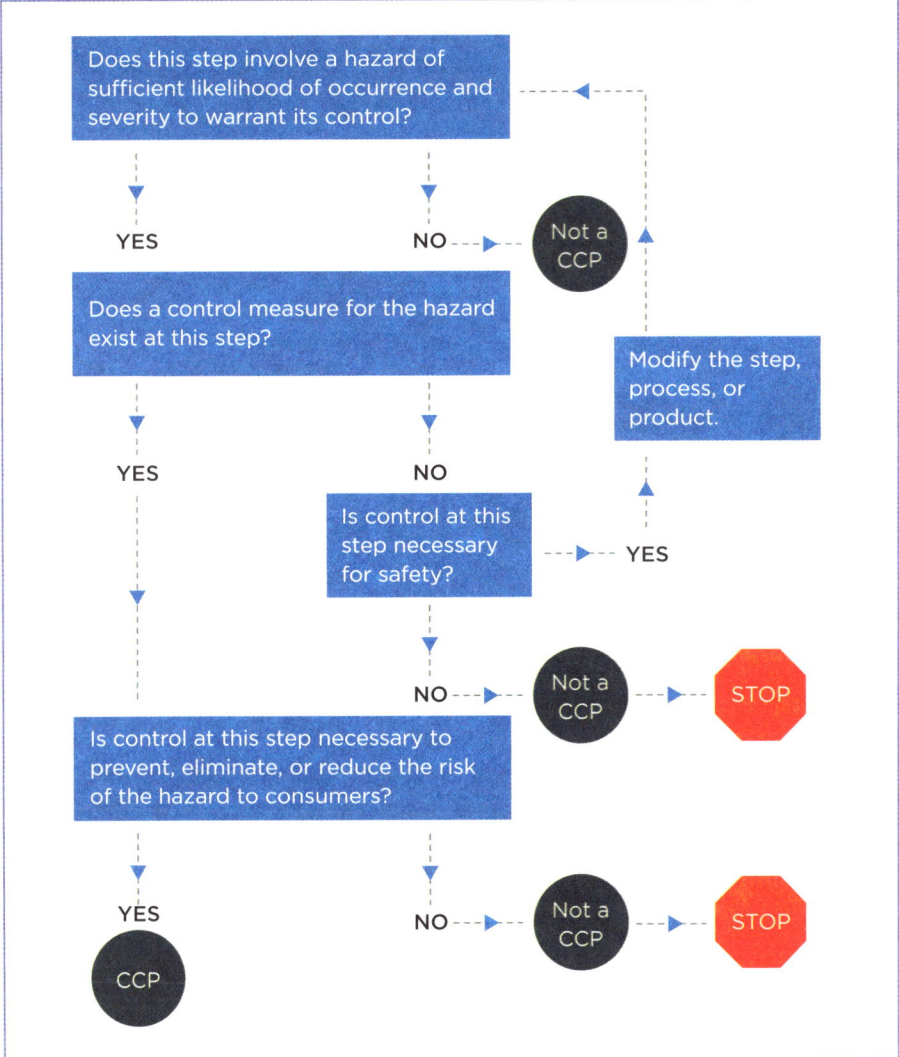

7. Establish a Record-Keeping System

A record-keeping system documents HACCP activities and includes time and temperature monitoring records. Use forms to document the flow of food products, time and temperature, and corrective actions. Maintain daily HACCP logs in a notebook accessible to all members of the food production team. The HACCP log may identify critical limits to check and include a place for employees to document corrective actions taken. Be alert to **dry lab**, the practice of entering time and temperature measurements without actually taking them. Dry lab will undermine the success of any HACCP program.

HACCP and Planning

When analyzing HACCP records, look for patterns that indicate a need for employee training and equipment repair or replacement. Sometimes HACCP information will indicate a need to change the kitchen layout, menus, ingredient selection, preparation methods, processes, or procedures. These records can provide a valuable tool for planning and refining a safe food production system. Consider the flow of food, and update the HACCP plan as changes are made.

GLOSSARY

Dry Lab
Recording temperatures without actually taking them

Figure 19.18
HACCP Verification Activities

- Establishment of appropriate verification schedules
- Review of the HACCP plan for completeness
- Confirmation of the accuracy of the flow diagram
- Review of the HACCP system to determine if the facility is operating according to the HACCP plan
- Review of CCP monitoring records
- Review of records for deviations and corrective actions
- Validation of critical limits to confirm that they are adequate to control significant hazards
- Validation of HACCP plan, including on-site review
- Review of modifications of the HACCP plan
- Sampling and testing to verify CCPs

Source: FDA

For example, HACCP logs may indicate that it is difficult to meet cooling recommendations for tuna salad. Upon review of the flow of food for tuna and mayonnaise, you realize that food preparation is starting with ingredients at room temperature. Corrective Action: Change the procedure and pre-chill potentially hazardous ingredients.

In another example, when reviewing the plans to redesign the kitchen, map out the flow of food for key menu items. The current layout presents opportunities for contamination that could be avoided: The trash room occasionally overflows into an area where fresh meats are received, and food waste from dining service is being processed very close to the cold food preparation area. Corrective Action: Work with an architect to specify that food receiving and preparation areas must be isolated from sources of contamination.

In another example, observations highlight the hazard associated with cross-contamination. Corrective Action: Use color-coded cutting boards to reinforce safe practices among employees.

The Process Approach to HACCP

In a food production operation, HACCP may take a different form than in a food processing or packaging environment. The FDA explains "The resources available to help you identify and control the risk factors common to your operation may be limited." The report advises that a "complete HACCP system" is ideal, but variations are acceptable, as long as the plan is designed to control risks and incorporate "some, if not all" of the HACCP principles. Because each set of procedures for production and service is different, "HACCP has no single correct application," according to the FDA.

7. Describe a HACCP plan for receiving frozen foods at your foodservice facility.

In a process approach, assign sets of food flow charts to process-related categories and manage them as groups. See Figure 19.19 in the Supplemental Materials for process examples. The FDA suggests three types of processes:

- **Process 1:** Food preparation without cooking, where the flow of food is: receive > store > prepare > hold > serve. Examples: salads, cold sandwiches.
- **Process 2:** Preparation for same-day service, where the flow of food is: receive > store > prepare > cook > hold > serve. Examples: baked chicken, meatloaf.
- **Process 3:** Complex food preparation, where the flow of food is: receive > store > prepare > cook > cool > reheat > hot hold > serve. Examples: casseroles in which meats or other ingredients are cooked and cooled the day before assembly, or leftovers that are reheated and served at another meal.

View the Supplemental Material for this chapter for Figure 19.19, Process Examples.

There can be variations in these processes, but they do characterize the foodborne illness risks fairly well; examples of the risks are outlined in the FDA Annex. Process 3 includes at least two trips through the hazard zone, since it carries the greatest risks. It clearly requires carefully managed temperature control, especially in the cooling and reheating steps. Date marking and storage are also important.

Target food-flow steps involving the hazard zone and apply controls to manage the hazards in all processes. For Process 1, where there is no cooking to destroy potential pathogens, controls focus more on purchasing specifications, receiving check-in, date marking, and storage time and temperature. For Process 2, cooking (endpoint temperatures) and holding will require your most active managerial control.

Processes may also emerge for menu items. A chicken salad sandwich, for example, may include elements of Process 3 (receive, store, prepare, cook, cool) and Process 1 (store, prepare, hold, serve). Figure 19.20 in the Supplemental Material illustrates examples of hazards and controls for foods prepared for same-day service.

View the Supplemental Material for this chapter for Figure 19.20, Examples of Hazards and Controls.

If foods are grouped according to their flow in the operation, mapping out a flow for each individual menu item is not required according to the FDA, adding that "a hazard analysis on individual food items is time and labor intensive and generally unnecessary." Managing the steps in a process as a SOP "achieves the same control of risk factors as preparing a HACCP plan for each individual product," suggests the report.

Summary

Food Safety is an important concern for the CDM, CFPP. Adequate training and care must be taken to ensure that food is served safely, especially to vulnerable populations. HACCP is a proactive method for managing food safety. It allows a CDM, CFPP to focus on resources where they are needed most at critical control points (CCPs) in the flow of food. Although not specifically required for most food production and dining services operations today, HACCP is a great model because it is an effective management tool for control. HACCP builds upon standard operating procedures. It requires documentation and monitoring and can be looked at as a process for the various types of facilities necessary to create a detailed HACCP flow chart for every food in order to implement.

8. Looking at Figure 19.19 in the Supplemental Materials, what is the HACCP process for a satellite kitchen?

Chapter References

RESOURCES	
Centers for Disease Control and Prevention *Food Safety*	cdc.gov/foodsafety/
FDA Food Code	fda.gov
Hazard Analysis Critical Control Points	fda.gov/food/retail-food-protection/fda-food-code
U.S. Food & Drug Administration (FDA)	foodsafety.gov/news/fsma.html

Safe Food Handling: The Physical Plant

Overview and Objectives

Active Managerial Control (AMC) is a preventive food safety management system. Food service managers use AMC to prevent the risk of foodborne illness rather than reacting when an inspector points out an uncontrolled risk factor. The manager becomes the inspector daily. This chapter outlines the active managerial control for regulations, employees, physical facilities, equipment maintenance, and environmental space. After completing this chapter, you should be able to:

- Identify the federal safety laws/regulations for a facility
- Prepare a safety inspection checklist and correct problems as needed
- Develop an emergency plan for disaster preparedness
- Identify materials and consideration for the physical facilities and purchase of small equipment
- Ensure the cleaning and sanitation of equipment and utensils
- Follow an Integrated Pest Management (IPM) system
- Organize the equipment workflow for use, placement and access to supplies, hand sinks, and lavatory facilities

> **GLOSSARY**
>
> **Active Managerial Control (AMC)**
> The act of incorporating procedures and/or actions used to prevent the risk of foodborne illness

Federal Safety Laws and Regulations

Regulatory inspections are part of the everyday life in food production and dining services facilities. Regarding sanitation, regulatory inspections will be assessing the control over the risk factors of foodborne illnesses. The FDA lists the elements of an effective food safety management system in its 2017 Food Code. **Active Managerial Control (AMC)** is important as the responsibility for controlling foodborne illness rests with the manager as well as the employees. An AMC program should include:

1. **Written Policies.** Policy statements set expectations for employees. For example, the policy for cold holding might be that all Temperature Control for Safety (TCS) food will be kept refrigerated below 41°F. Standard operating procedures (SOPs) are used for performing critical operational steps in the food preparation process.

2. **Training.** All staff should be trained on the policies on a regular basis. As part of a cold holding policy, all food preparation staff should be trained that TCS food should be 41°F or less. The person in charge should not be the only person who is aware of and responsible for following the policies.

3. **Monitoring** (a method for verifying that employees follow specific policies). Record-keeping should be up to date and equipment maintenance should be ongoing. Means of quality control and assurance should be in place. For example, a temperature log for checking temperatures of TCS foods throughout the day is one means of monitoring a cold holding policy.

4. **Corrective Action** (what to do if the monitoring shows that a policy is not met). The corrective action should be part of the policy statement. For example, does the cold holding policy tell staff what to do if the TCS food is out of temperature on the temperature log?

Food production and dining services operations must comply with many local, state, and federal regulations. Elements of the AMC program above are required for some state and federal regulations, although not all guidelines are always required because each state may interpret the federal laws differently.

Regulations

Each of the three branches of government is involved in protecting the safety of the food supply and public health. See Figure 20.1 for an explanation of each. Congress and the Senate comprise the legislative branch, passing laws on food handling and protection. Agencies like the FDA, within the executive branch of the government, develop regulations to implement the laws. The judicial branch reviews the policies and procedures of regulatory agencies to protect the rights of both private businesses and the public. Laws usually state broad objectives and need to be interpreted. Regulations are more specific and give guidance on how to comply with the law. Several regulations may be necessary to implement one law at the federal, state, and local level.

It is important for the Certified Dietary Manager®, Certified Food Protection Professional® (CDM®, CFPP®) to learn the standards and expectations of different

1. A global pandemic requires that foodservice establishments put in necessary safety protocols for food handling. Think of one example and develop AMC elements for that protocol.

regulatory agencies and to develop policies and procedures to achieve compliance. Local laws may be stricter than state laws. If so, the dining services operator must comply with the most stringent standard. When in doubt, the CDM, CFPP should consult a representative of the regulatory agency or their administrator to review the regulations.

Local or Municipal Laws and Regulations

Depending on the size of the community and the number of dining operations it has, the county or municipal government may have a department of health or food protection that enforces local laws.

State Laws and Regulations

Each state has a department charged with protecting the safety of food produced, served, and transported in its respective state. The office may be within the department of public health or the department of agriculture.

Federal Laws and Regulations

Federal laws and regulations exist to protect food safety by requiring inspection, controlling food additives, and regulating the transport of food across state borders.

FDA Food Code

The **FDA Food Code** is a framework on which an effective retail food safety program can be built. Today, the FDA's purpose in maintaining an updated Model Food Code is to assist in food control jurisdictions at all levels of government by providing them with a scientifically sound technical and legal basis for regulating the retail segment of the food industry. This includes the establishments or locations in the food distribution chain where the consumer takes possession of the food.

The Food Code is neither a federal law nor a federal regulation and it does not replace local regulations. Rather, it represents FDA's best advice for a uniform system of regulation to ensure that retail food is safe and properly protected and presented.

Although they are not the federal requirements (until adopted by federal bodies for use within federal jurisdictions), the Food Code provisions are still designed to be consistent with federal food laws and regulations, and are written for the ease of legal adoption at all levels of government. The most current FDA Food Code recommendations may or may not apply in the particular jurisdiction, so it is important to become familiar with all sanitation regulations that apply to the facility in which you work.

> **GLOSSARY**
>
> **FDA Food Code**
> A model that assists food control jurisdictions at all levels of government by providing them with a scientifically sound technical and legal basis for regulating the retail and food service segment of the industry

Inspections

One way agencies and governments assess compliance with regulations is through the inspection process. The FDA recommends that food production and dining service operations be inspected once every six months. An inspection often begins with an inspector or sanitarian identifying him/her self and presenting the appropriate identification. *If an inspector does not present identification, be sure to ask for it.* In most cases inspections are unannounced. In some areas of the country, inspections only occur in response to complaints. In other areas, routine inspections can be expected by every food operation. Some operations may be inspected by several different agencies.

Figure 20.1
Regulatory Agencies and Resources

U.S. FOOD AND DRUG ADMINISTRATION (FDA)

The FDA, an agency of the Department of Health and Human Services Public Health Service, is responsible for ensuring the safety and wholesomeness of all foods sold in interstate commerce except for meat, poultry and eggs, all of which are under USDA jurisdiction. FDA develops standards for the composition, quality, nutrition, and safety of foods. It collects and interprets data on nutrition, food additives, and environmental factors, such as pesticides, that affect foods. FDA also sets standards for certain foods and enforces federal regulations for labeling, food and color additives, food sanitation, and safety of foods. FDA monitors recalls of unsafe or contaminated foods and can seize illegally marketed foods.

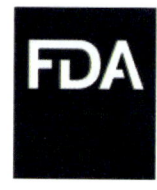

U.S. DEPARTMENT OF AGRICULTURE (USDA)

Through inspection and grading, the USDA enforces standards for wholesomeness and quality of meat, poultry, and eggs produced in the United States. USDA food safety activities include inspecting poultry, eggs, domestic and imported meat, and inspecting livestock and production plants. The USDA is also responsible for making quality (grading) inspections for grain, fruits, vegetables, meat, poultry, and dairy products (including cheeses). The USDA's education programs target family nutritional needs, food safety, and expanding scientific knowledge.

CENTERS FOR DISEASE CONTROL AND PREVENTION (CDC)

An agency of the Department of Health and Human Services, CDC is involved as a protector of food safety—including responding to emergencies when foodborne illnesses arise. It directs and enforces quarantines while administrating national programs for prevention and control of vector-borne diseases (diseases transmitted by a host organism) and other preventable conditions. It maintains statistics on foodborne illnesses.

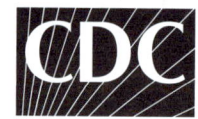

NATIONAL MARINE FISHERIES SERVICE (NMFS)

A part of the Department of Commerce, NMFS is responsible for seafood quality and identification, fisheries management, habitat conservation, and aquaculture production. NMFS has a voluntary inspection program for fish products. Its guidelines closely match regulations for which FDA has enforcement authority.

U.S. CENTERS FOR MEDICARE & MEDICAID SERVICES (CMS)

Centers for Medicare & Medicaid Services (CMS) The Centers for Medicare & Medicaid Services is a federal agency within the Department of Health & Human Services that administers the Medicare program. CMS works with state governments to administer Medicaid, the State Children's Health Insurance Program (CHIP) and Health Insurance Portability Standards.

LOCAL GOVERNMENTS

State and local government agencies cooperate with the federal government to ensure the quality and safety of food produced within their jurisdictions. FDA and other federal agencies help state and local governments develop uniform food safety standards and regulations and assist them with research and information. States inspect restaurants, retail food establishments, dairies, grain mills, and other food establishments within their borders. In many instances, they can embargo illegal food products, which gives them authority over fish, including shellfish, taken from their waters. FDA provides guidelines to the states for this regulation. Many states have their own fish inspection programs. The FDA also provides guidelines for state and local governments for regulation of dairy products and restaurant foods.

Areas that an inspector will probably address include:

- Food purchasing practices, including the use of approved sources of food and potable water.
- Food storage practices, including the cleanliness and temperature of the food storage areas, signs that proper stock rotation methods (FIFO) are being used, labeling and dating practices for food products, protection of food from cross-contamination, and the proper storage of chemicals. The latter must be stored away from the food preparation areas in clearly marked containers.
- Food preparation and service practices, including the thawing, cooking, holding, transporting, serving, cooling, and reheating of food. The inspector may want to review the temperature logs, measure food temperatures, review date-marking procedures, and observe the work habits of the staff.
- Personal hygiene of employees, including their cleanliness and use of disposable gloves and utensils to avoid hand contact with food. The presence of any staff with reportable symptoms or illnesses as well as the accessibility and use of handwashing sinks and supplies are also checked. The inspector may interview staff about their work habits and practices.
- Cleaning and sanitization practices, including manual and mechanical warewashing practices, proper dilution of chemical sanitizers, and proper water temperature. The inspector will tour the premises and inspect equipment to determine overall cleanliness. The inspector may request a copy of cleaning schedules.
- The inspector will likely evaluate the facilities, including safe water supply, proper sewage disposal and the backflow prevention with air gap or approved device, absence of pest infestation, and pest control methods and the techniques employed.

While the FDA Food Code provides a sample risk-based inspection form and guidelines, the form and criteria used locally may vary. Have food temperature logs and staff training records available for the inspector. Some facilities are required to have a manager certified in dining services sanitation on the premises at all times. Be sure that the proper records and evidence of certification are current and available.

An inspector who discovers minor infractions will establish a deadline for their correction. Correct violations immediately, and if possible, even before the inspector leaves the premises. The inspector may note that the correction has been made and remove the violation from his/her evaluation prior to leaving the facility. Take notes during inspection. These will help make any necessary improvements. They can also be a resource to prepare for future inspections. A health inspector can serve as a resource, too. If there is anything you do not understand—ask.

If a serious problem or imminent health hazard is noticed, the inspector may order the facility to close immediately. A food production and dining services operation that fails to correct problems by established deadlines risks fines and loss of the permit to operate.

2. Based on the areas of inspection, develop a self-inspection checklist for your foodservice facility.

HACCP-Based Inspections

Some local health departments have changed their inspection process to one based on the HACCP principles. Instead of traditional inspections that focus on the observed food operation, a HACCP-based inspection focuses on the flow of food. This style of inspection is more likely in a production kitchen or a location with satellite service of prepared food sent to a remote dining service (i.e,. a pre-plated cook-chill service). The inspector will review the HACCP logs during the visit, allowing the inspector to inspect food safety practices over a long period of time rather than just on the day of inspection.

Inspection Preparation

An inspector will usually leave a written report that notes the areas for improvement and any violations. Study the written report to determine why violations occurred and to develop an action plan to avoid having the same violation occur a second time. To improve compliance during inspections, follow these guidelines:

- **Plan and Prepare:** Obtain a copy of applicable regulations and review them in advance. For questions about the regulations, contact the regulatory agency that enforces them. Develop policies and work practices that comply with the guidelines.
- **Use Self-Inspection:** Conduct routine self-inspections to identify issues before they become a problem. Ask an inspector for blank inspection reports or create self-inspection forms specifically for the dining services operation. Several examples of self-inspection forms are included in this textbook. Correct the problems, if any, that are discovered during the self-inspections.
- **Network:** Through professional organizations, discuss regulations and compliance issues with peers. Identify common strategies and resources.
- **Train and Educate Staff:** Train all the staff members in safe food preparation practices and the regulations that are applicable to their own jobs.

Emergency or Disaster Preparedness

A disaster is a sudden change, often an unstable condition, that requires decisive action. Often an emergency endangers the health of a client or employee, or it jeopardizes the safety and security of the dining services operation. A disaster can occur in any type of dining services operation. Some examples of crisis situations are:

- Fire
- Flood
- Tornado or hurricane
- Utility (water or gas) loss
- Delivery driver strike
- Food tampering by client or employee
- Sudden illness of an employee or client
- Workplace violence
- Bomb threat
- Robbery or theft
- Vandalism
- Act of terrorism
- Epidemic or Pandemic
- Foodborne illness outbreak

3. Develop an emergency plan for a facility that has had an electrical outage. What are the different areas of food service that will be impacted as a result?

Emergency Plan

Imagine being the CDM, CFPP of a dining services operation that has been flooded and is without utilities. What if the dining services operation were at a hospital, nursing home, or other facility where the expectation is to continue providing meals? How can this work? How could you be sure that the food being served is safe? To handle such a situation properly, it is necessary to plan in advance. Anticipate the type of crisis situations that your operation might face and develop a plan of action. Examples of advance planning and preparation for crisis situations are:

- A nursing home maintains a supply of bottled water and a one-week supply of disposable dishes for use in the event the water supply becomes contaminated or that the water service is lost.
- A correctional facility maintains an emergency menu and food supply for use in case power is lost or the weather prohibits the delivery of food.
- A fire evacuation plan is established for a fine dining restaurant and employees are trained in the use of fire extinguishers.
- Employees at a hotel are trained in procedures to follow if they receive a bomb threat, such as what to listen for and what to ask the caller.
- A hospital has an agreement with a regional food supplier to provide a refrigerated truck.
- A fast food restaurant has an established procedure to follow if they receive a complaint about a foodborne illness.
- Emergency phone numbers for police, fire, and medical personnel are posted by each telephone in a college dining hall.
- Employees of a correctional facility are trained in non-violent intervention techniques.
- A resort maintains a crisis management manual with procedures to follow in the event of most emergency situations.

A CDM, CFPP should always have a written plan on how to feed clients in an emergency. Food preparation in situations where power is lost or food deliveries are impossible may require a preplanned menu that includes foods that do not require cooking, such as peanut butter sandwiches, fresh or canned fruit, and similar items. In creating a plan, consider what supplies are likely to be on hand, how to handle a severe staffing shortage if employees cannot get to work, and whether the operation will feed extra people. In some healthcare facilities, an emergency staffing plan may include drawing on employees from other non-client care departments. The staff needs to be aware of the emergency plan so they will be ready to activate it at any time.

> A hurricane preparedness plan is a standard when working at a large hospital in Jackson, Mississippi. There was no plan for the three days without water when the city pipes froze one winter. Although the basic problem was not the same, the fact that a plan had been thought out and contacts established within the community allowed the staff to act on parts of the plan instead of reacting to the crisis.

Foodborne Illness Outbreak

A dining services operation may, at some time, receive a complaint about foodborne illness. Every dining services operation should have a plan in place to deal with such complaints. Questions that should be asked of the complainant include:

- What is your name, address, and phone number?
- When did you eat at the dining services operation (day and time)?
- What were you served?
- When did you become ill?
- Have you sought treatment? If so, where?
- Was anyone else with you when you ate at the dining services operation?
- If yes, are they also ill and what did they have to eat?

Do not accept responsibility for the illness or agree to pay for medical care. Encourage the complainant to seek medical care if he or she indicates a need, but do not state that the facility will pay for the medical care. (This is a decision to be made by the Administrator and the facility's Risk Manager/Lawyer.) If the suspected food is still in service, immediately take it out and save it. In many hospitals and larger senior living communities, there is an employee health or infection control nurse to contact. This is your first step as he or she would know if other employees have reported similar illnesses. Alert the senior leadership team of the reported complaint, the possibility of others being affected, and the need for any immediate action. Senior leadership may decide to contact the liability insurance carrier and to interview the staff involved in preparation of the suspected food.

After receiving the complaint, contact the local department of health. Reporting the complaint to local public health officials should be done immediately to prevent any possible illness from spreading further. A laboratory analysis of the suspected food can help to confirm the presence of foodborne pathogens—or establish the safety of the food. Some facilities even have a procedure to save a plate of food from each meal.

The local health department will investigate the complaint of a foodborne illness. A team of investigators will likely interview the victim, visit the dining services operation to interview the management and personnel, take samples of suspected food items, and evaluate the food protection practices of the dining services operation. The HACCP logs can provide a record of food handling practices in the facility.

Pandemic

Our entire world has witnessed a global pandemic with the outbreak of Coronavirus Disease 2019 (COVID-19). Food safety, the safety of employees and the physical facilities is a big concern. The CDC, FDA, CMS, and other agencies are resources for providing timely recommendations, regulatory information, guidance, and technical assistance necessary to support rapid COVID-19 response efforts.

Managing Crisis Communications

In the event of a crisis situation, there should be one designated person responsible for contacting members of the media. All other staff should decline answering questions and refer members of the press to the designated spokesperson. Before answering any questions, the spokesperson should determine and understand the facts surrounding the emergency or crisis situation. In many cases, the spokesperson should consult with the organization's legal counsel before answering questions, if possible. During an emergency, the spokespersons are also encouraged to follow these do's and don'ts:

- Do provide factual information.
- Don't speculate, guess, or provide false information.
- Do develop a prepared statement of exactly what information you want to release and then follow through with your statement.
- Don't feel obligated to answer all of the questions you are asked.
- Do communicate in a clear and concise manner.
- Don't use jargon or shocking descriptions.
- Do ask technical experts to provide explanations of complex situations, if necessary.
- Don't allow pointed questions to alarm you.
- Do inform the media that public health and safety is your priority and that you are cooperating with the regulatory agencies.
- Don't appear uncooperative or intimidated.

Food Security

In today's world, food security is a growing concern. The FDA recommends that CDM, CFPPs consider the possibility of food tampering, or other criminal or terrorist actions that may result in unsafe food. Terrorist activity could occur at any point in the flow of food—on the farm, in a food processing facility, in a warehouse, or in a dining services operation. A manager should be alert to this possibility and definitely take proactive steps to help prevent or limit this kind of crisis in a dining services department. FDA advice for dining services operations includes the following:

- Train staff to report any unusual or suspicious behavior.
- Promote security awareness among employees. Ask them to look for and report signs of tampering.
- Supervise and observe dining services activities.
- Screen employees before hiring.
- Provide work assignments and schedules, and insist that each employee wear an identification (ID) badge.
- Restrict access by not allowing employees in work areas when they are off-duty, and do not allow others into food storage and food production areas.
- Prevent staff from bringing personal items into non-public food preparation or storage areas.
- Monitor the activity in self-service areas, such as salad bars.
- Limit access to and secure storage areas for chemicals used in the operation (e.g., no public access; secure with lock and key).
- Monitor the inventory and report unusual changes, such as the disappearance of products, or unauthorized appearance of products.
- Establish a chain of communication. Train the staff to inform a designated manager of any concerns.
- Have a crisis response plan and keep all emergency contact numbers for the community readily accessible. Include the FDA emergency number (866-300-4374) on your contact list. Also include the phone number of your state complaint coordinator.

Government agencies at all levels, from federal through local, participate in ensuring food safety. A CDM, CFPP should be familiar with regulations that apply to the dining services department and work diligently to comply with them routinely. While the FDA Food Code provides a model for sanitation regulations, each health jurisdiction sets its own standards. Routine inspections are a means through which government agencies help to ensure the safety of dining services clients, and additionally, the equipment used to prepare the food. The equipment and the physical facilities of the dining services operation have a tremendous impact on the safety of the food served. In the next section, we will consider what characteristics enable dining services equipment and facilities to support safe food.

Managing Physical Facilities

The design and construction of a commercial kitchen and dining services is a specialty niche in the builder's world. The regulations related to wiring, placement of outlets, equipment spacing, airflow, and hood space make the kitchen design both interesting and difficult. Equipment specifications and local regulations may make adding the desired equipment very expensive or even impossible to get. It is helpful for the manager to work with internal engineering staff to identify opportunities and placement for new equipment.

Equipment representatives may be able to assist in the selection of a new stove but a commercial kitchen designer is recommended for major projects or remodels. He or she can help design a space that is efficient, uses the most appropriate equipment for the type of service being provided, and help navigate the approval process with local authorities. The manager should never "just add" a major piece of equipment to a kitchen or dining room without first verifying that it meets the safety and mechanical regulations for the location.

The following comments are based on commonly used guidelines and recommendations. Local regulations and specifications may differ.

Construction Materials and Considerations

Floors, Walls, and Ceilings

The materials for floors, walls, and ceilings are selected on the basis of ease in cleaning, resistance, and durability. Utility service lines should not be unnecessarily exposed and they should not obstruct or prevent cleaning. Walls and ceilings are often light in color to distribute light and to make any soil more noticeable.

The floor in food preparation and utility areas should be easy to maintain, wear-resistant, slip-resistant, and nonporous. Common materials for floors are quarry tile, terrazzo, and sealed concrete. Other materials may be used in dining rooms. For instance, tightly woven carpeting would be acceptable in a dining room but not in a food preparation or storage area.

Vinyl tile is not recommended, even for dining rooms, because it is difficult to maintain and they wear out quickly. Ceramic tile is a common floor finish for public restrooms and other high traffic areas. Floor mats, if used, should be easy to remove and clean.

Floors that are flushed with water for cleaning or are subject to frequent liquid spills should have adequate drains to allow the liquids to draw off by themselves.

The best wall finish in food preparation areas is structural glazed tile or ceramic tile. Both can withstand heat, grease, and frequent cleaning. Structural glazed tile is also resistant to the impact from movable carts and equipment. This is important in preventing chips. Surfaces that are chipped or cracked allow microorganisms to attach themselves.

Coving is required at the juncture of floors and walls. Coving at a floor-wall joint facilitates cleaning by preventing accumulation of bits of food that attract insects and rodents.

A wide variety of construction materials is available for the ceilings, including: acoustical tile, painted drywall, painted plaster, and exposed concrete. Acoustical tile is a common choice because it is economical and has sound-absorbing qualities. Special nonabsorbent acoustical tiles have been developed. Tiles are easier to replace when needed.

Heating, Ventilation, and Air Conditioning Systems

Heating, Ventilation, and Air Conditioning (HVAC) systems should help maintain appropriate temperatures and air flow. The elements of an HVAC system—including hoods, vents, and filters—should be inspected and cleaned on a regular basis to ensure efficient operation and to prevent the risk of a fire from the grease build-up. Hoods can be commercially cleaned to eliminate grease build-up, a fire hazard. All preparation and work areas where odors, fumes, or vapors accumulate should be vented to the outside. Heating, ventilating, and air conditioning systems should be designed and installed so that the make-up air intake and exhaust vents do not cause any contamination with food, food contact surfaces, equipment, or utensils. Vents and hoods should be maintained in a clean condition and air filters, if used, should be changed regularly.

Lighting

Lighting should be adequate so that the dirt and soil are visible, the area easy to clean, and bright enough to prevent accidents from poor lighting. Lighting is measured in foot-candles. Work areas require 50 foot-candles of light. Storage areas and walk-in coolers require at least 10 foot-candles. In food preparation and warewashing areas, lighting, as in fluorescent bulbs, must be shielded and shatter-resistant.

Special Area Considerations

Dry Storage Areas

Storage areas should be dry, well ventilated, and constructed of easy-to-clean surfaces. Concrete or tile floors, cement block walls with epoxy paint, and acoustic ceilings are common for all storage areas except those in refrigerated places. Three- or four-level metal shelving is commonly used in storage areas. Slatted or louvered shelves are recommended for storage areas because they permit proper air flow. Storage areas should be maintained at 50°F - 70°F.

4. You are working with the facilities team on redesigning the kitchen. What are various areas and some considerations you would keep in mind during the team discussions?

Warewashing Areas

Warewashing areas should be designed so that they are easy to sanitize and can withstand wet conditions. Common construction materials include slip-resistant quarry tile floors, ceramic or structural glazed tile walls, and moisture-resistant acoustic ceilings.

Preparation Areas

A major consideration in preparation areas is the work surfaces. A common material used in the construction of work surfaces is stainless steel which is non-corrosive, non-absorbent, and non-toxic, making it a very suitable material for use in dining services operations. All food contact surfaces must be accessible for cleaning and sanitizing.

Toilet and Handwashing Facilities

Toilets should be conveniently located but are separate from food preparation areas. The number of toilets and sinks required will vary by the size of the dining services operation and is usually determined by state and local regulations. Separate restrooms for employees and clients are recommended. The doors to toilet areas must be tight-fitting and self-closing.

Dining Services Equipment

Equipment Standards

Many utensils and products intended for household use are not appropriate for use in dining services operations. A CDM, CFPP should purchase only equipment that is intended for use in the dining services industry. In general, dining services equipment should be designed to be easily cleaned, maintained, and serviced—either in the assembled or disassembled state.

Metal pieces such as slicer blades and mixer pieces should be made of heavy gauge metal and should be checked frequently for nicks or broken areas.

One way to identify professionally designed and constructed equipment is to look for the National Sanitation Foundation (NSF) International mark. (See Figure 20.2) The NSF International mark of approval is a recognized standard of acceptance for many pieces of equipment. This seal assures the manager that the equipment meets certain construction standards for sanitation and safety.

Another important standard is the Underwriter's Laboratories (UL) mark, which indicates compliance of the equipment with electrical safety standards. (See Figure 20.2) UL has developed nearly 20 safety standards for the commercial dining services industry. Only equipment meeting these standards can display the blue UL sanitation certification.

The following are examples of characteristics to look for when purchasing dining services equipment:

- Easy disassembly for cleaning.
- Durable, corrosion resistant, and non-absorbent.
- Materials that do not impart any significant color, odor, or taste to food.
- Smooth surfaces free of pits, crevices, ledges, bolts, and rivet heads.
- Coating materials that are resistant to cracking and chipping.
- Rounded edges and internal corners with finished, smooth surfaces.

Figure 20.2
Equipment Standards Marks

Refrigeration Equipment

Refrigeration equipment is important for food protection. To ensure maximum performance of refrigeration units, these steps should be followed:

- Check to see that gaskets and hinges fit tightly and that there is no air leaking out.
- Clean or replace the air filter.
- Clean the condenser.

Some dining service operations connect refrigerator thermostats to security or other monitoring equipment. Maintenance or management personnel can be notified immediately if the equipment fails—rather than discovering food spoilage several hours later. Thermal barriers made of flexible, overlapping, plastic (PVC) strips can be mounted on the doors of walk-in refrigerators and freezers to help maintain temperatures even when the door is opened. There should be room inside or on the door for a temperature log that is filled out three times a day. The manager should take the actual food temperature if there has been a disruption in service or if it appears that the thermometer is off.

Equipment Installation

The equipment that is fixed because it is not easily mobile should be installed so that it is placed to allow access for cleaning along the sides, behind, and above the equipment. Equipment that is not easily movable should be sealed to the floor or elevated on legs that provide at least 6 inches (6" or 15 cm) clearance between the floor and the equipment. Equipment mounted on concrete bases or on small steel legs can interfere with proper cleaning. Easier access for cleaning can also be provided by mounting the equipment on wheels so it can be moved or by using wall-mounted equipment.

Cutting Boards

Surfaces such as cutting blocks that are subject to scratching and scoring should be resurfaced if they can no longer be cleaned and sanitized effectively, or they should be discarded if they cannot be resurfaced. Wooden cutting boards may be prohibited in some areas. If used, they must be made of hard maple wood. Cutting boards made of food-grade seamless hard rubber or acrylic are recommended.

Color-coded cutting boards are available: red for meat, yellow for poultry, white for dairy, green for fruits and vegetables, beige for cooked poultry, and blue for seafood. Even a two-board combination (such as red for raw foods and beige for cooked foods) will reduce the risk of cross-contamination.

Thermometers

Monitoring proper storage, cooking, holding, cooling, and reheating temperatures is vital to food protection. The most common thermometer used in the dining services is the bimetallic stem type which are made up of two joined metal strips. The expansion and contraction of these strips move a pointer on the dial face of the thermometer. Bimetallic thermometers need to be calibrated on a regular basis to ensure accuracy. Technology offers some alternatives to bimetallic thermometers. As more dining services operations implement the HACCP food safety programs, other types of dining services thermometers are becoming more common.

Thermocouple and Thermistor

The probes of these electronic thermometers can measure the temperature of food and provide a digital display. Some have additional electronic features, such as the ability to store temperature readings. Most have interchangeable probes, which allows matching the probe to the food or equipment. A thermometer with a small, thin probe allows for greater accuracy in checking the temperatures of thin foods, such as ground beef patties, fish filets, or strips of meat for stir-frying. In fact, the Food Code stipulates using one of these for thin foods. (See Figures 20.3 and 20.4.)

An important consideration with any type of temperature-measuring device is cross-contamination. A thermometer used to measure the temperature of a raw food and then used to monitor a prepared food can contaminate the prepared food with bacteria. Probes should be sanitized with an approved sanitizer after each use. Dining services storage areas should be equipped with thermometers to measure the ambient temperature. Grill and oven thermometers may be used to verify the calibration of cooking equipment.

Clean-In-Place Equipment (CIP)

Clean-in-Place Equipment (CIP) must be self-draining and designed so that the cleaning and sanitizing solutions can circulate throughout a fixed system and contact all food-contact surfaces. Clean-in-place equipment that cannot be disassembled for cleaning should have access points to allow the inspection of interior food contact surfaces. CIP equipment and pieces that can be disassembled require the same steps for

Figure 20.3
Monitoring Temperature of a Thin Food, Like Salmon Steak

Figure 20.4
Verifying Temperature of Salad with Bimetallic Stem Thermometer

Images courtesy of Cooper-Atkins

cleaning and sanitizing: wash, rinse, sanitize, air dry.

Equipment Calibration

Storage equipment is essential for maintaining proper food temperatures. Cooking and holding equipment—such as ovens, grills, steam tables, and food warmers—should be calibrated on a regular basis. Equipment that is not calibrated may not cook food thoroughly or hold the food at a safe temperature.

Mechanical Warewashing Equipment

Dishwashers must be equipped with a temperature measuring device that indicates the temperature of water in each tank and the temperature of water during the sanitizing final rinse. Warewashing machines should be equipped with internal baffles, curtains, or other means to minimize any internal cross-contamination between the solution in the wash and rinse tanks. In mechanical dishwashing, adequate dwell time is also a consideration. Dwell time is the time that dishes spend in contact with heat during sanitization.

Manual Warewashing Equipment

A sink with at least three compartments must be provided for manually washing, rinsing, and sanitizing equipment and utensils. A temperature-measuring device must be provided for frequently measuring the washing and sanitizing temperature of the water. Dishmachine temperatures should be monitored and recorded. Test strips may be used to monitor the concentration of chemical sanitizing agents. Newer machines should be equipped to dispense detergents and sanitizers automatically. It should also have a visual signal or audible alarm to indicate a failure to dispense these chemicals.

Cleanability

Cleaning and maintenance are important considerations when designing a dining services facility and when purchasing equipment. A well-designed dining services operation utilizes materials that are durable, nonporous and easy to clean. Regulations for dining services operations have changed considerably over the last several years. It is important to check what new standards are there before making any construction, remodeling, or major purchasing decision. The sanitary design of a dining services facility is often governed by a number of laws, including public health, building, and zoning laws. The primary consideration for the sanitary design of dining services facilities is cleanability. **Cleanability** is the extent to which an item is accessible for cleaning and inspection, and ease with which soil can be removed by normal cleaning methods.

> **GLOSSARY**
>
> **Cleanability**
> The ability of a piece of equipment to be easily accessible for cleaning, soil removal, sanitizing, and inspection

Here are some examples of how food safety can be part of a facility design:
- Equipment is easily dissembled.
- Finishes are durable and easy to clean.

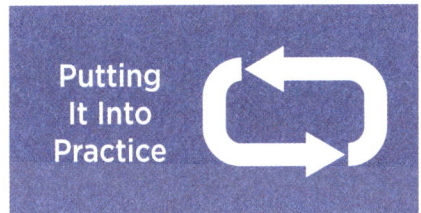

5. A new employee disassembles and cleans the slicer, takes the portable pieces to the dishmachine and runs them through. She then reassembles the slicer. What step(s) has she overlooked? How would you ensure that all steps have been followed?

- Equipment is attached to the wall, eliminating legs, which makes it easier to clean under the equipment.
- Equipment racks have a minimum number of legs.
- Garbage disposals are placed in work areas to facilitate waste removal.
- Shelves under tables are portable, so they can be easily cleaned.

Developing a Cleaning Program

Maintaining a clean environment for food preparation is an important part of food safety. The presence of bacteria and the likelihood of foodborne illnesses increase if a dining services operation fails to use appropriate cleaning and sanitizing procedures. Equipment, food contact surfaces, and utensils must be clean to sight and touch. The food contact surfaces of equipment should be free of any encrusted grease deposits and other soil accumulations. The plumbing under the dishmachine should be clear of rust and lime build-up. Non-food contact surfaces should be kept free of dust, dirt, food residue, and debris. A philosophy of clean-as-you-go should be instilled in all dining services staff. A cleaning program will most likely be effective if the CDM, CFPP incorporates a system of self-inspection and training.

Maintaining a clean dining services operation requires that the CDM, CFPPs use their skills in planning, organizing, staffing, training, and directing. They must first determine what the cleaning needs of the operation are and when these cleaning functions should be carried out. The managers should then determine who will be responsible for carrying out the cleaning. Some cleaning may be done by contract personnel, but most is completed by dining services employees. The managers should provide adequate staffing so that the employees will be able to carry out the planned cleaning activities. The managers should train the employees in proper cleaning techniques and the safe use of chemicals. Finally, the managers should evaluate the cleaning programs on an ongoing basis to ensure their effectiveness and to correct any identified problems.

View the Supplemental Material for this chapter for Figure 20.5, Sample Daily Cleaning Schedule; and Figure 20.6, Sample Cleaning Self-Inspection Checklist.

A written schedule, such as that in Figure 20.5, in the Supplemental Material, can be developed to outline the cleaning program and the staff responsible for it on a daily basis. When compared to the posted work schedule, identifying the individual employee from day to day is easily done.

A self-inspection checklist (Figure 20.6 in the Supplemental Material) can be used to evaluate the effectiveness of the cleaning program. Depending on the condition of the department, the self-inspection may be a daily or weekly job for the manager.

Detailed instructions on proper cleaning techniques should be incorporated into the employee training programs, both during the orientation phase and as part of the ongoing in-service education program. An example of this appears in Figure 20.7.

Cleaning Products

Detergents are powerful dirt-removing cleaning agents. Types of cleaning products are described in Figure 20.8. A cleaning supply vendor can assist in selecting the right chemical for the right job. Or, the local or state regulatory agency may be able to provide a list of approved chemical products. Factors in selecting a detergent include:

- Dissolvability: how well the detergent disperses with water.
- Wetting ability: how well it saturates the surface of the object to be cleaned.

Figure 20.7
Sample Cleaning Procedures for Floors

Equipment Needed:
- Broom
- Dustpan
- Two Mops
- Two Mop Buckets

Supplies Needed:
- Heavy-Duty Detergent

WHAT TO DO	HOW TO DO IT
STEP 1 Sweep	• Sweep the floor with a broom, making sure to get under equipment. • Minimize dust by using short, controlled strokes. • Use dustpan to pick up debris.
STEP 2 Set up mop buckets	• Fill each bucket 3/4 full with hot tap water. • Put the appropriate amount of cleanser in one of the buckets.
STEP 3 Apply cleaner to floor	• Dip first mop into cleanser solution and wring out. • Mop small section of floor using a figure-eight motion. • Allow detergent to loosen soil for a few minutes.
STEP 4 Rinse floor	• Dip the second mop into the rinse water, wring out, and use the mop to pick up the dirt and cleaning solution. • Change detergent solutions and rinse water often.

SAFETY CONSIDERATIONS

- Check product label and refer to the Material Safety Data Sheet (MSDS) for precautions and emergency procedures in the event of an accident.
- Follow manufacturer's directions on detergent label to ensure the proper dilution.
- Use "wet floor" signs to prevent accidental slips and falls.

- Emulsification ability: how well the detergent suspends the fats in water and keeps them suspended.
- Free rinsing ability: how well the detergent keeps soil from returning to the cleaned object.
- Deflocculation ability: how well the detergent puts lumps of food-soil in suspension in water.
- Non-toxicity: the extent to which the detergent is free of toxins and other elements harmful to humans.
- Corrosiveness: how great a corroding effect the detergent has on the surface of the item to be cleaned.

Wiping Cloths

Cloths used for wiping up food spills should not be used for other purposes. And they must be stored in a sanitizing solution. Dry or moist cloths that are used with raw animal foods must be kept separately from cloths used for other purposes and they must also be kept in a separate sanitizing solution.

Cleaning Sponges

If sponges are used such as in three-compartment sinks, they have to be cleaned, sanitized, and stored in dry locations. Sponges should not be used on any food contact surfaces.

Clean vs. Sanitary

Clean does not mean sanitary. **Clean** means free of visible dirt or debris. Cleaning is accomplished by physical and/or chemical means and is a two-step process:

1. Wash with an approved detergent
2. Rinse with clear water

Sanitary means free of harmful levels of microorganisms. It is almost impossible to sanitize equipment and facilities unless they are cleaned first. Clean dining services equipment may appear safe to use, but if it is not sanitized, then a hidden threat to food safety exists. Equipment and utensils must be sanitized after cleaning. The FDA Food Code defines a thermometer probe as a utensil, too, so it must also be cleaned and sanitized.

Sanitizing

Sanitizing is the process of making equipment and work surfaces sanitary. There are two major methods of sanitizing: heat sanitization and chemical sanitization.

> **GLOSSARY**
>
> **Clean**
> Free of visible dirt

Figure 20.8
Types of Cleaning Products

Alkaline Detergents	The most commonly used detergents. General-purpose alkalines are only mildly alkaline and are usually applied to walls, celings, and floors. Heavy-duty types are highly alkaline for use in dishwashing machines.
Abrasive Cleaners	Effective in scouring off rust, grease, and heavy soil but can scratch certain surfaces such as stainless steel. Use caution with abrasive cleaners, as scratches in food contact surfaces can harbor bacterial growth.
Acid Cleaners	Acid cleaners have more specialized uses, such as deliming dishmachines and removing water spots. Use acid cleaners with caution to avoid skin irritation.
Degreasers	Degreasers are highly alkaline and can remove grease build-up from floors, ovens, and vents. Degreasers are also known as solvent cleaners.

Note: To avoid producing a poisonous gas, never mix chemicals together.

6. Write out a training plan for dishwashing staff.

- Heat sanitization: The procedure is to expose an object to sufficiently high heat for a sufficient period of time to sanitize it. According to the FDA Food Code, cleaned food contact surfaces can be sanitized by immersion in water that is 171°F or above for at least 30 seconds.
- Chemical sanitization: **Sanitizers** are chemicals that destroy harmful pathogens. The dilution or strength of a sanitizing solution is measured in parts per million (ppm). Dispensing equipment for sanitizers should be calibrated on a regular basis and the strength of a sanitizing solution should be checked with a chemical test strip on a daily basis. Chemical test strips are often available from the chemical supply vendor. Keep in mind that the effectiveness of a sanitizer may be affected by the temperature, hardness, and/or pH of the water in which it is mixed. Also, some chemical solutions lose their strength over time. Chemical sanitizers are summarized in Figure 20.9.

> **GLOSSARY**
>
> **Sanitizers**
> Chemicals that destroy microorganisms

Dishwashing

Manual Cleaning and Sanitizing

Manual cleaning and sanitizing is generally done with a three-compartment sink. (Some municipalities are now requiring a four-compartment sink. The additional compartment is designated for pre-scraping.) If using a three-compartment sink, remember to pre-scrape utensils and cooking equipment before placing them in the first compartment sink. Here are the steps in manual cleaning and sanitizing using a three-compartment sink:

1. Pre-clean to remove loose food soil.
2. Wash in the first sink using an approved detergent with a water temperature of 110°F-120°F.
3. Rinse in the second sink using clear water.
4. Sanitize in the third sink using an approved sanitizer at the appropriate concentration and temperature.
5. Allow dishes to air dry and store in a clean, dry, protected area.

Remember to change the water as necessary to maintain the temperatures and to clean the sink after each use. Use cleaned and sanitized drain boards to stack the equipment and utensils during air drying.

Mechanical Cleaning and Sanitizing

While there are various sizes and types of dishwashers (see Figure 20.10), the following cleaning and sanitizing steps will apply to most operations. These six steps are necessary in any mechanical warewashing operation. Each step is equally important in obtaining clean and sanitary dishware.

Figure 20.9
Chemical Sanitizers

Product	Dilution in Parts Per Million (ppm)	Water Temperature	Immersion Time
Iodine	12.5 - 25	75°F - 120°F	30 seconds
Chlorine	50 - 100	100°F - 115°F	30 seconds
Quaternary Ammonium Compounds	180 - 200	75°F minimum	30 seconds

General guidelines only; follow manufacturer's directions or local regulations.

Figure 20.10
Mechanical Dishmachine Temperatures

Type of Machine	Wash Solution Temp.	Sanitizing Rinse Temp.
Stationary rack, single temperature machine	165°F	165°F
Stationary rack, dual temperature machine	150°F	180°F
Single tank, conveyor, dual temperature machine	160°F	180°F
Multi-task, conveyor, multi-temperature machine	150°F	180°F

NOTES:
- The temperature of the sanitizing rinse should not exceed 194°F.
- The actual temperature attained within a hot water sanitizing machine (at utensil surface) should be at least 160°F when measured by a thermometer or temperature test strip.

The steps are:

1. **Separate:** Separate the items that will require special attention, such as those that are heavily soiled or have burned-on residue.

2. **Pre-scrape or pre-flush:** Excess food soil and pieces of paper straws or napkins will clog the dishmachine, scrap trays, pump and wash arms—and reduce their effectiveness. Excess food soil in the wash tank also uses up more detergent and requires more frequent changes of water in the wash tank.

3. **Rack dishes:** Proper racking of dishes is essential for getting good results. All of the racks should be filled with similar items. A rack should contain cups only, or plates only, or bowls only, etc. Avoid mixing loads. The dishmachine works by spraying water at the dishes, and if the water cannot reach all of the dish surfaces, the dishes cannot get clean.

4. **Wash:** Washing dishes requires a properly operating dishmachine and the proper detergent usage. Be sure to use the right detergent and that the machine is set up properly. It should also be free of paper, straws, and excess food.

5. **Perform sanitizing rinse:** Rinsing is done automatically and requires only the proper flow of water, proper water temperature, and the proper rinse aid. Visually inspect the machine to ensure that the rinse jets are not clogged. Verify that the rinse temperature is reaching the appropriate point, that the rinse injector is supplied with the proper rinse aid, and that dwell time is adequate.

6. **Air drying:** Air drying the dishes requires nothing but time. Wait until the dishes are completely dry before putting them in a clean, dry storage area. Avoid stacking utensils within one another until they are completely dry.

Dish and Utensil Storage

After cleaning and sanitizing, all dishes and utensils must be stored dry, in clean, dust-free areas above the floor, and protected from other dust, splashes, spills, and other forms of contamination.

Equipment Inspection and Maintenance

Preventive maintenance of equipment and facilities is required as an ongoing process in order to keep food production and dining services facilities in good repair and condition. Preventive maintenance goes beyond the daily cleaning. Some preventive maintenance responsibilities will undoubtedly be carried out by the dining services staff, while others may be performed by the facility maintenance staff or through a contract with a commercial equipment maintenance company. It is important to determine what duties the dining services and the maintenance team will perform.

Preventive maintenance includes weekly, bimonthly, monthly, quarterly, and semi-annual cleaning responsibilities. Figure 20.11 shows a partial preventative maintenance cleaning schedule. When assigning these cleaning duties, it is important to include the who, what, when, and how that are part of any cleaning schedule. How do you decide who should do which cleaning duties? Obviously, no one wants to be assigned to clean the grease traps each time. Determining who does what cleaning can be a great topic for a department meeting. Get input from the staff as to how cleaning duties should be divided up. One facility uses a job jar and each week the employees each pull a job from the jar.

It is the CDM, CFPP's responsibility to make sure that cleaning is done properly and according to schedule.

A checklist should be used to ensure that equipment and facilities are properly cleaned and maintained, as shown in Figure 20.12, found in the Supplemental Materials for this book. Whatever the schedule is, make sure that proper tools, equipment, and cleaning materials are available when needed. The manager is also responsible for making sure that employees are thoroughly trained in the procedure and cleaning materials for each task. For example, one facility noticed a significant increase in the cost of sanitizers. Upon investigation, one of the staff believed that if some sanitizer was good, double the amount would be better. Training needs to include why the concentration of sanitizer is important.

View the Supplemental Material for this chapter for Figure 20.12, Equipment Cleaning Checklist; and Figure 20.13, Dishmachine Temperature Log.

Preventive Maintenance Records

There are different types of preventive maintenance records. Two are temperature logs and equipment repair records.

Temperature Logs

Temperature logs should be established for equipment where maintaining temperature is critical. These logs can be set up on a monthly basis and maintained by an assigned staff person. Temperature logs are essential to help determine the time when the equipment stopped working. Since time and temperature are important in maintaining food safety, temperature logs are part of preventive maintenance. Temperature logs can be useful during inspections if they are maintained and completed appropriately. Figure 20.13 in the Supplemental Materials for this book shows a sample of a dishmachine temperature log. Similar logs can be set up for coolers and freezers.

7. As part of the Active Managerial Control system, what are the different logs and forms you can use to ensure that equipment is continually looked at for preventive maintenance and record keeping is in place?

Figure 20.11
Preventive Maintenance Cleaning Schedule for Facilities and Equipment

What to Clean	When to Clean	How to Clean	Person Responsible	Initial When Complete
Drain Covers	Monthly	Remove and wash thoroughly with detergent or degreaser if necessary		
Walls	Monthly	Wash with detergent or degreaser if necessary		
Ceiling Vents	Monthly	Wash with detergent or degreaser if necessary		
Hood Filters	Monthly	Wash filters, replace if necessary		
Grease Traps	Every two months	Clean with degreaser		
Fans	Monthly	Wipe down blades and fan cover		
Ice Machine	Quarterly	Remove ice, clean interior surfaces with detergent, flush ice-making unit		
Cooler/Refrigerator	Bimonthly or more often as needed	Wipe down racks, clean floors and fan with detergent		
Freezer	B-annually	Empty, defrost, wash racks, floors, fans with detergent		
Steamer	Weekly	Use approved deliming agent		
Dishwashing Machine	Weekly	Use approved deliming agent		
Dish Racks	Weekly	Scrub with detergent		
Food Carts	Weekly	Scrub with detergent or use steam cleaner		
Garbage Cans	Weekly	Scrub with detergent or use steam cleaner		
HVAC	Every six months	Steam clean		

Equipment Repair Records

The CDM, CFPPs should maintain a record of repairs for each piece of major equipment. This equipment repair record that contains the number of repairs and the cost of each is essential when writing a justification for new equipment. The equipment repair record should be done as soon as a new piece of equipment is received. And in today's electronic age, there is unlimited data space for computerized equipment repair records, including setting up reminders for periodic maintenance. See Figure 20.14 in the Supplemental Materials for a sample equipment repair record form.

Equipment Replacement Decisions

As a CDM, CFPP, you will be expected to purchase or recommend for purchase new equipment. The equipment maintenance record will assist you in deciding what to purchase, when to purchase, and why. The steps in replacing or purchasing new equipment should include:

1. Conducting cost analysis.
2. Finding out when the cost analysis/justification for replacement was written.
3. Developing equipment specifications.
4. Installing the equipment and training the staff.

These steps will be explored in greater detail in Chapter 22: Manage the Capital Budget.

Water, Plumbing, and Waste Management

Working with maintenance or a local plumbing firm during construction times or after emergency situations, such as a flood or tornado, is extremely important. It is the manager's responsibility to make sure that maintenance staff know the local, state, and federal sanitation regulations. One example is the FDA Food Code requirement that a drinking water system will be flushed and disinfected before being placed in service after construction or an emergency situation.

Water can be a vehicle for transmitting harmful microorganisms. Part of the food protection process involves selecting appropriate sources of water, and managing how clean and waste water are handled in the operation through the plumbing system. In addition, food safety requires the proper management of refuse.

Water served in a dining services operation—as well as water used in food preparation, warewashing, and even handwashing—must be **potable**, or safe to drink. An approved source may be the local public water system. Or, it may be a non-public water system that meets the national, state, or local primary drinking water regulations. Water from a non-public source must be sampled and tested at least annually, and the report must be kept on file in the dining services operation. Water must be received through an approved water main or water transport vehicle. Bottled drinking water that meets appropriate standards is also permissible.

Ice is also a form of water and should be made from potable water. It is important to maintain ice machines in good repair and follow basic sanitation practices in serving ice to clients. Figure 20.15 summarizes some key practices to help ensure the use of safe ice.

Plumbing

Plumbing systems also cover handwashing sinks. The FDA Food Code requires that handwashing sinks provide water at a temperature of at least 100°F. Handwashing sinks must be maintained so that they are accessible to employees at all times. Employees may ONLY use chemical hand sanitizers as a substitute for handwashing when food exposure is limited and handwashing sinks are not convenient, such as in an approved temporary food operation like a mobile unit. An amendment to the FDA Food Code requires that toilets and urinals NOT be used for the disposal of mop water.

The plumbing system performs two very important functions. It brings potable water to the operation and it removes waste materials to a sewer or disposal plant. A major consideration for food protection is to avoid any connection between the two functions.

> **GLOSSARY**
>
> **Potable**
> Water that is safe to drink

> **GLOSSARY**
>
> **Cross-Connection**
> A dangerous link between an outlet of drinkable water with unsafe water
>
> **Backflow**
> When contaminated water flows back into potable water
>
> **Back-Siphonage**
> When water is siphoned back into potable water supply after loss in water pressure

View the Supplemental Material for this chapter for Figure 20.14, Sample Equipment Repair Record Form.

Fixtures and equipment that are used for food preparation, cleaning, or sanitizing cannot have a **cross-connection**—a dangerous link between an outlet of a drinkable water system and unsafe water. An unapproved link may allow contaminants to flow into potable water, making it unsafe. A cross-connection is a structural design issue.

Backflow is the process when contaminated water flows into potable water. For example: a faucet is located below the flood rim of a sink, when the sink gets too full dirty water may flow back into the faucet. Sometimes, rather than just flowing back into the potable water, contaminated water is actually sucked into the clean water supply. This type of backflow is called **back-siphonage**. It occurs after a loss in pressure in the water supply and water is siphoned back into the drinkable water supply.

To prevent backflow, plumbing lines should provide for an air gap. An air gap is an unobstructed air space between an outlet of drinkable water and the flood rim of a fixture or equipment. For example, the space between the flood rim in a sink and the outlet of a faucet is an air gap. If an air gap is not present, then an approved mechanical device to prevent backflow should be installed.

Plumbing should be kept in good repair. Be alert to leaks or drainage issues that might contaminate the food or food preparation areas. Make sure to know the local codes, as plumbing regulations vary. Always use the services of a licensed, qualified plumber for installing or repairing the plumbing systems.

Waste Management

Proper management of waste and garbage will help to maintain a clean, sanitary dining services operation and to prevent pest infestations. As quickly as possible, garbage should be removed from the food preparation and serving areas. Trash holding areas should be located as far as possible from food.

Figure 20.15
Ice Management Practices

- Close or cover the ice bin when not in use.
- Wash hands following established procedures before scooping or dispensing ice. Realize that hands can transfer microorganisms directly to ice, and freezing temperatures do not destroy all pathogens.
- Use a scoop or designated utensil to transfer ice (do not use glass). Touch only the handle of the scoop.
- Store the scoop in or near the ice bin in a protected manner, or in a sanitizing solution (per your local health regulations), with handle up.
- Clean and sanitize ice scoops regularly.
- Do not store any food products or beverages in or directly above the ice bin.
- Report any concerns about equipment malfunction to a designated supervisor.
- Assure that the cleaning compounds are stored and used in such a way that they cannot spill or spray into ice.
- Protect ice supplies from broken china or glasses. If glass breaks or a chemical spills in the vicinity of an ice bin, empty, clean, and sanitize the bin.
- Routinely clean and sanitize the ice collection.
- Follow the manufacturer's instructions for maintenance, which may include deliming the machines and replacing the filters.

Garbage cans should be sturdy and easy to clean. They should be equipped with tight-fitting lids and covered when not in use. Garbage cans should be cleaned on a routine basis, and garbage cans with cracks or leaks should be replaced immediately. Indoor trash areas should be cleaned on a regular basis and the garbage should be picked up at regular intervals to prevent excess odors and reduce food sources for pests.

If the facility has a recycling program, be aware of the local, state, and federal sanitation requirements regarding it. For instance, the FDA Food Code requires that recyclables be kept covered if the containers contain food residue or after a recycling container is filled.

Chemical Safety

The use of chemicals is an essential component of a dining services operation. Chemicals are used in cleaning and sanitizing, and sometimes in the office operations. Chemicals that are stored or used incorrectly pose hazards to food because they can contaminate food and make it unsafe. Chemical safety is an important part of a comprehensive food protection program. In addition, the federal government imposes regulations on chemical use for dining services operations. A related issue is the safe practice for chemically preventing and eradicating pests.

Chemical safety is addressed by the **Occupational Safety and Health Administration (OSHA)**, a government agency responsible for protecting the safety of employees, including those in dining services operations. OSHA has issued a regulation requiring employers to inform employees about the possible dangers of the chemicals they use to do their jobs and to train them to use these chemicals safely.

The regulation is called the **Hazard Communication Standard (HCS)**, or Right to Know Law. The purpose of the HCS is to ensure that all employers receive the information they need to inform employees about chemicals they work with, and to train their employees on how to properly use hazardous substances. It helps in the design and implementation of employee protection programs. It also provides necessary hazard information to employees so that they can participate in and support protective measures.

Safety Data Sheet

By law, a document called a **Safety Data Sheet (SDS)** must be made available by every chemical manufacturer (see Figure 20.16 in the Supplemental Material). An SDS should be available for every chemical used in your operation and placed in a location that is readily accessible to all employees. The SDS addresses the safe use of a chemical, as well as the hazards, safety precautions, proper disposal practices, and how to deal with accidents. In some cases, the SDS may suggest the use of personal protective equipment, such as rubber gloves or goggles.

Safety Data Sheets are not easy to read, so employees will require orientation in how to use them. Be sure that employees understand:

1. What to use each chemical for.
2. How to mix each chemical.
3. What protective equipment is required.
4. Where to find the SDS for a chemical.
5. How to read it.
6. What to do in case of an accident or spill.

GLOSSARY

OSHA
Occupational Safety and Health Administration, responsible for enforcing chemical safety standards

Hazard Communication Standard (HCS)
Law that requires informing employees about chemicals they work with and to design and institute employee protection program

View the Supplemental Material for this chapter for Figure 20.16, Sample Safety Data Sheet.

Suggested training content is summarized in Figure 20.17. To comply with the Hazard Communication Standard, you should:

- Review the Hazard Communication Standard.
- Develop an inventory of chemicals used in the dining services operation.
- Request a Safety Data Sheet (also available online for easy access and printing) for each chemical used in the operation, and make it available to all employees.
- Make sure that all chemicals are in labeled containers.
- Include safe chemical use in the new employee orientation and as part of annual training for all employees.

Figure 20.17
Hazard Communication Training Program Content

- Location of Safety Data Sheets (SDS) in the operation
- Inventory list of hazardous chemicals used in the operation
- How to read product labels to learn potential hazards and directions for safe use
- Proper handling, application, storage, and disposal of chemicals
- Use and location of personal protective equipment
- Emergency procedures in the event of a spill or exposure

Chemical Storage

For food safety, it is also important to store chemicals away from food. Chemicals should be clearly labeled and stored in their original containers. If transferring chemicals from one container to another it is necessary to transfer them only to durable, clearly labeled containers. Containers used to hold and dispense chemicals should be clearly marked and should never be reused for food storage. Likewise, discarded food containers should never be used for chemical storage as someone may mistake the contents for food.

Medicines

The storage of medicines are also regulated by the FDA Food Code, which requires that "only those medicines that are necessary for the health of employees" are allowed in the dining services department. They must have the manufacturer's label and are located to prevent contamination of food, equipment, utensils, linens, and single-service articles. Refrigerated medicines must be stored in a covered, leakproof container that is identified as a container for the storage of medicines. They must also be located so they are inaccessible to children.

8. After receiving quaternary ammonia, the receiving clerk stores it in the dry storage above the canned tomatoes. What should be done now?

Common Pests

A safe food operation is free of insects, birds, and other sources of contamination. Measures must be taken to prevent contamination of food, utensils, equipment, and linens by pests. Many pests carry pathogens that can render food unsafe for consumption.

Cockroaches

Cockroaches are common pests in dining services operations and they represent a significant threat. Cockroaches are carriers of disease and can multiply rapidly. Cockroaches are most active at night and in dark areas where there is less disturbance from people. While there are many different species of cockroaches, three types are frequently found in dining services operations. German cockroaches, the most abundant species in the U.S., are pale brown with two dark-brown stripes behind their heads. They seem to prefer warm places in the dining services operation. American cockroaches are the largest in size and are reddish brown. They prefer open, wet areas and spaces that are slightly cooler than the favorite spots of German cockroaches. Oriental cockroaches are shiny and dark brown to black. They prefer conditions similar to those of the American cockroach.

Houseflies

The common housefly is a great threat to food safety. Flies feed on animal and human waste and then transmit pathogenic organisms as they travel from item to item. Houseflies are numerous during late summer and early fall, since the population has been growing during the warmer weather.

Rats and Mice

Rats and mice can force their entry into a building through small openings. Both rats and mice are skilled swimmers and can enter a building through floor drains and toilet bowl traps. Rats and mice are both nocturnal creatures, being most active at night. One indication of an infestation is the presence of fecal droppings in dining services areas. Another sign is the presence of gnaw marks on food and food containers in storage.

Birds

Birds, such as pigeons, sparrows, and starlings, are other pests of concern. Birds can enter a building through doors and windows that do not have screens and through ventilation openings. Birds can be carriers of mites and harmful microorganisms such as Salmonella.

Pest Control

Pest control is the reduction or eradication of pests. Due to the variety and prevalence of pests in and around foodservice operations, a pest service operator is recommended, and in some jurisdictions, required. There are a number of interventions available.

One of the safest and most effective methods of controlling flies is the use of insect light traps. Light traps must be enclosed so that pests entering the trap are contained within and cannot fall out into the dining services operation. Mechanical traps can be used with birds and rodents.

Pesticides, insecticides, and repellents are other control techniques. Extreme caution should be exercised, however, when using the chemical control methods to prevent the contamination of food. Only chemicals approved for application in dining services operations may be used. Furthermore, only individuals with the proper training and knowledge should apply them. In addition, pesticide application must not occur during food preparation or service. Check local regulations for further restrictions on the use of pest control devices.

Pest control cannot be accomplished effectively unless proper cleaning has occurred. One method of pest control alone is not often effective. For this reason, many dining services operations use an approach called **integrated pest management (IPM)**. IPM uses a variety of techniques and focuses on prevention. CDM, CFPPs should implement an IPM program and include these elements:

- Routine inspection of incoming supplies and inspection of the premises for evidence of pests.
- Restrict access into the facility with screens and building maintenance.
- Reduce food sources for pests through good cleaning and sanitization practices.
- Control pests by working with a licensed pest control operator (PCO), someone who is trained and licensed in pest management and use of pest control chemicals and devices.

All openings to the outside of the building must be closed to restrict access to the rodents. Screens in doors and windows can help to restrict the access of insects. Self-closing doors and proper seals around doors will also reduce the accessibility of the dining services operation to pests. Some facilities are required to use fly fans or air curtains.

The manager should check all deliveries for signs of pest infestation prior to accepting them. All food storage and preparation areas must be kept in a clean and sanitary condition. Food spills are sources of food for pests. Food stored against the wall creates places for pests to hide, nest, and multiply. Proper garbage management can reduce the risk of pest infestation.

Live Animals

Generally, live animals are prohibited from dining services establishments. The FDA Food Code makes an exception for the following, if food, equipment, utensils, linens, and unwrapped single-service articles are kept sanitary:

- Decorative fish in an aquarium.
- Patrol dogs accompanying police or security officers.
- In areas that are not used for food preparation.
- Pets in the common dining areas of facilities such as nursing homes, assisted living group homes, or residential care facilities at times other than during meals if the following conditions are met:
    > Doors separate the common dining areas from food storage or food preparation areas.

> **GLOSSARY**
>
> **Integrated Pest Management (IPM)**
> A coordinated approach to pest control, food production, and dining services to manage pests

9. Why is it important to have Integrated Pest Management in any foodservice facility?

- > Condiments, equipment, and utensils are stored in enclosed cabinets or removed from the dining areas when pets are present.
- > Dining areas, including tables and countertops, are cleaned and sanitized before the next meal service.

Summary

Maintaining a safe food supply from the purchase to the time of service depends on established policies, employee awareness, and well maintained physical spaces. CDM, CFPPs have lists of regulations, inspections, and laws to help guide their policy development and validate their expectations and restrictions. Ultimately, the goal is a safe and sanitary dining service for employees and clients.

Chapter References

RESOURCES	
BLINK Safety Training for Food Service Employees	https://blink.ucsd.edu/safety/resources/training/food.html
Centers for Disease Control and Prevention	Cdc.gov
Centers for Medicare & Medicaid Services	CMS.gov
FDA Emergency Preparedness: COVID 19 Response	https://www.fda.gov/emergency-preparedness-and-response/coronavirus-disease-2019-covid-19/covid-19-related-guidance-documents-industry-fda-staff-and-other-stakeholders
FDA Food Code 2017	https://www.fda.gov/media/110822/download
Food & Drug Administration	Fda.gov
National Marine Fisheries Service	fisheries.noaa.gov
National Sanitation Foundation (NSF) International Mark of Approval	Nsf.org
OSHA Occupational Hazard Communication Standard	Osha.gov
OSHA Safety Data Sheets	https://www.osha.gov/Publications/OSHA3514.html
U.S. Department of Agriculture	usda.gov
Underwriters Laboratories (UL) Electrical Safety Standards	UL.com

Manage the Operating Budget

Overview and Objectives

Effective management of costs and revenues is critical to the success of a foodservice operation. The ability of the Certified Dietary Manager®, Certified Food Protection Professional® (CDM®, CFPP®) in maximizing revenue while minimizing cost is vital in helping their facility maintain the bottom line. This chapter focuses on the various aspects of financial control techniques—specifically, financial terms, foodservice budgets, and ways to control meal and labor costs. After completing this chapter, you should be able to:

- Explain financial terminology
- Analyze and prepare a department budget
- Understand the difference between an operating budget and a capital budget
- Calculate food cost and meal equivalents
- Understand labor costs
- Calculate meals per labor hour
- Compare actual costs to budget costs
- Examine factors affecting labor costs

Improving the bottom line in a foodservice department is an important task for a manager. Knowing the sources of revenue and expenses, and using tools such as a budget to manage the money, are keys to good financial management.

Review of Financial Terms

This information is the basis of a Professional Practice Standard for CDM, CFPP. Two very important tools for planning, monitoring, and adjusting the financial performance of a dining services department are calculating raw food costs and calculating labor costs. A CDM, CFPP may determine a cost per meal based on total cost divided by the total number of meals. Managers also talk about cost per client day or cost per patient day (cost/ppd).

> (Note: For purposes of this textbook, the word *client* is being used rather than patient, resident, inmate, student, or child. However, the industry measure for food costs in health care is referred to as cost per patient day. For this measure, patient also means client.)

Understanding key financial terms in Figure 21.1 is important when reviewing budgets and costs.

Budgeting

In any business, sound management dictates that there is a plan for financial performance. This is an essential component that protects an organization against suddenly running out of money. A **budget** is a written plan for income and expenses. Typically, it covers a one-year period. This period may follow a calendar year, such as January through December, or it may follow a different 12-month period, such as July through June. The 12-month period for which a budget applies is called a **fiscal year**. A fiscal year is set by the financial managers of the facility and applies to the entire facility.

A budget helps a CDM, CFPP plan and make decisions about purchasing food and equipment, hiring workers, scheduling overtime, and much more. In essence, a budget provides a road map for the accounting department. The two most basic components of a budget are:

- Revenue: Money coming in or income.
- Expenses: Money going out or costs.

In any organization, the budget is arranged according to a hierarchy, starting with revenue and moving on to various expenses. Each department or section of the organization has its own set of numbers. A composite of all the individual department financial projections becomes the budget for the facility as a whole. Thus, a dining services budget feeds into the comprehensive plan for the facility.

As an aid in both planning and implementing a budget, financial planners break it into smaller pieces, called categories. A budget for a dining services operation, for example, may list expenses as an annual total and then also list specific groups of expenses with a projected dollar figure for each. The same concept applies to revenues. Figure 21.2 illustrates how budget categories may be presented.

This is a simplified example of a dining services budget. In this example, revenues come from sales in two categories: a cafeteria and for outpatient education. The budget

---

GLOSSARY

Budget
A written plan or prediction for income and expenses

Fiscal Year
The 12-month or 52-week period for which a budget applies

Figure 21.1
Financial Terminology

TERM	DEFINITION	COMMENT/EXAMPLE
FTE—Full Time Equivalent	The equivalent of one person working full time at 40 hours per week. Or it may mean two or more people whose hours together add up to 40 hrs./wk. Labor budgets are usually based on FTEs.	To determine FTEs per year for one full time person: 8 hrs./day x 5 days/wk. x 52 wks./yr. = 2,080 hr./yr. or one FTE.
Pay Period	A defined cycle for documenting hours worked and processing the payroll to issue paychecks.	If you are paid every other week, your pay period is two weeks long.
Overtime	The time an employee works beyond a regularly scheduled work day or pay period.	An employee who works 83 hours in one pay period (40 hrs./wk. for 2 weeks) would be entitled to three hours of overtime.
Exempt Employee	An employee who is exempt from overtime pay. This person is on salary and receives a standard rate of pay.	In most organizations, managers are classified as exempt.
Non-Exempt Employee	An employee who is *not* exempt from overtime pay.	Most foodservice staff positions.
Census	The number of clients or client count on a given day. How this is determined depends upon the type of food service.	Healthcare, Corrections/Schools: Managers will receive a daily census count. Cafeteria or Restaurant: Census is determined from the point of sale (POS) records.
Cost Per Meal	The calculated total food, supply, and labor cost divided by the number of meals served.	Often, comparisons of food cost per day or meal are used between facilities.
Food Cost Percentage	Used to calculate the percent of food cost compared to the revenue of a retail operation (cafeteria). The food cost for a specified period such as a month divided by the total sales for the same month.	For example, total sales for the month of October were $32,159 and the monthly food cost was $11,473. 11,473 / 32,159 = .3567 or 36%
Gross Versus Net	Gross means a sum of money, before any deductions are applied. Net is the amount of money that remains after all needed expenses have been deducted.	$1,220/month: Net incomes might be $875 after all of the deductions.
Break-Even	When revenues and expenses are equal.	There is no loss or profit.
Subsidies	External funding for foodservice activities.	School Foodservice: Usually refers to funding and/or food received from the USDA. Healthcare & University: Meals for staff may be subsidized as a planned benefit that may be transferred back to Human Resources as a labor cost. More frequently the cost is left as an unreimbursed expense in dining services.

Some of these terms have been defined in preceding chapters.

represents a projection or estimate of the income the operation expects to receive from each of these. Meanwhile, expenses are grouped by labor, food, supplies, and repairs.

Note that in this example, each category in the budget has a number. Meat purchases, for example are in category #701. Numbering of categories is commonly referred to as subaccounts and helps financial planners identify categories clearly.

Types of Budgets

The two most common budgets that CDM, CFPPs may use are an operating and a capital budget.

Operating Budget. This is an estimate of costs incurred in the process of generating meals. So it would be an estimate of the food costs, beverage costs, and labor costs. The operating budget is a financial plan for the period of time it covers. That time period might be one month, six months, or one year.

Figure 21.2
Sample Budget Categories

REVENUES		
101	$1,200	Outpatient Education
102	$120,000	Cafeteria Revenue
	$121,200	**TOTAL OPERATING REVENUES**
OPERATING EXPENSES		
Labor		
301	$571,985	Salaries
302	$131,557	Employee Benefits
	$703,542	**LABOR**
Supplies		
701	$275,213	Supplies: Meat, Fish, Poultry
702	$234,521	Supplies: Other Food
703	$27,854	Supplies: Supplements
704	$9,853	Supplies: Cleaning Products
705	$5,733	Supplies: Office and Admin.
	$553,174	**SUPPLIES**
Supplies		
801	$15,000	**REPAIRS AND MAINTENANCE**
Total Expenses		
	$1,271,716	**TOTAL OPERATING EXPENSES**
NET OPERATING BUDGET (EXPENSES, REVENUES)		
	($1,150,516)	**NET REVENUE OVER EXPENSES**

Another common practice is to break expenses and revenues down into smaller time increments, which makes it easier to monitor. In a dining services operation, a typical unit of time is one month. There are two ways to determine a monthly budget. If expected revenues and expenses are to accumulate evenly throughout the year, prorate all the figures. This means adjusting each figure according to a specified increment of time. So, to determine a one-month budget, divide each figure of an annual projected dollar amount by 12. In the example in Figure 21.2, wages paid to employees in a one-month period should be approximately: $571,985 ÷ 12 = $47,665.

A more complex budgeting model says that revenues and/or expenses will not be the same from month to month. Imagine operating a dining service for students in a university. Knowing that the client/customer counts or numbers receiving meals will drop sharply for the summer months, when student enrollment is very low, results in lower revenues from student meal plans. At the same time, there will be less spending on food and labor in the dining rooms. In a budget such as this one, a specific figure is planned for each category for each month.

Capital Budget. A capital budget is a plan for building improvements and additions or replacement of equipment. In order to complete a facility capital budget, each department will need to submit their capital requests. Figures 21.3 A and B show a sample operation budget for a public school system that includes the capital budget line.

Developing a Budget

The budget is an estimate for the future financial performance of the operation. In almost any facility, managers in their respective areas are called upon to submit budgets for an upcoming fiscal year, often months in advance. How much of the process is done by financial managers, versus how much is done by department managers, varies from one operation to another. In some situations, the department manager is not actively involved in the budget process. The manager should always seek to be a participant in the planning and development of the budget they are going to be responsible for managing.

In general, though, the following steps are useful in budget preparation:

1. **Clarify the objectives within the framework of the facility.** Is the aim to operate at break-even or at a profit? If it is a profit, how great? What revenues are expected from the operation?
2. **Break the budget into sections.** For example, if a dining room is intended to operate at a profit, separate it into its own budget. It is easier to track the performance as a unique cost center for accounting purposes. This way, estimated costs and revenues for this area are independent of other department areas. Work with the financial officer to establish appropriate sub-account categories.

Putting It Into Practice

1. Using Figure 21.2, prepare a mock budget for a nursing home foodservice department. Make sure the fiscal year is indicated and the revenue and expenses are put into various categories.

3. **Estimate the revenues.** Compare current performance to the existing budget and examine each source of revenue. What changes are anticipated? Estimate revenues from any new services or any predicted changes in volume or pricing of existing services.

4. **Estimate operating costs.** This can be one of the most time-consuming aspects of budget preparation. In this step, examine food and labor costs. For food costs, most CDM, CFPPs plan for a modest increase. How much this should be varies by product, by season, by market conditions, and by revisions in the purchasing agreements. Speak with vendors, research food price trends, and examine the prime vendor agreement to gain further information.

Most operating costs relate directly to client counts or census. Consult with others in the organization to obtain census estimates for the coming year. Identify time periods where segments of the facility may be closed for renovation, new units may be coming online, service may be added to the campus, or reductions in scope are anticipated. Scale operating costs accordingly.

In health care, colleges and universities, corrections, and K-12 schools, often a defined amount per person per day is budgeted. In this situation, it is especially critical to control cost per meal to fit within the parameters defined. The meal counts may be set and the income per meal defined.

In a typical dining services operation there is a level of unreimbursed catering or revenue to include in the operating budget. Using a cost per meal or cost per day method to develop a budget that includes these services is less predictive. Consider this example related to food cost:

- Senior Leadership has given a budget of:
  > $6.75 Food Cost per client day
  > $1.20 Supply Cost per client day
  > $12.67 Labor Cost per client day
- The Food Cost per Client Day helps define the client menu only:
  > Annualizing the Food Cost based on a client count of 100, the Food Budget calculates to: $6.75 x 100 x 365 = $246,375
  > The problem is that this calculation does not adjust for services in non-client activity such as:
    - An increase in the meals served internally through catering that is not part of the client count but increases food cost.
    - An increase in cafeteria meals (which may generate revenue) which is not part of the client count but increases food cost.
    - Addition of a service, i.e., adding meals for a daycare, which is not part of the client count but increases food cost.

Figure 21.4 illustrates some of the calculations that may be required to project changes for a new food budget based on projected changes. The method of simply adding an inflation factor assumes that the current budget is appropriate and does not need to change other than to reflect price adjustments. If, however, the current food cost per client day is high, then senior leadership may define a percentage or dollar amount by which to reduce the budget. Major adjustments during the budget process directly affect the operating plan for the department and impact the menu, purchasing options, and the use of labor (more scratch, less convenience).

Figure 21.3a
Sample School Food Service Fund
Fiscal Year July 1, 2019-June 30, 2020

EST. CASH RESERVES JULY 1, 2019	**$8,170,934**
2019-2020 Budgeted Revenue	
USDA Meal Reimbursements	$ 26,566,154
Lunch Sales	2,696,082
Breakfast Sales	252,852
A la Carte Sales	4,578,351
State Matching	320,130
Interest & Miscellaneous	70,862
Estimated Commodities	1,753,920
TOTAL BUDGETED REVENUE	**$ 36,238,351**
FUNDS AVAILABLE FOR 2019-2020	**$44,409,285**
2019-2020 Budgeted Expenditures	
Salaries	$ 12,271,362
Social Security & Medicare Match	858,995
Retirement Match	1,671,003
Employee Insurance Match	3,697,783
Food Purchases	11,946,237
Warehouse and Vendor Supplies	952,933
Other Supplies	104,976
Equipment	757,674
Equipment Maintenance	393,501
Freight and Storage	367,839
Uniform Rental & Laundry Services	166,270
Mileage	85,995
Other Expenses	255,263
Utilities	954.600
Estimated Commodities	1,753,920
TOTAL BUDGETED EXPENDITURES	**$ 36,238,351**
2020 EST. CHANGE IN CASH RESERVES	**$ —**

Source: Metro Nashville Public Schools. Adapted with permission.

Figure 21.3b
Sample School Budget Fiscal Year 2019-2020
Calculating Based on Previous Year's Projections

Account Number		Account Name	2018-2019 Positions	2018-2019 Budget	2019-2020 Position Changes	2019-2020 Budget Changes	2019-2020 Proposed Positions	2019-2020 Proposed Budget	Remarks
1440					**FOOD SERVICE**				
1440	0	Salaries, Certifications	3.0	$ 237,638		$ (2,731)	3.0	$ 234,907	Food Service Certified Coordinators
1440	1	Salaries, Clerical	10.0	343,575	1.0	(12,364)	11.0	331,211	Senior Secretary, Senior Account Clerks, Account Clerks
1440	2	Salaries, Support	768.0	11,972,206		(266,962)	768.0	11,705,244	Director, Coordinators, Field Managers, FS Managers and FS Workers
1440	3	Food		11,781,619		164,618		11,946,237	Dairy, Produce, Frozen Food and Food Staples
1440	4	Supplies and Materials		1,097,352		(39,773)		1,057,579	Vendor & Warehouse Purchases, Fuel, Truck Repairs, Office Supplies
1440	5	Other Expenses		2,215,539		(77736)		2,137,803	Equipment Repair, Telephone, Commodity Freight, Uniforms, Laundry, Training Permits, Utilities, Technology Vendor Support
1440	6	FICA, Pension & Insurance		5,698,978		528,803		6,227,781	Pension, Insurance, FICA
1440	7	Equipment		739,038		18,636		757,674	Large Equipment, Smallwares, Technology Hardware
1440	8	Travel/Mileage		78,583		7,412		85,995	Mileage
Function Total			781.0	$ 34,164,528	1.0	$ 319,903	782.0	$34,484,431	
USDA Commodities				1,369,545		384,375		1,753,920	
Total Budget and Commodities			781.0	$ 35,534,073	1.0	704,278	782.0	$38,238,351	

Meal Prices	2018-2019	2019-2020
BREAKFAST		
Elementary and Secondary Adult Priced by A la Carte Item	$1.25	$1.25
LUNCH		
Elementary	$2.00	$2.00
Secondary	2.25	2.25
Adult (MNPS staff or working volunteer)	3.00	3.00
Adult (parent/visitor)	3.50	3.50
Adult (parent/visitor holiday meal)	4.00	4.00

Source: Metro Nashville Public Schools. Used with permission.

For labor, consider any major changes that may have an impact, such as an upcoming contract negotiation with the union, an across-the-board pay increase for employees, the opening of a new restaurant across the street and similar information. Also consider the FTEs. Is there any change in services planned that might affect this number?

Although supplies are only about 5-8% of the total spend in the department, significant changes in the budget can impact the supply costs as well. If the organization decides to cut 1.5 FTE's from the dishroom and use all disposables in the cafeteria, the supply cost for chemicals will go down but the supply cost for paper goods will dramatically increase.

5. **Estimate capital expenses.** Capital expenses may include new equipment, a different meal delivery system, or renovations and supporting supplies that fall into unique categories for budgeting purposes. The financial decision-making around capital expenses are determined by different processes and will be discussed further in Chapter 22.

Calculating Costs

Calculating the cost of food can be simple math that provides a basic figure or it can be a more analyzed calculation that is a better "documented" number. In the most straightforward terms: How much money was spent on food last month? However, that sum total of purchases does not account for what was already in the storeroom at the first of the month nor what was left on the shelves at the end of the month. Adding up the invoice cost of food purchased is the food cost, but that is not just the client food cost. The invoices also include the unusual purchases for the annual medical staff gala or the turkeys bought as an employee "gift" each November. For budgeting purposes, a more detailed food cost is needed that divides out client meals from staff meals, catering, and guests.

Figure 21.4
Annual Budget Preparation

CATEGORY	CURRENT BUDGET	PROJECTED CHANGES	NEW BUDGET
Staples	$ 146,000	+1.5% (multiply by 1.015)	$ 148,190
Meals	132,000	+2% (multiply by 1.02)	134,640
Bakery	12,000	no change	12,000
Dairy	27,000	+0.5% (multiply by 1.005)	27,135
Produce	69,000	+3% (multiply by 1.03)	71,070

2. Using the mock budget developed for the nursing home, project revenue and expenses for the following fiscal year with remarks to justify increases/decreases.

Inventory Methods

This method requires a month-end physical inventory each month with the dollar value extension for each item. It is the most accurate method of determining monthly raw food costs. Food cost percentage is calculated by taking the cost of goods sold and dividing that by the revenue or sales generated from that finished dish. Cost of goods sold is the amount of money you've spent on ingredients and inventory in a given time period. The formula for calculating monthly raw food costs using this method is:

Beginning Inventory Value (the ending inventory value from the pervious month) + Purchases (for the month) - Ending Inventory = Monthly Food Costs (what was actually used during the month). This divided by food sales for the month will give you the food cost percentage.

Beginning Inventory = $15,000
Purchases = $4,000
Ending Inventory = $16,000
Food Sales = $10,000
Food Cost Percentage = (15,000 + 4,000 - 16,000) ÷ 10,000
Food Cost Percentage = 3,000 ÷ 10,000
Food Cost Percentage = 0.30 or 30%

Computerized inventory systems have made calculating monthly food costs much easier because purchases are recorded automatically. A physical inventory will still need to be completed monthly in order to calculate the ending inventory.

Recipe Method

Food cost can also be calculated per recipe or dish made. This method is based on determining the total cost of food for each standardized recipe.

The cost of each ingredient is added together and divided by the number of servings to calculate the cost per client of the recipe. Recipes must be used exactly as written (ingredients carefully measured and recipe portioned exactly). Most facilities need computer software to assist in this method. (The Recipe Cost versus the Menu Cost was discussed in Chapter 3, along with the impact of the yield factor.)

How to Calculate Food Cost per Serving (or food cost per menu item):

Food Cost per Food Item = Food Cost of Ingredients x Weekly Amount Sold
Total Sales Per Menu Item = Sales Price x Weekly Amount Sold

Now that you have calculated your food cost per dish, here's the formula for calculating food cost percentage: Food Cost Percentage = Total Cost Per Dish ÷ Total Sales Per Dish

Total Cost Per Dish = $2,500
Total Sales Per Dish = $10,000
Food Cost Percentage = 2,500 ÷ 10,000
Food Cost Percentage = 0.25 or 25%

> View the Supplemental Material for this chapter for Figure 21.5, Sample Food Cost Calculations.

Putting It Into Practice

3. Calculate food cost percentage for an operation that has a beginning inventory of $6,275, purchases of $3,840, ending inventory of $2,371.14, and sales of $20,800.

Menu Cost Report

A menu cost report is another very valuable tool. This report shows what it costs to produce a particular menu. A menu may be pre-costed, which means its costs are calculated during the planning phase. A tool such as this ensures that menu planning realistically meets the budget.

In addition to a pre-cost report, some operations run a post-cost report, or one that shows what the menu actually cost when production and service have been completed. This helps to identify operational variances. It shows where the planning may have fallen short, where food is unaccounted for, or where other factors need better control.

There are many formats and options for a menu cost report. An example of a menu pre-cost report appears in Figure 21.6. This report indicates that, as planned, the menu for regular diets served on day 1 of a cycle breakfast menu costs $1.32 per client. The cost of each item has been calculated based on the portion size used and actual food costs.

Some of these costs have come directly from purchasing records. For example, a CDM, CFPP examining pricing for skim milk has determined that the facility pays $0.17 per four ounce carton of skim milk. Other numbers for a report such as this one come from a calculation of costs for each serving of each standardized recipe.

A manager may also extend a report such as this for additional meals and (if applicable) additional special diets. A more complete costing report for the cycle day also indicates how many clients are actually being served on each diet. A sample menu cost report showing these extensions appears in Figure 21.7.

What is the impact on the budget compliance if one diet costs more or less to serve than anticipated? Based on a report such as this one, the answer depends on how many clients receive this particular diet. In this example, a variation in meal cost for regular diets will have the greatest bottom line impact because there are more clients receiving this meal. (Notice that the food cost for the Pureed Diet is higher than the other meals. This is due to the increased cost of thickened liquids which are a part of the diet.)

Meal Equivalents

The number of **meal equivalents** per labor hour is a primary measure of productivity and production. To calculate meal equivalents (MEQ), one must convert different meal services (i.e., breakfast, supper, and snacks) and non-program food sales that include the cafeteria service, floor stock (food taken to other locations for clients), catering to outside groups, staff meals, tube feedings, coffee and snack times, and nourishments to the equivalent of one meal equivalent for comparison.

Meal equivalents can be used for tracking food costs, budget performance, or other Key Performance Indicators, as well as for benchmarking within or outside the organization. It is important to always use the same calculation and be consistent so the comparison from one point in time to another is valid.

There are several different systems for counting the number of meals served. Each calculation has its benefits and supporters, as well as potential errors. The patient (or client) day has a more widely accepted standard definition of the midnight count of clients "in house" while a meal has a variety of different definitions. Due to these various definitions, Total Meal Counts are hard to track and verify.

> **GLOSSARY**
>
> **Meal Equivalents**
> A calculated estimate of the number of meals prepared or served

Figure 21.6
Menu Pre-Cost Report for One Meal

MEAL: Breakfast Menu, Cycle Day 1, Regular Diet		
Menu Item	Portion Size	Cost per Portion
Orange Juice	6 oz.	$ 0.31
Cheese Omelet	1 each	0.35
English Muffin	2 halves	0.12
Margarine	2 pats	0.05
Jelly	1 pack	0.04
Coffee	12 oz.	0.19
Skim Milk	4 oz.	0.17
Condiment Pack	1 each	0.09
	TOTAL	$ 1.32

Figure 21.7
Menu Cost Report for All Diets, One Day

Diet	PER CLIENT FOOD COST					Number of Clients	Total Food
	Breakfast	Lunch	Dinner	Snacks	Total Cost		
Regular	$ 1.32	$ 1.77	$ 2.14	$ 0.32	$ 5.55	100	$ 555.00
Diabetic	1.36	1.65	2.11	0.35	5.47	43	235.21
Heart Healthy	1.47	1.55	2.08	0.19	5.29	23	121.67
Pureed	1.38	2.11	2.70	0.61	6.80	13	88.40
Tube Feeding					6.12	21	128.52
					DAILY TOTAL	200	$ 1,128.80

Labor Costs

In a food production and dining services department, there is an assumption that food purchases are the majority of the budget. However, labor costs, especially employee benefit costs, have increased dramatically. Employees are the greatest assets and greatest expense. Food costs typically run around 40%, while labor costs are closer to 55% of the total department budget (before benefits).

Estimating Labor Costs for Budget Purposes

For facilities that have a daily census (hospitals, long-term care, corrections, schools, universities), it is a useful planning tool for estimating personnel costs. Use the average census, since it may drive labor costs, to help estimate personnel expenses for the operational budget. The human resources department might be able to provide the necessary salary information to assist in this calculation.

There are other factors that impact the labor hours in a dining services department. When planning the labor budget, consider the following:

- Number of menu items.
- Type of menu.
- Type and extent of services offered.
- Type of equipment.
- Layout of equipment and department in relation to dining rooms.
- Seasonal variations in staffing.
- Number of hours the dining services department is open for business.

Once the factors affecting labor have been identified, begin estimating the costs. Review Chapter 9 for information on calculating staffing positions, labor hours, and FTE's. Figure 21.8 shows a sample budget with salary and employee benefit categories.

Managing labor expenses means monitoring it on a very regular basis. Overtime hours can quickly get out of hand if not monitored consistently. When first starting, monitor the labor usage to budget every week to understand the ups and downs. If the budget is computerized, access the financial reports with the year-to-date figures.

Figure 21.8
Sample Budget With Salary Categories

SALARIES	2020	Year-to-Date	2021
Administrative	$ 53,257	$ 45,001	
Managers	84,412	78,581	
Employees (includes waitstaff, kitchen staff, sanitation staff)	183,645	165,247	
Call-in Staff	2,780	2,649	
TOTAL SALARIES	$ 324,094	$ 291,478	
EMPLOYEE BENEFITS	2020	Year-to-Date	2021
Health/Life/Dental	$ 139,360	$ 139,760	
Retirement	18,797	19,001	
FICA	20,418	20,067	
Unemployment	3,214	2,978	
Workers Compensation	6,482	5,189	
TOTAL EMPLOYEE BENEFITS	$ 188,271	$ 186,995	
TOTAL LABOR COSTS	$ 512,365	$ 478,473	

Labor Financial Measurements Used in Foodservice Operations

Labor Costs Per Meal. Just as in calculating food costs PPD or per meal, you should also calculate labor costs per meal. Use the formula listed below:

> **Example:** Use the Total Labor Costs from Figure 21.8 and a sample Total Meals Served of 191,118
>
> $512,365 ÷ 191,118 = $2.68 Labor Cost per Meal

Labor Costs per Meal Served = Labor Costs ÷ Total Meals Served

Figure 21.9
Including Meal Equivalents In Labor Cost per Meal

Total Meal Equivalents Costs for March:

Other Meals
Cafeteria Sales for the Month of March. $18,562.00
Floor Stock Requisitions for March 415.00
Catering for Coffee, Snacks, Activities 219.00
Staff Meals for March 1,405.00
Tube Feedings and Nourishments 5,637.00
TOTAL. $26,238.00

Average Price for a Typical Cafeteria Meal (Market Basket Method) $3.21

Meal Equivalents for March: $26,238 ÷ $3.21 = $8,174 Meal Equivalents

Total Meals 191,118 ÷ Meal Equivalents 8,174 = 199,292

Divide the Labor Cost by the Total Meals Served: $512,365 ÷ 199,292 = $2.57

Note: While a decrease in labor cost per meal by 10 cents may not seem dramatic, it can make a huge difference in your overall labor costs. What if your administration said your labor cost per meal could not be more than $2.50 per meal? You could lower the cost by 10 cents per meal just by counting all of the meals you are producing.

It is important to control both food cost and labor cost per meal to meet the fiscal objectives of the facility.

Other Labor Cost Considerations

Part-time Staff. Another way to lower costs in food service is through the use of part-time employees. The use of part-time staff to replace full-timers has increased significantly in the past 10 years. Often part-time staff can dramatically decrease labor cost. How much savings is dependent upon the wage differential from full-time staff and the benefit package offered to part-time employees. Let's look at an example of a university food service that currently employs 10 full-time cooks over 14 shifts per week. The university employees receive an average wage of $16/hr. plus employee benefits equivalent to an additional 30%.

```
Wages:     10 cooks x 40 hrs. x $16 per hr.  = $6,400
Benefits:  $6,400 x 30%                      = $1,920
           Total Labor Cost                  = $8,320/wk.
```

If the university decides to cover some of the shifts with LTEs or Limited Term Employees who work only part-time for $10/hr. and qualify for only 20% benefits.

```
Full-time Cooks:
Wages:     6 cooks x 40 hrs. x $16/hr.  = $3,840
Benefits:  $3,840 x 30%                 = $1,152
           Total Labor Costs            = $4,992

Part-time Cooks:
Wages:     8 cooks x 20 hrs. x $14/hr.  = $2,240
Benefits:  $2,240 x 20%                 = $448
           Total Labor Costs            = $2,688
           New Total Labor Costs        = $7,680/wk.
```

If the organization decides to increase the number of part-time employees, make sure they feel a part of the department and are included in all of the training.

Labor Legislation. The effect of labor legislation can be significant when considering the staffing budget. Unfortunately, labor legislation varies from state to state. There are some general terms that apply to all states: minimum wage and provisions for overtime. Both of these are set by the Fair Labor Standards laws that were discussed in Chapter 10.

Working With Human Resources (HR) Department

If the CDM, CFPP is fortunate enough to have an HR department, many of the tasks regarding labor will be completed by that department. For instance, HR personnel will help determine where to place an employee on the salary schedule. HR will keep all employee records. They will provide the insurance, tax, and other forms for personnel.

If there is no HR department, the manager may be expected to maintain salary records. Insurance and tax forms along with other information may also need to be provided to personnel. Work with administration to determine what forms are required and what salary should be offered.

Working With Labor Unions

Labor contracts will always be an important factor affecting staff costs. Labor contracts impact wages, benefits, and other aspects of human resources management. Unionization provides certain advantages to employees. It also imposes certain requirements on the CDM, CFPP who must comply with a union agreement.

The decision for employees to form or join a union is made through a voting process. A **union** forms an agreement with an organization on behalf of the group of employees. Employees may form or join unions in order to attain better working conditions, improved safety, better pay, or specific benefits. However, membership in a union is not a guarantee that employees will receive everything they want or expect.

GLOSSARY

Union
An organization of workers intended to represent their co-workers in labor agreements

Reasons for an employee desiring to join a union sometimes relate directly to relationships with management. Following sound management practices may minimize the employee's perceived need for a union. Implementation of procedures to address employee concerns, and a manager who keeps in touch with employees' needs and wants, helps create a collaborative environment. Some techniques used to do this include a suggestion box, employee survey(s), employee relations rounds conducted by the HR department (or by the manager in small facilities), employee meetings, and effectively conducted employee appraisal programs. Whenever these or other techniques are used to assess employee concerns, management needs to then act on the concerns and suggestions seriously and attempt to make improvements.

Other reasons for joining a union include a desire to be heard, the appeal of a formal means of expressing concerns to administrators, and a feeling that group attachment brings security. A formal group of employees is perceived as stronger than an informal group.

Impact of Unions On Administration

Once employees are represented by a union, administration will probably have to alter some operations. Follow the contract for salary rather than decide at what level to place a new employee. Regardless of an employee's ability or skills, each must be treated equally if he or she is in the same (or similar) job classification. Frequently, seniority—rather than other factors which might distinguish employees' qualifications and performance—may become the most important factor in matters affecting personnel-related decisions.

There can be advantages to unionization. The presence of a union prompts development and/or improvement of policies or procedures that affect relationships with employees. A facility that does not have well-developed policies and management tools is likely to benefit. On certain issues, administrators will also be able to deal with only one representative of unionized employees rather than with various individual staff members. Finally, top levels of administration may need to recover much decision-making responsibility that had previously been delegated to supervisors, since the actions of a single supervisor may have facility-wide implications in a unionized environment. To the extent that centralized decision-making is beneficial, it is another advantage to union affiliation.

The Collective Bargaining Process

Many people define collective bargaining as negotiations between union and facility representatives leading to a contract. More generally, however, the term **collective bargaining** applies to routine communications and negotiations involving contract agreements, interpreting contract clauses, and resolving disputes (grievances) between union and administrative officials. A great deal of time can be spent in negotiating a union agreement. It is common for union contracts to apply for a period of three or more years. To prepare for the negotiation, administrative officials in a facility must obtain information about prevailing wage and salary rates and fringe benefit provisions. They must also assess the facility's financial position, resources, and ability to commit to specific wages and other terms. Furthermore, they must analyze existing contracts, communicate with union representatives, and consider probable union concerns.

Through discussion and negotiation, the union, representing the employee and the facility administration reach a final agreement about relevant issues, including wages

GLOSSARY

Collective Bargaining
Generally refers to communication between administration officials and union representatives

and salary. This agreement is signed and formalized, with each party committing to honor it for the time period specified.

How can the CDM, CFPP prepare and budget for increasing labor contract costs? When administration is negotiating a new contract, a manager should make sure that the labor costs provided by the administration are accurate. If possible, have the HR department survey other union foodservice departments to determine recent changes in their wage scale. This information will also be helpful.

Utilize Guidelines for Salary Scales and Merit Raises

Every facility should have a salary schedule. If the staff is represented by a union the facility is bound by the contract to follow that salary schedule. If there is no union in the facility, there should still be a salary schedule and policies about merit increases. The HR department should maintain a database or have access to a regional database of salary guidelines for the industry. They may have access to local wage rates for positions similar to those in the dining services department. This will help determine the prevailing local rate for cooks, dining room attendants, storeroom clerks, and other positions in the department.

Another resource that might help with salary guidelines is the Association of Nutrition & Foodservice Professionals Annual Salary Survey. Figure 21.10 , found in the Supplemental Materials, shows the 2022 Salary Survey results. While this information focuses on salaries for CDM, CFPPs, it can still be a reference for your facility because it contains benefit information and represents the entire United States.

View the Supplemental Material for this chapter for Figure 21.10, ANFP Salary Survey 2022.

Chapter References

RESOURCES	
Labor Costs	https://www.foodservicedirector.com/operations/food-labor-budgets-most
Labor Relations	https://www.dol.gov/general/topic/labor-relations
Meal Equivalents	https://schoolnutrition.org/uploadedFiles/2_Meetings_and_Events/Presentation_PDFs/ANC_2018/Case-Study-Benchmarking-Meals-Per-Labor-Hour-(MPLH).pdf

Manage the Capital Budget

Overview and Objectives

The Certified Dietary Manager®, Certified Food Protection Professional® (CDM®, CFPP®) is expected to know their department space and equipment to anticipate the needs for replacements or renovations. They also have to present the case for large dollar investments for the future. The capital equipment budget planning process is significantly different from the operations budget and often includes a more difficult approval process. After completing this chapter, you should be able to:

- Review capital equipment needs and requirements
- Evaluate existing capital equipment condition and life expectancy
- Evaluate options for replacement of capital equipment
- Write budget justification for new capital equipment
- Recommend specifications for new capital equipment

GLOSSARY

Capital Expense
The cost of a single item that exceeds a finance defined limit with an expected use, or life, longer than the general operating budget

View the Supplemental Material for this chapter for Figure 22.1, Sample Equipment Log.

The Capital Budget

In most organizations, the Finance Department has set a maximum spending level for any one purchase item. Often the top price the manager can spend without additional authorization is $1,000, and up to $5,000 in some facilities. Purchases larger than that amount for a single item are considered to be a **Capital Expense** with an expected use, or life, longer than the general operating budget. To control large ticket purchases and manage the depreciation of equipment from an accounting perspective, capital budgets are developed using a totally different process.

Often the capital budgeting process includes an estimate of items that will be needed in the next year, 2-5 years, and even out 5-10 years. The estimates help senior leadership to project the need for investment funds in the coming years and to spread out the cost of replacement purchases. The annual capital budget is essentially an estimate of the equipment that will be needed in the next 12 months.

In food production and dining services, capital expenses are typically related to the large kitchen equipment or meal delivery systems. Replacement of the dishmachine is often a $75,000 to $250,000 expense and has a lifetime use of many years. Updating the dishmachine may seem obvious, but without thorough documentation and justification kitchen updates are typically the result of irreparable equipment failure instead of planned replacement. Often the need for new operating room equipment takes priority over the purchase of a stove or replacement of the walk-in compressor.

Managing the capital equipment process starts with maintaining a complete list of all items within the department. Frequently, Engineering has a comprehensive list that they use for preventive maintenance (PM) on major pieces of machinery. The Information systems department keeps track of all the computers, printers, and software systems. The finance department should have a list of all items within the department that are considered to be capital equipment and the current depreciation status of each. Compare the respective lists to make sure all items are covered, and add to it any equipment that needs to be monitored such as food processors, meat slicers, and utility carts. An example of an Equipment Log is shown in Figure 22.1, found in the Supplemental Material for this book.

Use the list of equipment to monitor the repairs and service expenses related to the equipment. See in Figure 22.2 in the Supplemental Material for an Equipment Repair Log. Note the frequency of down time and the cost of repairs, including substitute process expenses (the use of disposable serviceware when the dishmachine is down) and the cost of the company rep service calls. Each year, when preparing the capital budget, review and update the status of every piece of equipment on the list including the estimated remaining "life." Add items that have been purchased and remove items as they are disposed of or retired. Note that the equipment purchased today will likely have a shorter "life cycle" than older, more heavily designed pieces.

Often, contacting the local equipment company for recommendations of models and features will be enough information for the overall forecasting process. Most vendors will provide a "reasonable" estimate (usually fairly high to cover all costs) of the purchase price, along with the likely cost of installation. Typically, the capital budget requires or recommends that a copy of the product cut sheet be included as a reference. This is also available from the equipment vendor or online.

What Goes Into the Capital Budget

The list of items that fit into the capital budget can be endless. Common food production and dining services items include:

- Stoves, ovens, fryers, grills, steamers: cooking equipment
- Grinders, food processors, mixers, slicers: preparation equipment
- Coolers, walk-ins, freezers, reach-in: cold food holding
- Hot box, warmer, bain marie, steam tables, conduction tables: hot food holding
- Soft serve, coffee machines, beverages: dispensers
- Prep tables, utility carts, speed racks, storage racks, racks: work space
- Serving line, plate warmers, induction systems and pellets, delivery carts, trays, dishware and silverware (as part of the initial line purchase, replacement pieces are considered operating expenses)
- Software systems, computers, printers, cash registers, many pieces of office furniture
- Dishroom equipment, pot and pan sinks and equipment, carts, racks
- Ice machines
- Dining room tables and chairs
- Design and build out of new space or renovations

This is not an all-inclusive list, and some organizations may not include everything that is here, but this is representative of the items that fall under the capital budget versus the operating budget.

What Goes Into the Capital Budget Request

Once a piece of equipment has been identified for purchase, the manager needs to organize the supporting material to justify the expense, which may not be obvious when the piece of equipment is limping along. Let's use a dishmachine as an example to demonstrate what information is needed.

- The current equipment is 20 years old.
- The repair record shows that in the past year it has been down 4 different times from 1-6 days.
- The service rep has been in for repairs 3 of those times ($1,500 plus travel expense of $800).
- The chemical service rep has commented that the use of detergent and drying agent is unexpectedly high because the wash and rinse tanks have a continuous leak of water (estimated added cost of $2,200 annually).
- The engineering department has been monitoring the water usage and is concerned about the energy cost of the hot water used and lost (estimated addedd cost of water and gas of $2,700 annually).
- The labor cost associated with the downtime was 45 hours above budget in the last year (an estimated $1,000).
- The cost of disposables used to provide serviceware during downtime was $2,750.
- Patient survey results during the months affected in the last year all reflect comments regarding cold food and poor presentation, which in turn could impact the facility's reimbursements from Medicare.

View the Supplemental Material for this chapter for Figure 22.2, Sample Equipment Repair Log.

- In recent years the dishmachine design has been upgraded to use far less water than previously, run faster, and to be more economical in the chemical usage
  - > Replacement of the current unit would save more in water, gas for heating the water, drying agents, and chemicals through newer technology than even the amount lost through the leaks.
  - > Often the newer machines also use less floor space, allowing for better access.

The annual cost of repairs and overrun expenses is almost $11,000 a year. Suddenly, replacing the poorly functioning dishmachine becomes more financially reasonable.

Using the information collected, the capital request becomes easier to complete. The request form generally requires detailed information about the piece of equipment and installation, including the following:

- Specification cut sheets for one or more models
- Competitive price quotes from one to three vendors
  - > The Materials Management (Purchasing) Department can help source this information
- Delivery costs and timetables
- Installation costs
  - > Verify with Engineering the availability and accessibility to needed utilities.
  - > Estimated costs of utility upgrades if needed.
  - > Space needs and access (will it fit through the door and under the hood)?
  - > How much downtime of the current equipment will be needed and how will needs be met in the interim?
- Removal and disposal cost of the old equipment.
- What is the need for potential space redesign and cost to accommodate the new equipment?
  - > For example, a new garbage disposal, new scrapping tables, a heat booster for the hot water, water softening equipment, new racks and drying table, etc.

Often, the equipment vendor can assist with organizing the printed materials needed to support a capital request. They have access to materials developed by the manufacturers to calculate replacement costs, benefits, and features of different equipment and data to complete the **Return On Investment (ROI)** forms that are part of the request. The ROI is the length of time it takes to get your money back for an investment in the future.

Developing the capital budget forces the CDM, CFPP to look annually at all of the equipment and supporting systems within the department that are needed on a daily basis. The manager has to assess the current status and estimated useful life of the equipment and decide if replacement is needed this year, next year, or sometime further out.

GLOSSARY

Return on Investment (ROI)
The length of time it takes to get your money back for an investment in the future

Putting It Into Practice

1. Write out a Capital Budget Request for a range oven detailing the reason for the request and justification for the new purchase. What information would be most important?

Equipment Replacement Decisions

Eventually every manager is expected to recommend equipment for replacement or addition as department needs change. The equipment maintenance record will assist in deciding when to repair or purchase new, what to purchase, and why. The steps in replacing or purchasing new equipment include:

1. Develop Equipment Specifications: When the decision is being made to repair or replace equipment, the CDM, CFPP should develop a specification for the equipment. Considerations for purchase specifications include:
   - Will the equipment provide the time and temperature control that is necessary for safe food?
   - Is the equipment properly sized for the volume of food that is prepared?
   - Is the equipment reliable or is it prone to frequent breakdowns?
   - Is the equipment designed so that it can be easily cleaned and sanitized?
   - Is the equipment easy to use?
   - Will the equipment fit into the assigned space?
   - Further discussion of equipment specifications is explored in Chapter 23.

2. Conduct **Cost Benefit Analysis**: A cost-benefit analysis compares the relative value (quality and expense) of upgrading a piece of equipment with the downtime and cost of repairs.
   - A repair log can provide you with the history of breakdowns, lost time, and expenses.
   - Consider the current features that would be lost versus the new capabilities:
     > Will the cost of replacement allow for an upgrade, exact match, or maybe a reduction in features?
   - Consider the repairability of any new equipment including:
     > Access to moving parts, electrical panels/gas lines/water pipes.
     > Availability of manufacturer's repair reps (a three-day lead time for repair parts may disqualify a potential purchase for "mission critical" equipment).
   - When the cost of materials and labor to repair equipment is near to or greater than the cost of replacement, the equipment should be replaced.

3. When writing a cost-benefit analysis or justification for replacement, estimate repair costs by comparing the warranty information against the life of the equipment. Consult with equipment representatives and other food operators who have had experience with the equipment and/or the brand.

4. Installation and Staff Training: Often, the manufacturer or supplier will assist in ensuring that the new equipment is properly installed and provide training to staff. Vendors may charge an additional fee for hard copy equipment manuals, particularly if the online version of the manual is readily available. Managers and other purchasers should attempt to negotiate the price of equipment operation manuals, staff training, and other support into the purchase price of the equipment.

5. Typically, purchasing requires three competitive bids to compare purchase costs, delivery and installation charges, timeliness of delivery, and service warranty options.

> **GLOSSARY**
>
> **Cost-Benefit Analysis**
> Compares the relative value (quality and expense) of upgrading a piece of equipment with the downtime and cost of repairs

Alternatives

The purchase of major equipment is expensive and can be time-consuming. Often, manufacturers or distributors offer the option for long-term leasing of the equipment for a fee. Coffee equipment is readily available for an upcharge of a few cents per pound of coffee purchased. Dishwashers can be leased from the manufacturer or sometimes the chemical supply company has leasing agreements.

The downside of leasing is the lack of ownership, therefore, no equity value of the equipment, the commitment to purchase their products exclusively, and the ongoing cost no matter how long the item is in use. The upside of leasing is little or no out-of-pocket cost, since the manufacturer or distributor is responsible for all repair costs, and quicker access to newer technology than what is in current use.

Summary

Capital budgets are very different processes than the typical operations budget. The planning and preparation for capital investments requires different types of information and usually depends upon a well-documented, persuasive presentation to gain approval. When a piece of needed equipment is broken, repair or replacement is obvious. However, when the piece of equipment is not beyond the point of repair, often replacement is seen as discretionary spending—that can wait.

When money is tight and funding for new equipment and projects is limited, plan to prepare a formal presentation with a slide show, statistics to back up the recommendations, cost projections, and the value of implementing the proposal. Keep the needs of the clients, and the safety of staff and clients in focus when preparing the proposal and presentation. Review the suggestions in Chapter 15 for effective speaking, and design a presentation to convince senior leadership of the need to approve not just the capital budget, but also to release the funds for purchase.

Chapter References

RESOURCES	
Cost-Benefit Analysis	https://en.wikipedia.org/wiki/Cost%E2%80%93benefit_analysis
Return on Investment	en.wikipedia.org/wiki/Return_on_investment

Department Design and Layout

Overview and Objectives

The design and layout of the kitchen and dining area in any foodservice operation has a direct impact on its function. The Certified Dietary Manager®, Certified Food Protection Professional® (CDM®, CFPP®) is asked to plan a kitchen redesign and justify the layout and equipment purchased. This chapter helps prepare for those tasks. After completing this chapter, you should be able to:

- Identify factors influencing the layout and design of a foodservice facility
- Evaluate purchase of essential equipment relative to designs
- Develop equipment specifications
- Train staff on preventive maintenance of equipment, cleaning schedules, and using repair logs

Both design and equipment have a direct impact on the efficiencies of a food production and dining services operation. Effective design and equipment choices allow for operational objectives related to the menu, customer/client service, quality, schedules, budget, and safety. Whether planning a new operation or remodeling an existing operation, designing the physical layout is a critical step. Any change to menus or service models can trigger a need to revise design, equipment, or both.

Factors Influencing the Physical Layout

The layout of a facility can impact food quality and the ability to produce meals according to established timetables. It can also affect labor efficiency and staffing schedules. The task of designing a food production and dining services department is complex and should involve the team effort of a CDM, CFPP along with a project architect, foodservice design consultant, in-house engineering expert, and staff who use the equipment. Efficient flow of products through the food production area and work stations that maximize employee work activity is central to a well-designed work space. The flow of work varies from one operation to another.

Typically, facilities are designed by considering workload requirements. Then, work centers are developed based on logical groupings of menu items and tasks. Generally, the layout of a food production and dining services area should enable a logical, economical flow of foods from receiving through storage, production, additional storage (if required), and service. It should support separation of clean, sanitized products from soiled products. Concerns that must be considered include:

The Menu. The relationship between the menu and the production equipment is a "push me—pull me" one. Menu items such as "fry only" french fries are ill-advised in a production kitchen with no fryers. The menu defines the types of food products to be prepared and the equipment needed. The equipment present defines what can be written into the menu.

The space available has to accommodate the inventory, pre-prep, preparation, holding, and service defined by the menu. Limited storage space requires either a limited menu or daily deliveries.

Use of Convenience Foods. As the number and quality of convenience items increases, the need for food production space and equipment decreases. However, requirements for refrigerated and/or freezer storage space will typically increase. Conversely, if many items are being made from scratch, on-site needs for preparation space and equipment increase.

Quantity of Food to Prepare. Equipment and work space must be sized to accommodate the number of meals being produced for on-site as well as any off-site feeding and catering.

Production and Service Systems. Both production and service models influence the need for space and the use of space over time. In a decentralized system, much of the required work space and equipment shifts to remote units, such as serving pantries.

In a centralized system there is a much greater need for work space and equipment in the central location. In a cook-chill system, there may be greater opportunity to control scheduling of work; it is important to use space and labor time efficiently since food preparation is not intended for immediate service.

Each system also dictates varying needs for storage. For example, a cook-chill system requires large refrigerated storage areas along with blast chillers and rethermalization equipment. A decentralized service system needs refrigerated storage, transport equipment, and rethermalization units. Space for equipment and a layout that supports efficient work flow are essential. Over time, an established design and layout may need to be adjusted. For example, any of the following could occur:

- A 30-year baker is retiring, and the CDM, CFPP might determine it would be more economical and better for quality control to purchase more convenience items for the bakery.
- A replacement oven may have different space requirements than the existing oven or different electrical service requirements.
- A new service may require the operation to double its production of salad and soup products.

Space. Space allocated for food production and dining services affects both the facility layout and the amount, and type, of equipment that can be considered. Based on the needs of a facility, compromises in space, design, and budget are common. Square footage limitations or unusual layout may drive decisions to select space-efficient equipment options, and/or to choose single pieces of equipment that can perform multiple functions.

Funds. Budget funds allocated for equipment have an impact on plans. Food production and dining services often need to compete with other departments for limited space and budgetary resources for remodeling and/or new building activities.

Energy Efficiency and Sustainability. Over the lifetime of a piece of equipment, operating costs related to gas or electricity usage can be staggering. The food production and dining services department makes up a large percentage of a facility's energy bill. In 2001, an energy efficiency program called Energy Star® was launched to designate equipment that is highly efficient. An Energy Star® rating meets the minimum efficiency criteria. How do you begin controlling energy costs? Start with contacting your local energy companies. They may offer consulting services to help you design and order equipment for maximum efficiency. A local energy company may also conduct kitchen equipment test reports, giving you specific information about the energy usage of cooking and food preparation equipment. Your energy company may also conduct an on-site survey, resulting in a list of recommended actions to cut energy use and costs.

Figure 23.1 shows energy conservation tips to consider for your facility.

Sustainable and green building concepts are becoming more common in the industry. An emerging certification called LEED (Leadership in Energy and Environmental Design), developed by the U.S. Green Building Council, is encouraging buildings that are "designed and built using strategies aimed at improving performance across all the metrics that matter most. Some of these strategies are: energy savings, water efficiency, carbon dioxide emissions reduction, improved indoor environmental quality, and stewardship of resources and sensitivity to their impacts." Many facilities are adding composting, rooftop gardens, and herb gardens to further support the green initiative.

Water efficiency is also an aspect of green buildings. A number of facilities are looking at saving and reusing water. One example of water efficiency is a water-cooled ice machine. Other facilities are utilizing biotechnology. At least one university is using food scraps for bioenergy.

Figure 23.1
Energy Conservation Tips

1. Switch from incandescent EXIT lights to LED EXIT lighting. They last 10 times longer with an average annual savings of $40, excluding maintenance costs.

2. Switch from incandescent light bulbs in exhaust hoods and walk-ins to Energy Star® Light-Emitting Diode (LED) lamps. Replacing a single 60 watt incandescent lamp, operated 12 hours per day over 365 days, with a 12 watt LED lamp will save approximately $20 in annual operating cost at a utility rate of $0.10/kWh.

3. Turn off door heaters on reach-in refrigerators and freezers. Commercial reach-in refrigerators and freezers have door heaters to help prevent condensation build up around the door frame; however, in dry climates condensation may not be an issue and many refrigerators and freezers have door heaters which can be manually turned off. A single heater has an approximate annual operating cost of $50 at a utility rate of $0.10/kWh.

4. Use strip curtains or plastic doors on walk-in coolers and freezers to prevent warm air infiltration and reduce compressor runtime. Utility studies have shown an annual savings of $100 for a typical 10 x 10 walk-in freezer equipped with a strip curtain assuming a utility rate of $0.10/kWh.

5. Fix all water leaks. A seemingly innocent hot water leak with a flow rate of half a gallon per hour can have an annual cost of $90 if left unabated. Cost assumes a natural gas cost of $1.00/therm and a water/sewer utility cost of $8.00/CCF.

6. Clean dirty refrigeration system–evaporator and condenser coils. They should be inspected monthly for dust, lint, and other obstructions and cleaned if necessary.

7. Set water heater to proper temperature. Only heat water to the temperature required for specific tasks in your operation. Facilities with a high temperature dish machine typically require 140°F supply hot water and those with a low temperature machine can require supply hot water as low as 125°F. A water heater set 10°F too high in a typical casual dining restaurant using 2,000 gallons of hot water per day will cost an extra $900/year, assuming a natural gas utility cost of $1.00/therm.

8. Replace high flow pre-rinse sprayers with high performing, low flow sprayers that have a flow rate no higher than 1.6 gallon per minute. Retrofitting a high flow nozzle rated at 5.0 gpm with a low flow unit rated at 1.2 gpm in a dish room where operated one hour per day over 365 days will save approximately $1,700 in natural gas and water costs.

9. Implement a strict start up and shut down schedule for all cooking appliances. Fryers, ovens, griddles, and charbroilers require no more than 20-30 minutes to pre-heat. Pay special attention to charbroiler and manually controlled griddles—shut them entirely off, partially off, or down during slow service periods.

10. Install and/or maintain programmable thermostats to manage heating and air conditioning systems. Properly program the thermostat so that during unoccupied periods, cooling is set to 85°F and heating to 55°F. During occupied hours set the cooling set point as high as possible and heating set point as low as possible, but still being mindful to maintain staff and customer comfort. As a rule of thumb, for every cooling degree set point increase and heating degree set point decrease, system operating cost lowers by 3%-4%.

Incorporating energy efficiency in the capital planning for equipment replacement is looking ahead. Perhaps the state or local utility has a rebate program to help cover the cost. Or maybe when the freezer needs to be replaced a larger Energy Star® model will provide more storage and better efficiency. As with any plan, review it annually to update with the latest information on efficient commercial kitchen equipment.

Ergonomic Factors. Ergonomic factors influence the comfort, efficiency, and safety of a work environment, and are of great concern in food production and dining services. Designs that control physical fatigue and help prevent injury related to repetitive motion are important. These concerns are recognized as designers reduce distances employees must travel, adjust heights of work areas to fit the needs of employees, and develop comfortable (thickened) handles for small utensils.

Noise. There can be a great deal of noise in food preparation areas. Use of soundproofing materials and the selection of less noisy equipment can help reduce these problems. Excessive noise can distract employees, leading to accidents and injuries. Likewise, when equipment noise carries into the dining space, clients and guests are affected.

Lighting. Adequate lighting is critical for safety as well as for managing the quality of work in food production and dining services department. Lighting is separated into ambient, task, and accent lighting.

- Ambient or general lighting provides overall illumination—often, florescent ceiling bulbs are used in food production areas. The level of brightness is intended to provide light without glare or significant shadows.
- Task lighting is intended to provide illumination for specific work areas. Often, pendant drop lights or ceiling spot lights are used in dining areas to provide focused light.
- Accent lighting adds drama or interest in a space. The light is focused on a design point of interest, such as artwork or architectural features.

Lighting is another area where energy savings can be realized. For instance, check out LED lighting for commercial freezers.

Heating, Ventilation and Air Conditioning (HVAC). Work in food preparation areas can be very hot with high levels of humidity. Concerns about temperature are appropriate as air conditioning needs are considered, and as cooking and cleaning equipment selection decisions are made. Today, most food preparation kitchens have a level of air conditioning to maintain an appropriate work environment.

Typically, the food production and preparation area is a large open space with large volumes of air that need to be continuously circulated (the ventilation component of HVAC). Access to "make-up air" directly relates to how much equipment, particularly heat-producing items like grills and fryers, can be designed into a space.

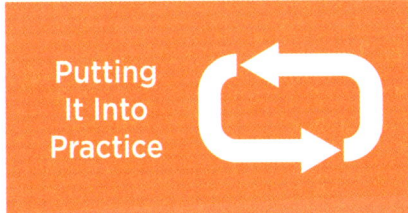

Putting It Into Practice

1. You are redesigning the kitchen for your hospital food service. Using the factors outlined here, justify your plan in layout and equipment purchase.

Safety and Sanitation. Health regulations dictate cleanability of equipment, temperature and humidity requirements for dry storage and lighting requirements, along with the design and venting of heat, ventilation, and air conditioning systems, and much more. These concerns are important and must meet all applicable federal, state, and local codes.

Local Construction Codes. Building codes may stipulate many aspects of design. In some locales, special regulations apply to healthcare facilities. Working with a foodservice kitchen designer, for major projects in particular, will ensure compliance to the building codes that are different for kitchen construction. The general construction designers often are not aware of the specific codes related to dining rooms and kitchens.

Security. Security concerns are always a top priority in the design. For example:

- Should storage areas be located close to the back door? No, because this may increase the opportunity for theft.
- Should receiving and preparation areas be under the view of the CDM, CFPP? Yes. Thus, an office design may use glass partitions that allow a manager to monitor operations from a desk.

While the list of questions can continue, the point is that the control of food and materials during production and service is influenced by the amount of security built into the facility.

Design of Receiving and Storage Areas

Receiving areas should typically be as close as practical to storage areas. They should also be large enough to house incoming deliveries, so that employees can follow effective receiving practices. Additional space should be available for related equipment, such as scales and dollies.

To limit access by unauthorized persons, storerooms should be designed with walls that extend from the floor to the ceiling and with ceilings that cannot be entered from an adjoining room through a drop ceiling, pipe chase area, or other connecting area access points. Locked doors are usually required. If an ingredient room is used, it should be planned close to dry storage areas and to the food preparation areas.

Design of Food Preparation and Service Areas

In production areas, cooks need storage space for pre-preparation items, aisles to accommodate carts and space for small equipment, such as scales, slicers, and food processors. To organize work efficiently, they need counter space and prep areas close to their production equipment (stoves, steamers, grills, etc.).

For decentralized service in which products are prepared in a remote location and reheated or finished close to the point of service, consider what additional equipment and space requirements are needed. Service needs may require less space but more specialized equipment and utility service.

In a cafeteria, it's important to structure a design that fits the service model. For example, a design for a straight-line service is much different from one used for a scramble service. In addition, it's important to consider client's entry and exit points, and to allow space for clients to move around comfortably while serving themselves, without getting in each other's way.

If food items are to be prepared on an as-ordered basis, utility connections, ventilation systems, and space to house cook-to-order equipment in service areas must be considered. Equipment to hold hot and cold food items near the point of service will be needed. Sometimes cafeteria operations use a hot and/or cold food pass-through so that production staff can make items readily available for service without having to go into public food production and dining services areas. A pass-through is a connecting area between the kitchen and the service area.

If cafeteria operations are to collect cash, space for cashiers, point-of-sale equipment, and other necessary items must be included. Electrical and computer networking requirements are part of this planning component.

An important consideration in design of production and service areas is Flow. Flow refers to the movement of product or people in an operation. It is ideal to have a straight-line flow from receiving to warewashing. This minimizes cross traffic and prevents accidents at the workplace. Dining area planners must consider not only the number of persons to be served at one time, but also the flow of soiled dishes back to dishwashing areas and the removal of trash from the public spaces. Commonly, food production and dining services operations use a conveyor system to transport soiled dishes. The servery and dining space need to be practical for the clients being served, comply with sanitation guidelines, and also be aesthetically comfortable.

Dining areas greatly influence the clients' impression of an establishment. The atmosphere of the facility itself, the cleanliness and condition of dining room furniture, fixtures and equipment, lighting, and a wide range of other concerns are important to these impressions. Planning a dining area requires consideration of questions such as:

- How many clients must be fed at one time?
- How much space should be allocated for each diner?
- Does space for walkers or wheel chairs need to be planned?
- Who else will be present (service staff, nursing staff, family, etc.), and how much additional space will be needed?
- What other activities besides dining services will occur in dining areas? (In many skilled nursing facilities, dining areas become multi-purpose rooms at other times of day.)
- What specialized equipment is needed to ensure client comfort?
- How will food be served in the dining area, such as a salad bar or food cart?

2. Your facility is moving from traditional "made from scratch" production to a heat and serve operation. Determine three pieces of equipment that are required to be purchased.

Design of Other Food Production and Dining Services Areas

In addition to food storage, production, assembly, serving, and dining areas, other spaces also merit planning. Consider the need for:

- Office space for the manager and supervisors.
- Space for dish and pot washing, holding of refuse until pickup, space for washing carts and shelving equipment, and so on.
- Cleaning and other chemicals storage.
- Refrigeration equipment for walk-in units.
- Space for mobile transport equipment.
- Location of handwashing and prep sinks consistent with local, state, or federal codes.

Many healthcare facilities provide snacks for unit-based nourishment centers. The CDM, CFPP should lend expertise about how nourishments are stored, rotated and protected until the time of service.

Space Allocation

The proportions of space used for receiving, storage, production, service, and clean-up can vary depending on menus and service models. Figure 23.2 is an example of the breakdown and space allocations for a traditional 6,000-square-foot kitchen. This is one that essentially cooks food and then serves it.

How might this allocation vary for other kitchens? A cook-chill kitchen would require much more refrigerated storage space. A kitchen relying intensively on convenience foods or a no-cook kitchen might require a great deal of storage space, but very little production space.

Design Principles and Employee Input

A great source for getting input into redesigning or building a new kitchen will come from the current employees. They are the experts who use the equipment and the current kitchen design every day. Allow them to provide suggestions about work flow and essential equipment relative to new department designs or construction. Involve employees with each step of the redesign/design project for valuable, insightful information for planning meetings.

Keep a record each time an employee complains about a piece of equipment or a design element in the kitchen. When ready for the redesign/design process, simply access the history of issues already documented. An easy way to document these complaints/suggestions is to have an email file labeled Kitchen Design and send yourself a quick email each time an employee provides a suggestion or a complaint.

Remember to include needs such as wiring for computers. More areas of the food production and plating services need network connectivity, docking stations, and remote printing capability.

Figure 23.2
Space Allocation for a Traditional Kitchen

Subsystem	Space Allocation (sq. ft.)	
Receiving	120	3.00%
Storage	1,120	28.00%
Preparation	1,100	27.50%
Cooking	470	11.75%
Serving	800	20.00%
Clean-up	390	9.75%
Subtotal	4,000	100.00%
Fixed Space*	2,000	
Subtotal	6,000	

*Includes janitorial storage, restrooms, lounge areas, etc. Source: John B. Knight, Ph.D, Purdue University

Specifying and Purchasing Equipment

In many facilities, a CDM, CFPP has direct purchasing authority for ongoing supplies and small purchases but must seek approval to purchase capital equipment, so the purchasing procedure may be different. As discussed in Chapter 22, a capital budget justification is likely required. In addition, a manager may need to review plans and specifications with a maintenance or engineering expert to plan installation and to assure compliance with all relevant codes and regulations. Because capital equipment does require significant investment and will become a part of the operation for a long time, purchasing decisions are very important.

Before making a purchasing recommendation for capital items, follow these basic background procedures:

Step 1: Determine a need.

Step 2: Consider the capital budget. (Review Chapter 22 for information regarding the capital budget.)

Step 3: Investigate options.

Step 4: Consult with others (Engineering, Information Systems, Purchasing, etc.) in the organization.

Step 5: Obtain price quotations.
- For very large purchases, a CDM, CFPP may use a process called **request for proposal (RFP)**. This is a formal document stating the requirements for the purchase. It is distributed to potential suppliers, each of whom indicates their ability to meet each requirement along with a price. In some facilities, purchasing staff may be involved in requesting price quotations from suppliers, comparing quotations, and undertaking supplier negotiations.

GLOSSARY

Request for Proposal (RFP)
A written description of large dollar items that is then sent to a supplier to obtain a competitive bid

Step 6: Prepare a capital budget request.

Step 7: Make a decision.

Step 8: Award the bid and schedule delivery.

Keep senior management updated regarding issues or concerns during the purchasing process.

Selecting Food Production and Dining Services Equipment

To make a decision about an equipment purchase, review a number of factors:

Suitability for Intended Use

Since a wide range of equipment products is available for almost any purpose, it is important to consider the suitability of each product. Suitability issues include how well the equipment can perform the required job in the intended setting. The volume of output a piece of equipment can handle may not match the need.

Consider a pizza oven for an example. How many pizzas will need to cook at a time to meet service requirements and how long it will take to cook them? Specified equipment must accommodate the load, as well as any anticipated increases in volume. Some equipment is described in terms of a duty cycle, or how many operations it can perform within a specified period of time.

Ease of Operation

Equipment should be as easy to use as possible, requiring minimal steps for operation, and providing a user-friendly design. To evaluate this, it is wise to test equipment while involving any employees who will be responsible for using it.

Durability and Warranty

It is necessary to confirm that the product will stand up to its intended use. A warranty provides some indication of durability, as well as financial protection if the product cannot withstand use. Study a warranty carefully to determine any conditions that apply. Review what is and what is not covered by the warranty and whether service charges may apply.

Construction and Safety

Closely aligned with durability is the integrity of the equipment's construction. Equipment must be easy to clean and safe to operate. Compliance with established standards for safety and sanitation are indicated by seals and certifications from various organizations, such as NSF and UL. (See Figure 23.3 for a summary.) Many pieces of food production and dining services equipment today are treated with antimicrobial protective compounds that discourage growth of bacteria and mold. These products are incorporated into construction materials and last the lifetime of the equipment.

Compatibility With Existing Equipment

It is important that equipment be compatible with existing systems. For example, trays being purchased must fit into the current carts, and attachments for electric mixers must fit existing equipment. As applicable, be sure equipment being purchased will fit into available space, integrate into existing structures and utility systems, move through doorways, and is compatible with current wiring. Is equipment compatible with ADA (Americans with Disabilities Act) regulations?

Assistance Provided Before and After Purchase

Before a purchase, some suppliers provide design analysis, technical analysis, creative suggestions, and a plan for operational integration. After a purchase, suppliers may provide delivery, installation, on-site testing, demonstration, training, and maintenance. Evaluate and clarify tasks such as these. In cases where a supplier is not providing these services, it is also important to determine how each will be accomplished, and what costs will be incurred.

Price

A detailed clarification of price incorporates the items above. In comparing prices from alternate suppliers, be sure to compare the bottom-line figure that reflects all associated costs and discounts.

Operating Cost

This is different from price but is critical in the evaluation of what a piece of equipment will cost. Operating expenses include the cost of energy to use the equipment, as well as the cost of supplies. Some equipment uses proprietary, disposable supplies available only from the manufacturer. Pricing for such supplies must be evaluated carefully. To evaluate costs, it can be useful to project supply costs over a period of one year.

Figure 23.3
Approval Agencies for Foodservice Equipment

NSF International
(approval designated by the NSF seal): Provides standards for materials, design, construction, performance, cleanability, and foodservice sanitation.

Underwriters Laboratories
(approval designated by the UL mark): Provides testing and certification to verify that electrical or gas equipment is safe to operate. Appliances are tested to ensure they comply with fire safety requirements and won't emit shock.

American Gas Association
(AGA certification): Provides safety testing services for gas appliances through the International Approval Service.

International Standards Organization
(ISO): ISO standards address quality in manufacturing. Through compliance with established standards, a manufacturer can become ISO certified.

Agencies providing energy information for foodservice equipment Energy Star® Provides a listing of Energy Star® commercial equipment.
www.energystar.gov/products

North American Association of Food Equipment Manufacturers
(NAFEM): A trade organization that provides links to equipment companies.
www.nafem.org

The Food Service Technology Center
(FSTC): Provides fact sheets and other publications such as energy efficiency calculators on commercial equipment.
fstc@frontierenergy.com

Federal Energy Management Program
(FEMP): Provides up-to-date information on energy efficient federal procurement, including the latest recommendations.
www.energy.gov/femp

Service and Reputation

As with food purchasing decisions, ultimate success with a purchase depends on a supplier's reliability in meeting commitments and the quality of services and repairs provided.

Types of Equipment

The menu served, the style of service, and the number of meals served daily will have the greatest impact on the types of equipment needed. Figure 23.6 summarizes equipment options for preparing a variety of menu items. Each type of food production and dining services will need different equipment.

The figure outlines preparation equipment suitable for a school food production and dining services operation based on number of meals served daily.

Equipment Specifications

Any piece of equipment chosen for a food production and dining services department is available with alternatives and options. In preparing a capital budget or even making a small equipment purchase, develop an **equipment specification**. This is a detailed description of the product. When multiple suppliers are asked to quote equipment prices, as in an RFP, the specification is important for ensuring that the same features are referenced in each quote. The specification nails down what is essential for ensuring that what is purchased will meet the defined needs precisely.

To develop a specification, it helps to do some product research first to identify realistic expectations. Answer questions about the product needs, such as:

- What size or capacity is required?
- What time constraints must the product meet, e.g., cooking time for a particular product, number of dishes per hour, etc.?
- What construction materials are desired, e.g., stainless steel (___ gauge), glass, aluminum, antimicrobial treatment, etc.?
- What exterior finish is needed?
- For power equipment, gas or electric, and to what specifications (e.g., 220 volt, single phase or 3-phase)?
- What size motor is needed (e.g., ___ HP)?
- What technologies should the equipment use, e.g., convection, conduction, pressure-less steam, etc.?
- What water treatment systems or filtering systems are required?
- What safety seals are required (UL, NSF, etc.)?
- Where will this unit reside—floor model, countertop, under counter, etc.? Does it need legs or wheels?
- What space dimensions are available (specify length, width, depth, and height)? What door size or hood height does it need to fit into?
- If the unit has doors that open, in what direction will they open, and what amount of space is available?
- What pan or tray sizes should this equipment use (if applicable)?
- What user features are needed, e.g., control panel features, manual or automatic functioning, multiple speed options, etc.?

GLOSSARY

Equipment Specification
A detailed description providing information needed to purchase a piece of equipment

Figure 23.4
Food Preparation Equipment for School Foodservice

PREPARATION EQUIPMENT	MEALS PREPARED PER DAY		
	<400	401-700	701-1000
Convection Ovens	(1) double	(2) double	(3) double
Tilting Braising Pans	(1) 23 or 30 gallon	(1) 23 or 30 gallon & (1) 40 gallon	(2) 40 gallon
Kettles	(1) 10 gallon	(1) 20 gallon	(1) 10 gallon & (1) 20 gallon
Steamers	(1) 2-compartment	(1) 2-compartment	(2) 2 compartment
Ranges	(1) 2-burner	(1) 2-burner	(1) 2-burner
Mixers	(1) 60 qt. with 30 qt. attachments	(1) 60 qt. with 30 qt. attachments	(1) 30 qt & (1) 60 qt.
Slicers	(1) automatic	(1) automatic	(2) automatic
Food Processors	(1) tabletop	(1) tabletop	(1) tabletop
Heated Cabinets: Pass-thru or Reach-in	1 section	2 section	3 section
Refrigerators: Pass-thru or Reach-in	1 section	2 section	2 section

Source: Adapted from Institute of Child Nutrition. University of Mississippi. Guidelines for Equipment to Healthy Meals. NFSMI-R-25-96. Used with permission.

- What special features are needed, e.g., HACCP data logging, programmable memory, optional accessories, etc.? (A range is typically sold with one oven rack or no oven rack—do you need more?)
- What features will enhance cleanability, e.g., easy disassembly, self-cleaning options, etc.?
- What safety and ergonomic features are required, such as auto shut-off when not in use, guards for sharp components, etc.?
- How will equipment be installed and by whom?
- Where should utility connections be provided (back, side, etc.)?
- What are the warranty requirements (parts and/or service, for what period of time)?
- What energy-saving or energy efficiency requirements are required (KW or BTU usage)?
- What training needs are specified?

A sample equipment specification appears in Figure 23.5, found in the Supplemental Material for this book. Consult with suppliers for information, and with in-house

View the Supplemental Material for this chapter for Figure 23.5, Sample Equipment Specification.

engineering staff to be sure that the specific power requirements and installation needs are correct. Once the specification is complete, provide it to suppliers and ask them for a quote. While a specification needs to be detailed enough to ensure expectations are met, leave some space for flexibility with qualifiers like "equal to or better than…" In the final analysis, the specification should be realistic and attainable for a number of competing products in the marketplace.

Financing Capital Equipment Purchases

Financing may be a special concern, especially if adequate funds are not immediately available. In some situations, a facility may lease equipment. Leasing can also be a way to test feasibility of a new idea. For example, a facility desiring to test a satellite delivery program may use leased equipment for a short-term trial.

In another payment scenario, the supplier may finance the purchase. With a typical financing arrangement, an initial down payment is necessary at the time equipment is ordered to protect the supplier against costs incurred if the order is canceled. Another payment may be required at the time of delivery and the remaining balance may be financed by the supplier at a defined interest rate.

Sometimes suppliers offer special deals related to equipment in conjunction with food purchases. For example, a supplier of waffle batter may offer the specialized iron required to make waffles on a free-use basis for as long as the operation is purchasing the batter. This can be helpful with cash flow. However, it's important to evaluate a decision to bring in this equipment by all established criteria and to evaluate the overall costs of using the supplier's products.

In another payment scenario, the supplier may finance the purchase. With a typical financing arrangement, an initial down payment is necessary at the time equipment is ordered to protect the supplier against costs incurred if the order is canceled. Another payment may be required at the time of delivery, and the remaining balance may be financed by the supplier at a defined interest rate.

Equipment Maintenance

The best way to maintain equipment is through in-depth training on the use and upkeep of the piece of equipment. (See Figure 23.7 for a list of common equipment training needs.) Initial training for use, cleaning, and maintenance for complex equipment is typically provided by the supplier. Some equipment bears clear labels with instructions and safety precautions. A CDM, CFPP may also create a simple cheat sheet or poster outlining operational steps.

Maintain operating manuals and associated literature such as purchase price, vendor, and maintenance records in organized equipment files, accessible to all who may need it.

All equipment requires basic care such as routine cleaning and sanitizing after use. On another level, many pieces of equipment require periodic preventive work to limit

3. Develop specifications for a dishwashing machine for your kitchen.

Figure 23.6
Equipment and the Menu

	OVENS			STEAM EQUIPMENT					BROILERS	
	Ranges	Convection	Cook & Hold	Steamers	Kettles	Braising Pans	Fryers	Griddles	Cheesemelters	Char-Broilers
Breakfast										
Eggs	•	•		•	•	•		•		
Pancakes	•				•			•		
Biscuits	•	•	•							
Bacon	•	•				•		•		
Hash Browns	•					•		•		
Appetizers										
Soups	•				•	•				
Pizza	•	•	•							
Shrimp	•	•		•		•	•	•		•
Fish	•	•		•		•	•	•		•
Scallop Gratin	•	•	•						•	
Potato Skins	•	•	•						•	
Entrées										
Steak	•	•				•		•		•
Roast Beef	•	•				•				
Whole Chicken	•	•	•		•	•				
Meatloaf	•	•	•			•				
Lamb	•	•						•		•
Veal	•	•				•				
Burgers (4 oz.)	•	•				•		•		
Ribs	•	•	•	•	•	•				•
Chicken Parts	•	•	•	•	•	•	•	•		•
Shellfish	•	•		•	•	•	•	•		•
Salmon	•	•		•		•		•		•
Vegetables										
Grilled	•							•		•
Steamed	•		•	•	•	•				
Boiled	•				•	•				
In Cream Sauce	•	•			•	•				
Au Gratin	•	•	•						•	
Sautéed	•					•				
Sides										
Sauces	•				•					
Gratin Potatoes	•	•	•						•	
Baked Potatoes	•	•	•							
Mashed Potatoes	•	•	•	•	•	•				
Fries		•					•			
Rice	•			•	•	•				
Desserts & Bakery										
Breads	•	•								
Soufflés	•	•								
Pastries	•	•								
Cakes	•	•								
Crème Brûlée	•	•	•						•	

breakdowns and ensure maximum lifetime. Even well-maintained equipment can experience breakdowns that require immediate repair.

Preventive Maintenance

Beyond cleaning, a CDM, CFPP should plan a preventive maintenance schedule for all equipment. **Preventive maintenance**, an organized routine of cleaning, inspecting, and maintaining equipment, is essential to ensure that:

- Equipment operates at maximum efficiency, often with savings in energy costs.
- Equipment works correctly.
- Equipment attains its maximum life expectancy.
- Unscheduled downtime is minimized.

Several basic steps can be used to develop preventative maintenance programs.

1. Identify and list all equipment in the food production and dining services facility that need periodic inspection and maintenance. This includes equipment not only in the kitchen, but also in serving areas, clean-up areas, decentralized kitchens or pantries, and other areas.

2. Set up a schedule of preventive maintenance. Depending upon the equipment item, maintenance work may be necessary on a weekly, semi-annual, or other basis. Figure 23.8 illustrates a preventive maintenance schedule used for this purpose. This sample summarizes required preventive maintenance activities for a six-month period. Some operators track preventive maintenance activities through computerized systems—with a simple spreadsheet or a software application designed expressly for equipment management.

3. Review maintenance requirements. Typically, this information is developed by the manufacturer and provided with the equipment at the time of purchase. You can incorporate manufacturer's recommendations about equipment maintenance into a preventive maintenance and repair log, as illustrated in Figure 23.9, found in the Supplemental Material. The log should identify routine maintenance functions and how often they need to be completed. This may include items such as oiling a motor or replacing a fluid. The form should also identify the equipment name, model, manufacturer, serial number, and purchase date. As routine maintenance and/or repairs are conducted, the log should document each activity.

4. Maintain complete documentation of all maintenance and repair activity. More than just paperwork, this documentation helps in identifying and justifying decisions to replace equipment. A piece of equipment whose repair overhead becomes excessive is often a candidate for replacement. With documentation, a CDM, CFPP can determine when replacement will be cost-effective.

Certain preventive maintenance tasks may require the work of individuals outside the food production and dining services department. For example, in-house engineering or maintenance staff may handle maintenance on a conveyor system, a small engine, or ventilation hoods and fans. Some facilities make use of maintenance or service

GLOSSARY

Preventive Maintenance
An organized routine of cleaning, inspecting, and maintaining equipment

View the Supplemental Material for this chapter for Figure 23.8, Preventive Maintenance Schedule.

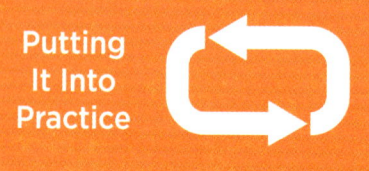

Putting It Into Practice

4. Write out a repair log for the freezer. How would you train your staff on preventive maintenance for the equipment?

Figure 23.7
Common Equipment Training Needs

- Overview—what this equipment is for
- How to turn equipment on and off
- Basic operational steps
- Safety precautions
- Protective equipment to use if required
- How to identify and use special attachments and what each is for
- Auto shut-off features
- Routine disassembly/reassembly (for cleaning)
- Procedures for cleaning and sanitizing (and what products to use)
- Food safety precautions (e.g., how to avoid cross-contamination when using a slicer)
- Use of self-cleaning features
- Use of programmable controls
- How to ensure adequate functioning
- Use of data logging, temperature monitoring, or related systems
- How to add consumable supplies
- Preventive maintenance
- Signs of trouble and reporting procedures

contracts with suppliers. Under this plan, eligible suppliers bid on the facility's maintenance needs. Quotations may be based upon time and materials, which means the client pays for labor and supplies each time he or she orders repair service. Or, a contract may be structured to provide any needed services and parts for a set monthly fee. Arrangements such as these may apply to repairs as well as preventive maintenance, and often the two are bundled into a service agreement.

Regardless of the players involved, a CDM, CFPP has responsibility for ensuring that all preventive maintenance tasks are defined and tracked. In addition, it is important to ensure that preventive maintenance meets manufacturers' recommendations, both to ensure effectiveness and to preserve the validity of any equipment warranty.

View the Supplemental Material for this chapter for Figure 23.9, Equipment Maintenance and Repair Log.

Cleaning Schedule

Part of a CDM, CFPP's responsibility is to manage all phases of maintenance. The first step is to define a cleaning schedule and assign tasks to employees. A cleaning schedule must flow from the production and service timelines, so that cleaning takes place when equipment is not in use, and is completed before a cook needs to use equipment. To make cleaning timely and effective, prepare a schedule and hold employees accountable. Most operations ask employees to sign off on cleaning tasks. On a daily basis, it's important to inspect this work and talk with employees about their responsibilities. Employees should also be encouraged to report any problems or concerns about equipment to their supervisor or the manager.

Specific cleaning procedures vary greatly from one piece of equipment to another, so it is important to develop guidelines from the manufacturers' instructions. As cleaning products are required, it is also important to name them specifically by product name for employees, rather than using generic terms. Cleaning instructions should be readily available to the assigned employees and the subject of employee training and periodic review. An example of a cleaning procedure appears in Figure 23.10.

View the Supplemental Material for this chapter for Figure 23.10, Sample Policy and Procedure: Equipment Cleaning.

Managing the Cost of Supplies

Chemical products are needed to clean dishes, pots and pans, and work areas. A wide range of products are available. Check with suppliers for ideas about available items and recommended uses, and use the supplier representative as a partner to help resolve cleaning and sanitation problems in the operation.

Cleaning supplies should be kept in non-food storage areas. As is true with other food production and dining services inventory, cleaning supplies must be properly controlled. Since these products are expensive, a formal issuing system similar to that used to control expensive food products may be in order. The rate of product usage, particularly for dishmachine chemical, is frequently tracked by managers as a controllable expense.

Product selection also plays a role in supply cost management. Sometimes, a cost-benefit study is necessary to confirm which product is the most potentially useful. To undertake this study, first define what the product is to do. Then, ask suppliers for suggestions about and samples of products that they believe will be useful. Using the instructions provided by the manufacturer, test each product. Then, objectively determine which meet your requirements. Keep in mind that the recommended chemicals for one facility may be different from another due to the equipment in use and the hardness of water quality available.

From that group of products, next examine cost. For example, one gallon of a cleaning agent may cost $50 but clean twice as many square feet, compared with a less expensive product. Calculate the defined cost per square foot, rack of dishes, load of laundry, and so on, to make a fair comparison. This boils down to a usage cost, rather than a purchase price.

Another cost control consideration relates to how employees use products. Sometimes, employees are tempted to over-use cleaning products, in a belief that more is better. This not only costs money, it may also pose safety concerns. Training and ongoing supervision are in order. As applicable, also assure that the correct measuring or portioning devices are on hand to eliminate guesswork.

For certain equipment, supply usage is largely controlled by the equipment itself for self-cleaning. High-pressure cleaning systems with applicable chemicals are also used for cleaning many items. Monitoring supply usage can help identify when there is a malfunction. Prompt service, in turn, can get supply usage under control.

The need for selecting a reputable supplier is just as important for the purchase of chemicals as it is for the purchase of food products, capital equipment items, and other purchases. The supplier may be included in the purchasing program and vetted by the GPO. Chemicals are a unique segment of the department requiring a vendor that is knowledgeable about the product needs of food production and dining services. Access to competitive pricing consistent quality and quantity, and timely delivery of the needed supplies are essential characteristics of a good chemical supplier.

Chapter References

RESOURCES	
Food Service Technology Center (FSTC) Energy Wise Foodservice Equipment Rebates	https://www.nationalgridus.com/media/pdfs/bus-ways-to-save/ee7111-instant-rebate-foodservice-program-brochure.pdf
Life-Cycle & Energy Cost Calculators	https://caenergywise.com/calculators/
University of Mississippi Guidelines for Equipment to Prepare Healthy Meals	https://files.eric.ed.gov/fulltext/ED432882.pdf
U.S. Green Building Council Leadership in Energy and Environmental Design (LEED)	https://www.usgbc.org/leed

The Purchasing Process

Overview and Objectives

Procurement or purchasing in a foodservice operation is the process of obtaining both food and non-food products for the organization. While Certified Dietary Manager®, Certified Food Protection Professional® (CDM®, CFPP®) may not have to write purchase specifications, they will be involved in purchasing food and supplies for their facility, and should know how to obtain the right products for the best value. This chapter reviews all aspects of the purchasing process. After completing this chapter, you should be able to:

- Identify considerations when purchasing products
- Understand purchasing specifications
- Use the ordering and bidding process
- Evaluate facility needs, budget restrictions, and products available
- Gather and evaluate product information
- Be familiar with computer applications and create a purchase order
- Check inventory and identify purchase needs
- Complete purchase order requisition forms
- Maintain inventory records
- Recognize inventory management practices (FIFO, par stock, physical, perpetual)

Purchasing is a highly specialized process and the topic alone is the subject of many books. This chapter covers only a few of the decisions in the process. Purchasing has changed significantly in the past 20 years, with most facilities completing the process online through a computerized ordering system with their prime vendor. Often, smaller healthcare facilities belong to multi-unit purchasing co-ops and enjoy the benefits of cooperative purchasing to leverage better prices.

The main focus of purchasing is to buy the products needed at the best cost and appropriate quality—and get them delivered when (and where) they are needed. Through effective purchasing, a CDM, CFPP achieves objectives related to quality, quantity, price, supplier, and schedule.

Quality. The purchaser must obtain the right quality products and services. This is not always the highest quality available. Instead, it matches the needs and budget of the facility. The relationship between quality and price is called value.

Quantity. Products must be purchased in the right quantity. Otherwise, the operation can run out of products, delaying or altering food production and service. Or, the operation can carry excess inventory, with resulting cash flow and loss implications.

Price. The buyer has a responsibility to obtain required quality products at the best overall price. Price shopping individual items across multiple vendors consumes time and rarely results in a lower net cost. Typically, a prime vendor relationship leads to a better total invoice bottom line.

Supplier. It is important to select product sources with thought, analysis, and comparison, rather than simply to select a supplier based on random factors.

Schedule. Delivery times should be coordinated with the vendor so needed staffing is available when deliveries are made. While occasional problems must be anticipated, supplier selection should include reliability of delivery schedules.

In large facilities, purchasing may be the responsibility of a specialized food buyer or purchasing agent. In smaller facilities, it is often the responsibility of the CDM, CFPP, supervisor, or food production and dining service director.

The purchasing task is ongoing. Through experience with suppliers, products, and services, the CDM, CFPP can develop a very effective system to help control costs and to assure that quality requirements are met.

Specifications for Equipment

As discussed in Chapter 23, specifications are also written for equipment and disposable items such as paper and plastic. Equipment manufacturers usually provide a spec sheet with their equipment that details the specific features of the equipment such as type, model number, standard features, etc.

This information can be very helpful when writing specifications for the purchase of new equipment. The specs should be as generic as possible and include what the equipment needs to do, i.e., Performance Specifications, and not so tightly written that only one item can meet the stated specs.

Specifications for Food

Management of the purchasing process begins with a specification for each product. A **specification (spec)** is a quality statement that spells out what requirements must be met in order for a product to be acceptable. It really describes the suitability of a product for its intended use in the operation. There may be multiple specs for the same general product depending upon the intended use. For example, if olives are used for garnishes as well as for the salad bar, two different products may be needed. Large olives that are perfectly shaped and are of uniform size (and expensive) are not necessary if the olives will be chopped for a salad.

The purpose of a specification is quality control. "You get what you ask for. If you don't ask for it, you are not likely to get it!" A product spec is used when requesting prices or bids from a list of possible suppliers. A spec helps assure a comparison of apples to apples, so to speak. In turn, this helps to compare prices meaningfully. It also defines a clear, mutual expectation of what will be received at delivery.

Writing specs comes after the decision about what general products will be needed for the menu as planned. Once the recipes are selected and the ingredients defined, the specific quality characteristics can be written.

Specification should be:
- Accurate and objectively describe quality aspects.
- Realistic.
  > Quality definitions cannot be so strict that few or no products will be acceptable.
- Stated in clear terms.
- Provide some flexibility for both the supplier and the buyer.

Technical Specifications: To write a product spec, begin with a product name (not the brand name but the product identifier). Include an intended use descriptor if it affects the choice of product, i.e., sliced olives for the salad bar. Provide a description of the product with quality information. Note any special requirements. An example of a specification format appears in Figure 24.1. Along with these details, identify required food safety controls, such as delivery temperatures, acceptable product dating, and any other essential characteristics.

What characteristics can be listed in the specs? These vary by product. For certain agricultural products, a USDA grade is an essential tool. A **grade** describes the quality of the product. A grade may describe uniformity, texture, fat content, flavor, maturity, and/or other quality factors. Grade assignments are based on standards established by the USDA for each applicable food. They provide an objective measure or standard which can be used for comparison. For example, a Fancy grade of canned vegetables indicates the best flavor, color, and tenderness. It also indicates the product is uniform in size.

> **GLOSSARY**
>
> **Specification (Spec)**
> A quality statement that lists what requirements must be met in order for a product to be acceptable. There are technical and brand specifications
>
> **Grade**
> A rating that describes the quality and appearance characteristics of a product

1. Write out specifications for eggs to be purchased for a hospital food service.

Figure 24.1
Product Specification Format

[Name of Foodservice Operation]

1. **Product Name:** _____

2. **Product Used For:** Clearly indicate product use, such as olive for garnish, hamburger patty for grilling, etc.

3. **Product General Description:** Provide quality information about desired product. For example, "iceberg lettuce; heads to be green and firm without spoilage, no excessive dirt or damage. No more than 10 outer leaves; packed 24 heads per case."

4. **Detailed Description:** State other factors that clearly identify the desired product. Examples of specific factors, which vary by product being described, include:

   - Geographic Origin
   - Variety
   - Type
   - Style
   - Grade
   - Size
   - Portion Size
   - Brand Name
   - Density
   - Specific Gravity
   - Container Size
   - Edible Yield, Trim
   - Inspection

5. **Check-In Procedures:** Describe what a receiving clerk will do to verify acceptability of the product. For example, products to be delivered at or below 41°F will be tested with a thermometer. Portioned meat patties will be randomly weighed. Lettuce packed 24 heads per case will be counted.

6. **Special Instructions and Requirements:** Any additional information needed to clearly indicate quality expectations can be included here. Examples include bidding procedures, if applicable, labeling and/or packaging requirements, and delivery and service requirements.

In addition, portion and count can be critical. For fish fillets, decide what weight is required for each fillet in order to match the needs of the recipes and menus. As another example, canned pear halves may be packed with varying counts in a #10 can. Container size may vary slightly from one vendor to another. However, if requirements are rigid due to space or usage quantities, specify them. For example, if a product will only be used in very small amounts for individual orders on demand, do not accept products in large units. Common can sizes appear in Figure 24.2. For ideas about other factors to include in specifications for particular products, search for the USDA Commercial Item Descriptions, available at http://www.ams.usda.gov.

In some facilities, the packaging itself is also specified. For example, glass may be prohibited for safety reasons. Today, processing methods may be important as well. Some facilities are also developing specifications that relate to food additives and allergens (factors likely to cause allergic reactions in sensitive individuals). If specific factors are important to the client group, include them.

2. Identify three products that may need brand specifications.

Figure 24.2
Common Can Sizes

SIZE	NET WEIGHT	MEASURE	COMMON PACK	PRINCIPAL PRODUCTS
#10	6 lbs. 9 oz.	12 - 13 cups	6 per case	Fruits, vegetables, some other foods
No. 3 Cyl	2.9 - 3.2 lbs.	5-1/4 cups	12 per case	Condensed soups, some vegetables, meat and poultry products, fruit and vegetable juices
#2-1/2	1 lb. 13 oz.	3-1/2 cups	24 per case	Fruits, some vegetables
#2	1 lb. 4 oz.	2-1/2 cups	24 per case	Juices, ready-to-serve soups, some fruits
#300	14 - 16 oz.	1-3/4 cups	24 per case	Some fruits and meat products
#1 (Picnic)	10-1/2 - 12 oz.	1-1/4 cups	48 per case	Condensed soups, some fruits, vegetables, meat, fish
8 oz.	8 oz.	1 cup	48 or 72 per case	Ready-to-serve soups, fruits, vegetables

Source: Food for Fifty

Figure 24.3
Purchase Specification Factors

MEATS	SEAFOOD	POULTRY	FRESH FRUITS & VEGETABLES	PROCESSED FRUITS & VEGETABLES
• Inspection (mandatory) • Grading (if desired) • IMPS/MBG Descriptions • Weight/Thickness Limitations • Fat Limitations • State of Refrigeration • Miscellaneous (tying, boning, packaging, etc.)	• Type (fin fish or shellfish) • Market Form (whole, eviscerated fin fish, alive, whole, shucked, etc.) • Quality Requirements (describe flesh, eyes, skin, gills, etc.) • Grade (if desired) • Inspection (voluntary) • Processing Requirements	• Kind (chicken, turkey, duck, goose) • Class (typed by age) • Grade (if desired) • Size (weight limitations) • Style (weight limitations) • Inspection (mandatory) • Style (whole, breasts, breasts with ribs, etc.) • State of Refrigeration	• Grade (if desired) • Variety • Size • Type of Pack • Count per Container • Growing Area	• Grade (if desired) • Drain Weight • Packing Medium • Can (container) Size

Examples of factors that may be included in a quality statement appear in Figure 24.3.

To identify additional details and options, talk with several suppliers. Many food distributors can provide a specifications manual. Some may also provide their own quality ratings that will help match products to needs. Realize that using known brand-name ingredients is not essential. A distributor's house brand may prove more economical, and may even be the very same product under a different label.

Use of branded menu items is a growing trend. A school system may serve French fries produced by a recognized fast food chain or chocolate chip cookies manufactured by a well-known company. A cafeteria may serve doughnuts, pizzas, or tacos that have national brand-name recognition.

Brand Specifications: When using branded menu items, a food production and dining service operation enjoys marketing clout as well as quality control. Costs may be higher, but sales may be too. Thus, a facility needs to base decisions to use branded products on value, impact on the financial bottom line, and where the product name will be seen. When offering unlabeled bulk salad dressing on a salad bar, a house branded dressing will likely be more economical and of equal quality (and flavor profile) to the nationally branded item.

Usually the specification should not include the brand of the food or equipment item. However, in some cases where the chef may want specific products such as ABC ketchup, the brand would be included in the specs. If specifying a brand, be prepared to defend why that brand must be purchased. Ready-to-use pasta sauce may seem like a standard item. However, flavor profiles differ significantly from one brand to another. In one university setting, the pasta sauce that had been purchased had a tomato paste aftertaste. The product did not meet the expected flavor profile. That data was used to justify a change in product brand.

Finally, if writing specs for specialized dietary products, involve a Registered Dietitian Nutritionist in developing specifications. Simple product names for low-sodium soup, heart healthy convenience entrées, or enteral nutritional supplements do not tell all. A dietitian can specify nutritional content for these products.

This has been a detailed discussion about the writing of specifications and what to include. In today's marketplace, the writing of food specs is rarely so detailed for each item in the inventory. Typically the standards have been defined by the broadline vendor purchasing managers through what they bring into inventory, the Group Purchasing Organizations, through what they spec for contract pricing and industry standards, through what similar facilities are willing to buy. Organizations driven primarily by budget concerns may choose to purchase lower grade products and, as such, may need to define their specs.

Evaluating Products

As suppliers suggest products to match the needs, the next step is to taste and test the products. It is important to taste products under consideration. Sometimes, it is also important to test it through the recipe production process, in order to verify quality and taste. When relevant, ask the supplier to deliver samples of several products that meet the specification for comparison. If the standard has been XYZ Peanut Butter, and the same product is available from a new vendor, then a sample is not necessary. However, when the recommendation is for a different brand, a taste and performance comparison is advised.

Foodservice Management—By Design

Some operations use the term **can-cutting** to describe the process of sampling products for possible purchase. To perform a successful taste test, involve several key members of the operation. At least one person involved in food production should attend—a manager, chief chef, or head cook. In addition, the person responsible for purchasing should be involved, and should review the product carefully. Use a simple rating card to allow panelists to rate taste, appearance, texture, and other pertinent characteristics. After each person has made an independent evaluation, ask panelists to compare notes and discuss the products. Can-cutting can be done for one product and multiple vendors or multiple grades and products from one vendor.

Comparing product yield and waste is part of the evaluation process. Generally, there is a difference between package weight and net weight for products. Net weight is the weight of the food product itself, after all packaging is removed. For canned products, consider the drain weight, or how much usable product is present after draining away the liquid. Ultimately, it affects both yield and price. Figure 24.4 shows an example of how this can make a difference.

GLOSSARY

Can-Cutting
A procedure for sampling products for possible purchase

Figure 24.4
Impact of Drain Weight

You are comparing two different products for canned peach slices, each packed in #10 cans.

Product #1: Minimum drain weight = 63 oz.
Price: $3.00 per can

Product #2: Minimum drain weight = 75 oz.
Price: $3.10 per can

All other factors being equal, which product represents a better value? To determine this, calculate the price per ounce of usable product:

Product #1: $3.00 ÷ 63 oz. = $0.0476 per oz.
Product #2: $3.10 ÷ 75 oz. = $0.0413 per oz.

In this example, Product #2 is actually a better value if the quality is equal.

View the Supplemental Material for this chapter for the Focus on Formula video on Calculating Drain Weight.

Purchasing Decisions

The person responsible for purchasing is expected to purchase the required products for the best price. There are several buying techniques that may help the purchaser: using bid pricing, purchasing groups and cooperatives, manufacturer's rebates, valuing inventory, and make or buy decisions.

There are essentially four styles of purchasing systems commonly in use: local grocery store, independent specialty product vendors, multi-vendor bid process, and Group

3. Describe a competitive bid process for a pizza vendor for your school food service. What do you hope to achieve with this process?

Purchasing Organization (GPO). Facility need and access to the various services will determine which system, or combination of processes, is best for the facility.

Independent Specialty Products Vendor

The Independent Specialty Products Vendor is the source of a narrow scope of products or items not commonly found through the larger vendors. The niche these vendors serve is commonly related to dairy products, fresh bakery goods, hand-cut meats, fresh seafood, locally grown produce or fresh produce. The CDM, CFPP needs to carefully manage the purchasing through the specialty vendors to ensure that the specialty nature of the products being purchased, often at a specialty based cost, delivers the value for the price paid.

Multi-Vendor Bid Process

The **multi-vendor bid process** goes back to a time when group buying contracts were not readily available. The concept behind a multi-vendor bid process is to obtain price quotes from a number of different vendors for each item being purchased. Requests for pricing on a list of items may be monthly or quarterly. Expecting vendors to "lock in" pricing for a year denies the vendor the ability to react to market variability.

To obtain price quotations from any supplier, a CDM, CFPP can use a competitive bidding process. **Competitive bidding** allows multiple vendors to submit bids or price quotations for products based on defined specifications. The manager can then accept the lowest appropriate quoted price resulting in cost savings to the facility.

Competitive bidding will help the manager in getting a lower price when:

- The volume of purchases is large enough to justify the time and expense involved for the vendor.
- Specifications are clearly known by all suppliers.
- Several suppliers desire to quote prices on the order.

Competitive bidding can be done through an informal or a formal process. In an informal process, the terms of the bid may be discussed or agreed upon by phone, email, or other form of open communication. In a formal process, the CDM, CFPP or purchasing agent invites suppliers to submit sealed bids on a detailed, written prospective order. The manager reviews written responses and makes a selection.

Keys to success for a bid purchasing system include:

- The quoted price and other terms of the agreement must be clearly understood.
- The price quoted by the supplier must remain firm for the length of time needed by the purchaser to make a decision.
- All suppliers must quote according to the same specifications for any given product.
- All eligible suppliers should be allowed to quote on the order.
- Parties document the agreed-upon price and all other terms.

The multi-vendor bid process is often related to a concept called **cherry picking**. In this model, a CDM, CFPP purchases each individual product from the vendor with the lowest price. Thus, one facility may place a relatively small number of purchase orders with many different suppliers. An advantage of this method is that the manager presumably obtains the lowest possible price for each item. However, normally the disadvantages outweigh the possible saving:

GLOSSARY

Competitive Bidding
Asking multiple vendors to submit price quotes for products or equipment based on defined specifications

Cherry Picking
A purchasing concept where individual products are purchased from individual vendors, usually based on price alone

- The manager forms weaker relationships with vendors and may dilute the facility's clout with suppliers.
- The time and administrative commitment to monitor each bid, assess the pricing options, and hold numerous vendors accountable to their price quotes is significant.
- Time is spent with multiple vendor reps resolving issues, reviewing new products, processing invoices, and multiple checks.
- The workload for receiving staff to deal with multiple deliveries also increases.

Group Purchasing Organizations (GPOs)

The **Group Purchasing Organizations (GPOs)** are typically groups of facilities banded together to negotiate both prime vendor contracts and manufacturers rebate agreements. In one model, the facilities work together through a separate organization called a purchasing group, representing multiple clients. The GPOs generally represent a market segment of similar facilities: health care, schools, resorts and casinos, hotels and hospitality.

The GPO is often organized around committees of operators representing a common service such as Pharmacy, Housekeeping, or Food Production and Dining Services. The operators bring to the committees their knowledge and experience in products and purchasing. The group defines or approves the specs for products to be included in the bid process, standardizes use of many products, reviews bid quotes, conducts product evaluations, and selects vendors. The group uses its volume to exert buying power and obtain preferred pricing. A purchasing group may involve all supplies to the facility, not just food.

In another model, CDM, CFPPs work together through a purchasing cooperative (co-op) to achieve volume and buying power. Generally, members of the group work together to specify and select products and suppliers.

If the facility belongs to a purchasing group or cooperative, it is important to participate as fully as possible, buying products on the contract. Otherwise, the clout of the group is diluted. It is equally important to participate in selection of products and vendors to assure they meet the needs of the group.

The Bid Process

Whether at the GPO or multi-vendor level, once specifications are ready, the next step is to obtain bids from suppliers. The key purpose of this process is to obtain the best value (the cost-quality relationship) and selection of products based on the needs of the buying group.

Commonly, a food production and dining service operation will select one main vendor for the majority of its food items. This primary supplier is referred to as the **prime vendor.** In a prime vendor arrangement, an operation agrees to purchase the majority of its products from a given supplier in exchange for guaranteed pricing for a defined period of time. Typically, this is about 80 percent.

Today, a prime vendor agreement is usually managed beyond the level of individual facilities. Instead, it is negotiated at a corporate level and passed on to the CDM, CFPP. The parties responsible for negotiating a prime vendor contract may be the corporate purchasing agents of a healthcare chain, a contract management company, or other organization. Meanwhile, a corporation or individual operation may select additional vendors, often locally based suppliers, for certain perishable items like fresh meats, produce, and dairy products.

> **GLOSSARY**
>
> **Group Purchasing Organizations (GPOs)**
> A contract buying program that negotiates favorable pricing for its members
>
> **Prime Vendor**
> A primary supplier who usually provides about 80% of the products purchased

Figure 24.5
Purchasing Options—Pros

GROUP PURCHASING	MULTI-VENDOR	LOCAL GROCERY	SPECIALTY PRODUCTS
• Easy access to pricing • The greater the purchases, the better the pricing • Less work for the manager • Specs are set by "the committee" • Rebates and incentives typically available • Someone else manages the contracts and vendor compliance • Value-added services are often available	• More product and branding options available • More delivery options • Rebates and incentives may be available • May have some value-added services	• Keeps the business local • Able to purchase items in smaller quantities • Able to purchase items in smaller pack size • Local access with immediate availability • Often has specialty items needed on an occasional basis	• Each vendor has a specific list of products • Product listings may be very deep for a limited scope • May provide rotation onsite of product for freshness • May provide locally grown items

Note that in a competitive bid process for a prime vendor, it is important to provide vendors with projected usage figures for each product because they will base quotations on the total volume. Then, as bids are received, examine the bottom line of each vendor. Prices for individual products may vary, with one lower or higher from one bidder or another. However, the real price comparison is made based on the sum total of all items. This figure helps drive the decision of which vendor to select.

Prime vendor purchasing offers a number of advantages:

- It improves the consistency of food purchased.
- It locks in predictable pricing.
- It makes the receiving process more efficient.
- It often generates improved vendor performance because of the value of the contract and the commitment of the client.
- It may provide an opportunity to enjoy value-added services. These are services a distributor adds to its line at a free or reduced cost for customers. Examples include computer software for ordering, inventory tracking, leveraged purchasing, or training materials.
  > Provision of standardized menus, computer hardware or menu software, at no cost to a facility, could be considered an **Anti-Kickback Safe Harbors** violation and could result in charges by the U.S. Department Health and Human Services.

Prime vendor purchasing can have disadvantages too, including:

- The loss of a reliable backup vendor.
- A limited variety of products.

GLOSSARY

Anti-Kickback Safe Harbors
A U.S. Department of Health and Human Services regulation to prevent a kickback or bribe for providing a service

- An increase in prices of specific products or brands that are not under preferred contract pricing.

While price is important, it is not wise to base vendor selection entirely on price. Here are some additional questions to ask before selecting a vendor:

- Does the vendor carry the majority of products needed, including any specialized items for modified diets?
- What is the vendor's ability to meet scheduling needs for delivery?
- What ordering procedures or technology does the vendor provide (such as interfaces with a computer system, or online ordering)?
- How reliable is the vendor's service? Can references be checked among other customers?
- How willing is the vendor to commit to established food safety guidelines?
- What access will be available to a service representative or sales person to assist with any problems that arise?

Manufacturer Rebates

In today's food production and dining service environment, many CDM, CFPPs have been pressing the limits of budget cuts. As a result, the margin of profit enjoyed by food distributors has decreased to a very minimal level. As managers continue to look for price breaks, a new avenue has evolved—manufacturers' rebates. A manufacturers' rebate is a refund offered directly from the producer of the product. For example, the manufacturer of ABC coffee gives a refund of $5 for every case purchased. Typically, the relationship between the manufacturer and the GPO or buying group identifies the potential for a product-specific rebate.

This opportunity can provide a significant impact on operating expenses. However, it also requires tracking commitments to see that purchasing levels are met and rebate checks are received. Often, the GPO, or buying group, works with the distributor to track the qualifying purchases through an online ordering system and automatically claim rebates.

Distributor Incentives

In an effort to secure purchasing commitments, many distributors have included access to discounts and incentives based upon reaching purchasing or payment targets. Although discounts vary from distributor to distributor, they often include:

- Drop Size—based on the average dollar value of the deliveries:
  > Total dollars divided by the number of deliveries.
  > Reducing deliveries to one, two, or three times a week can increase the average drop size.
- Early Payment—based on how quickly the invoices are paid.

4. Your foodservice operation has been using multiple vendors for purchasing and would like to make a change to a Prime Vendor. How would you make the change and what advantages would you gain from a Prime Vendor?

- House Brand Percentage—based on the percent of purchases that are from the distributor's house brands.

Additional discounts may be available or customized to the buying group.

As noted, there are many factors that need to be balanced when deciding which distributor to align with as a primary vendor that go beyond individual product price or local convenience.

What is On the Shelf—Inventory Management

Valuing Inventory

An essential tool for financial management in food production and dining services is an inventory valuation. This is a dollar figure representing the value of all inventory on hand at the moment. This figure is not only useful in completing operating statements reflecting the department's financial performance, it can also provide helpful information to use in managing the purchasing process. Based on accounting procedures in the facility, an **inventory valuation** may be required at the end of each month, or at other defined intervals.

To calculate value, track food prices (what was paid) for each product, per purchase unit. Multiply the number of purchase units on hand by the price for that product. Then, add all product values together. An example of a form for valuing inventory appears in Figure 24.6, found in the Supplemental Material for this chapter. Note that in computer-based systems, purchase prices are often maintained in the system. Then, a user enters a physical count for each product, and allows the computer to calculate value.

Inventory Management Tools

Some items are needed only for immediate and one-time use. However, most inventory products for a food production and dining service operation tend to repeat themselves. Planning what to purchase for each of these needs requires a different process.

For example, planning a Volunteer's Dinner for next week calls for beef tenderloin. This is an item not routinely used in any menu cycles. Hence, the filet mignon is a one-time need. To determine requirements, count the expected number of clients, pad this figure as appropriate, and then order according to the needs dictated by the recipe to be used.

Routinely, though, the vast majority of products on hand are used over and over, based on the menu cycle. There are several ways to manage ongoing inventory needs, including the minimum/maximum system, the par level system, the perpetual inventory system, and just-in-time purchasing. Each of these is described below.

Minimum/Maximum System

A minimum/maximum inventory system is one in which inventory levels are maintained within established ranges for each product. It is based on two reference points for each product in the inventory:

1. The minimum quantity for the product is the least amount that should be available; inventory levels should not fall below this figure.
2. The maximum quantity for the product is the most amount of this product that should be carried in stock at any given time; inventory levels should not rise above this figure.

GLOSSARY

Inventory Valuation
The dollar figure or value of all inventory on hand at a given time

Minimum/Maximum System
An inventory system where levels are maintained within established ranges

View the Supplemental Material for this chapter for Figure 24.6, Physical Inventory—Valuation Form.

Quantities for inventory products are expressed in purchase units. To determine how much to order, take a current count of purchase units on hand for an item in inventory (physical inventory). Then subtract the current count from the maximum quantity. Here is a simple example:

- The maximum level for canned peaches is four cases.
- The operation currently has two cases on hand.
- The order would be: 4 - 2 = 2 cases.
- Order two cases.

However, the system can become a bit more complex, based on how long it will take an order to arrive, and how much product may be used in the interim. In the above example, what happens, if while waiting for the two cases of peaches just ordered, an additional two cases are used? Now, there are no peaches available. Whether this is a serious issue for any given product depends on:

Lead time: how long it takes from the time an order is placed until it actually arrives, and

Usage rate: how much product is typically used during a defined time interval.

To account for these factors, calculate the lead units. Lead units are a special factor representing the number of units needed to subtract from current inventory to determine how much to order.

Each time the inventory is counted, subtract the number of lead units from the amount on hand. If the answer is below the minimum, order more. If it is not, re-evaluate at the next order date. Figure 24.7 illustrates how several key terms relate to each other, and Figure 24.8 illustrates how to calculate lead units and purchase quantity.

A minimum/maximum system of inventory management works well for non-perishable products, or products that can remain in storage for extended periods of time. Examples of such products include canned goods, dry goods, spices, condiments, and the like. In addition, it is appropriate for items routinely kept in stock, not for an occasional item ordered for a special event.

Figure 24.7
Terminology in a Minimum/Maximum System

The following terms and established values apply to each product you manage in a minimum/maximum system.

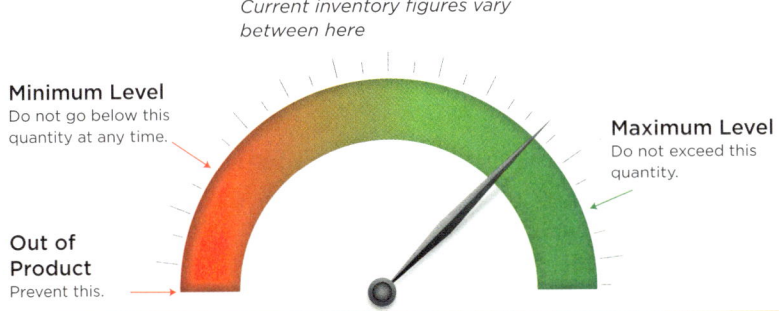

Figure 24.8
Calculating Lead Units and Purchase Quantity

Background: You are setting values for canned, stewed tomatoes in a minimum/maximum inventory system. Tomatoes are purchased in #10 cans, 6 cans per case.

Purchase Unit: Case

Based on predictions, volume of usage, and experience, you have set the following figures:

Maximum Quantity	6 cases. Do not want to carry more than this amount at any time.
Minimum Quantity	4 cases. Do not want to fall below this minimum, or you may risk running out.
Lead Time	3 days. It takes 3 days to receive the product.
Usage Rate	1 case per day. General use is about 1 case of stewed tomatoes every day.
Lead Units	This is lead time multiplied by usage rate or 3 days x 1 case/day = 3 cases. If the order for stewed tomatoes is placed today, expect to use another 3 cases of stewed tomatoes while waiting for the order to arrive.
Purchase Quantity	Take an inventory count today. If there are 5 cases of stewed tomatoes in stock, calculate purchase quantity as follows: Maximum Quantity - (Current Quantity - Lead Units) = Quantity to order, or 6 cases - (5 cases - 3 cases) = 6 - 2 = 4 cases. Order 4 cases of stewed tomatoes today.

Notice that in this system, how the minimum and maximum quantities are set can have a great impact. If the minimum quantity is set too low, there is a risk of running out of products. If the maximum quantity is set too high, excess inventory may be on the shelf. Excess inventory poses several disadvantages. It incurs storage costs, ties up cash flow, and increases the risk of losses through spoilage, theft, or product expirations.

Today, most CDM, CFPP attempt to maintain the smallest quantities of inventory products feasible, while still assuring that supplies will be adequate to produce and serve food reliably. Look carefully at lead units and also consider the reliability of the supplier. Sometimes, a supplier runs out of products, fulfillment of orders may be delayed, or a weather emergency may prevent deliveries. As with menu forecasting, inventory forecasting requires ongoing monitoring and refinement. The minimum level is set too low if product runs out when there are no unusual delays or other circumstances.

Par Level System

A simpler inventory management concept is the **par level** concept. Par levels, or minimum quantities, are set for each inventory item. Take physical inventory on a scheduled basis. After each count, compare the amounts on hand with the established par. If the on-hand figure is lower, order more to bring it up to par. This system can work for facilities with very stable menus and forecasts. For example:

- The green beans are packed 6/#10 cans to a case.
- The par for canned green beans is 10 #10 cans (or 1 case and 4 cans).
- Inventory count is 3 cans.
- The amount to order is 7 cans (1 case and 1 can).
- Due to pack size (6 cans/case), order 2 cases.

The par level needs to reflect the typical usage rate between deliveries and account for any needed lead time on special order or unique products. In the example of the green beans, a product always available from the distributor, the par is set at the amount needed through the next delivery. However, if an item is a special order and requires a three week lead time, then the par level needs to include the usage over a longer period of time.

Typically, the par system sets both the minimum amount to be on hand and the maximum amount is basically the par level plus one case or unit of purchase. The Par Level System is probably the most commonly used inventory ordering process.

Perpetual Inventory System

While minimum/maximum and par systems require a frequent **physical inventory**, a perpetual inventory system, in theory, does not. A **perpetual inventory** represents a running count of products on hand. In many respects, it operates just like a bank checkbook. The process works like this:

- Begin the system with a balance for each product. The balance is how many purchase units are on hand.
- When product is purchased and received, add this to the balance.
- When product is issued for use, subtract it from the balance.
- At any given time, a review of the balance will determine purchases required to replenish supplies. Generally, the total withdrawals over the period since the last order are used to order for resupply.
- Periodically, reconcile the perpetual balance by taking a physical inventory. Compare the actual figures for amounts on hand with what the perpetual inventory calculates should be on hand for each item.

This is just like balancing a checkbook. An example of a form for maintaining perpetual inventory appears in Figure 24.9, found in the Supplemental Material for this book.

Good practice dictates that one person take responsibility for maintaining the balance sheet, while someone else conducts the physical inventory for reconciliation. Just as in an accounting system, a reconciliation is a type of audit. Involving different people imposes control and helps prevent the opportunity for theft.

An advantage to the perpetual inventory system is control. Based on orders received and units issued, you know what should be in stores. If the figures do not match, you may have valuable information that can help control inventory shrinkage.

GLOSSARY

Par Level
A minimum quantity to maintain in inventory

Physical Inventory
A physical count of items in inventory that occurs weekly, monthly, quarterly, or annually

Perpetual Inventory
A running count of inventory that is updated continuously

View the Supplemental Material for this chapter for Figure 24.9, Maintaining Perpetual Inventory Form.

> **GLOSSARY**
>
> **Shrinkage**
> A decline or loss in inventory counts through anything other than withdrawals

Shrinkage

Shrinkage is a decline in inventory counts through anything other than withdrawals that have been accounted for. What can cause shrinkage? Here are some examples:

- A cook is opening a jar of pickles and drops it. The product is cleaned up and discarded.
- A visitor or employee walks through a storage area and pockets a product for personal use.
- A storage clerk does not rotate product effectively, following a first-in, first-out (FIFO) system. A case of sandwich meat becomes outdated and is thrown away.
- A purchaser buys food in excess quantities, and again, food expires and is thrown away.
- The salad maker decides that the fruited gelatin salad needs more fruit cocktail than what the recipe calls for, so she grabs another can off the shelf.

Furthermore, discrepancies may arise from documentation errors in the receiving process. For example:

- A purchase order specifies 40 pounds of ground beef.
- The delivery is only 38 pounds, but no one notices and documents this fact.
- The figure of 40 pounds is added to the perpetual balance. In fact, though, only 38 pounds have been added to the physical inventory. The running balance for ground beef is now incorrect.

In a related example, the distributor runs out of a product and is unable to supply it. If no one documents this error, the anticipated delivery may be added to the perpetual balance. In fact, though, no product was added to the physical inventory.

Any discrepancy discovered through reconciliation merits investigation. Often, by following up on discrepancies, a CDM, CFPP can pinpoint problems, make improvements, and better control inventory. Through this process, the manager may contain unnecessary expenditures as well.

A perpetual inventory system is most effective in a setting where the storeroom and walk-ins are closed, locked, and access is limited to the storeroom clerk. This usually includes staffing to pre-measure, tray up and prep all items requisitioned by the production team, thereby, controlling access to the inventory. Just like managing the checkbook, when one person is responsible for writing the checks and keeping the numbers up-to-date it works quite well. However, when 15 people are in and out of the checkbook every day it is hard to keep the numbers accurate. Control and limited access are key to a successful perpetual inventory.

5. Your reconciliation between the perpetual and physical inventory shows shrinkage. What are some steps you would put in place to minimize shrinkage?

Just-In-Time Purchasing

As mentioned above, there are many advantages to limiting supplies on hand for each product. The challenge though, is to keep inventory totals low while assuring adequate supplies are available as they are needed. A growing trend today is to shorten the timetable from purchase order to use. This is called **just-in-time purchasing (JIT)**. In this concept, a CDM, CFPP purchases products just in time for use.

How does this work? When frequent deliveries are available or menus are planned with specialty or fresh product usage within hours of delivery, JIT purchasing can be beneficial. Items such as hand cut steaks, custom vegetable mixes for stir-fry, or fresh ground beef can be ordered one day and delivered the next morning for use at lunch or supper that day. This allows for reduction in the inventory held on hand since the product delivery and usage are so close together.

Some large volume production centers have established JIT ordering so the products needed for everything made on Tuesday afternoon are delivered Tuesday morning. This requires a highly stable menu in terms of items and quantities, and tight coordination between the distributor and the production center. This concept also functions best when the production site is close to the distributor in the event a back-up item is needed.

Inventory Control Tools

The Receiving Process

It is essential that the right products, in the right quantity, at the right price, and from the right supplier be received at the right time. Thus, attention to the receiving process is critical to controlling inventory. (Review Chapter 18 for the food safety indicators in the receiving process.)

There are several components in an effective system. Trained staff must be available to perform required tasks. Employees with receiving duties must:

- Know quality specifications for each product.
- Recognize required quality.
- Recognize food safety indicators to assure food received is wholesome.
- Know how to handle discrepancies in quality or quantity.
- Know how to complete receiving records.

In small facilities, the CDM, CFPP may perform the receiving tasks. In larger facilities, there may be one or more employees whose duties are devoted to receiving and storage. A basic receiving process follows the steps described below.

Step 1: Check against purchase records:
- The quantity of all items must be verified against what was purchased; count items that come by count and weigh items that are ordered by weight.

Step 2: Inspect against specifications:
- Compare products against written specifications, especially meat products.

> **GLOSSARY**
>
> **Just-In-Time Purchasing (JIT)**
> Purchasing items as needed just in time

Step 3: Accept or reject products and contact the manager for the following:
- Wrong product is delivered or product does not meet specifications.
- Product was not ordered.
- The supplier has made an unacceptable substitute.
- Food safety indicators are unacceptable.
- Product was not delivered on time.

Step 4: Request or receive a credit memo if necessary:
- This occurs if only a partial order is delivered, OR
- The required items are not available (see Figure 24.10 in the Supplemental Material for a credit memo example).

Step 5: Inspect against delivery invoice before signing it:
- It is important that items appear on the delivery invoice in the correct quantity and at the correct price.
- Contact the CDM, CFPP if an unauthorized substitution is made or corrections are needed.

Step 6: Complete the receiving report:
- Large facilities that have a designated person receiving the products will require a signed, completed receiving report.

Prompt storage secures the inventory and keeps cold or frozen foods out of the danger zone. Conversely, deliveries left standing in hallways become invitations to theft. Depending on the layout of the facility, a delivery may be stored in an area where many people are walking, some may not even be food production and dining service employees.

Equipment for Receiving

A receiving area must have adequate space for completion of the steps outlined above. In a large facility, there may be a receiving dock connected with a special entrance for trucks. Generally, the receiving area should be located near the delivery door.

Necessary equipment may include: tools to open containers, an accurate scale, carts or dollies, containers to hold ice removed from fresh poultry or seafood, a thermometer, a calculator, marking and tagging equipment, and any needed office equipment (computer, file cabinet, clipboard, etc.).

Inventory

To be effective in placing an order, you have to understand the items in the inventory. In Chapter 4 (Standards and Specifications for Preparing Foods), the quality of the products to use was discussed. Earlier in this chapter, the specific standards (specifications) for the products were identified. Understanding the items in the inventory also means knowing the amount of items in inventory and the par levels.

Foodservice Management—By Design

Inventory Basics

To understand inventory, it's helpful to know a few basic terms:

- **Inventory item.** This is any product routinely supplied to the facility. Both food and non-food products can be inventory items. The food products are generally ingredients for recipes, or items that will be served directly to clients, such as individual cartons of milk or pats of margarine. Just as with a recipe, each inventory item has a unique identity or its own title. In computerized inventory or menu systems, each inventory item also has a unique number or identifier.

- **Inventory category.** Inventory may also be managed under categories just as recipes are. A category is a grouping that is logical and useful to the food production and dining service operation. For example, some CDM, CFPPs categorize items according to where they are stored. Thus, a category called frozen foods may refer to foods stored in the freezer. Subcategories may include names like: frozen foods—chicken, frozen foods—ice cream, and others.

- **Purchase unit.** A purchase unit is the package, container, or unit in which a product is purchased. For example, canned peaches may be purchased by the case of 6/#10 cans. Each case contains six cans. The purchase unit is a case. Other purchase units include: pounds (as in pounds of meat), bags (as in large bags of flour), drums (as in drums of fat for deep-fat frying), and others.

- **Issue unit.** An issue unit is the package, container, or amount in which a product is issued from the inventory storage area. Sometimes the issue unit is identical to the purchase unit. Other times, it is different. For example, the canned peaches purchased in whole cases of six cans each are issued by single #10 cans to food production staff. So, the issue unit for this example is: #10 can.

- **Storage areas.** Storage areas are defined locations where products are stored. Each product in an inventory list should have a defined storage area or location for easier control. Storage areas include freezers, refrigerators, deep-chill units, pantries, storerooms, and small supply carts kept in the kitchen or serving areas.

- **Inventory list.** A complete and up-to-date list of inventory is recommended. The inventory list defines the products specified as ingredients for recipes and direct-serve products for menus. A typical inventory list identifies: name, inventory number, inventory category, storage location, purchase unit, issue unit, and source (supplier from whom it is ordered).

- **Physical inventory.** A physical inventory is an actual count of products on hand at the current time. Counting products is often called taking inventory. A physical inventory is an essential control tool. How often a physical inventory is completed depends on the method used and the guidelines set by the finance department, which is often only at the end of the fiscal year. For tight control of inventory and purchasing dollars, once a week may be indicated. If theft is suspected, a nightly, inventory of high-ticket items (roasts, shrimp, barbecue ribs, turkey, hams, etc. should be rechecked every morning and throughout the day. In general, a good target for a price extended inventory is once a month.

View the Supplemental Material for this chapter for Figure 24.10, Credit Memorandum.

Putting It Into Practice

6. When receiving the order from a vendor, the receiving clerk finds an expired date on the canned tomatoes. What steps need to be taken next in the receiving process?

Most distributors also offer a downloadable spreadsheet with the listing of all items purchased and the most current pricing. Often, the spreadsheets can be edited to add items from other vendors so all inventory is tracked in one file. The sheets can be printed for use during inventory or the count can be entered directly into the computer for quick calculations. Review the sample form in Figure 24.6 in the Supplemental Material if access to a distributor's version is not available. In a physical inventory, each item on the shelf (not including opened items in the production area like flour in the bin or spices on the rack) is counted by the whole and partial purchase unit. A count of eight cans of peaches would be 1.3 cases.

One computer-based tool for taking an inventory uses bar codes to identify products. A handheld scanner reads a bar code representing each item on the inventory list and then the user keys in a number to indicate quantity on hand. This can speed up the process of taking inventory. When it is complete, the user can then apply the figures to determine inventory requirements. In addition, a user can typically print a report showing the current physical inventory.

ABC Analysis

Most CDM, CFPP recognize that the greatest dollar value of an inventory investment is represented by a relatively small number of items. If a facility purchases 400 products, perhaps only 100 or fewer of these items, such as meats, represent the greatest cost. The concept of **ABC analysis** helps a manager focus inventory controls where they are most needed. In an ABC analysis, follow these steps:

- Study purchases to determine which products are most costly.
  - > Categorize these as "A" items.
  - > Then group products that are next most costly. Categorize these as "B" items.
  - > Finally, identify items that are least costly, and categorize them as "C" items.
  - > Here, the idea of cost refers to the price of an individual item in a typical usage unit, not the total dollars spent on any item during the course of a week or month. In other words, while breads, cereals, and dairy items may represent a significant cost because of the quantity used, it is the use of costly "A" items that is of interest in ABC analysis.
- Categorize items in this manner to set priorities in purchasing, receiving, and storing. Costly "A" items must be carefully controlled; less expensive "C" items need less control.

In an ABC approach to managing inventory:

- Expend time and efforts to control the most costly inventory items.
- Minimize inventory investments, carrying smaller quantities of "A" products in inventory.
- Develop specific policies and procedures to control, purchase, receive, and store top-priority items.

How can the concept of ABC analysis be used in storage? Small facilities might designate one section of a reach-in refrigerator or freezer for storage of most expensive items. These units can be kept locked and inventory levels visually checked daily, if needed, to monitor the quantity of "A" items in these areas. The *precious room concept*—locked storage within a locked storage area—can be useful to store the most expensive dry items, including chafing dishes, buffet utensils, alcoholic beverages, and other expensive supplies and materials.

> **GLOSSARY**
>
> **ABC Analysis**
> Helps a manager focus inventory controls where they are most needed

Ways to Reduce Inventory Costs

Cash flow problems can occur when inventory levels are too high. Steps to reduce inventory costs include the following:

- Reduce the quantities of products purchased. To make the transition when stocks are too great, "live on inventory" for some time period and reduce the inventory on the shelf.
- Reduce turnaround time on deliveries. Only purchase what is needed and reduce dead inventory on the shelf. Computerized ordering systems can greatly support this practice.
- Adjust inventory pars when practical.
- Be sure that purchase units are well suited to usage needs. For example, a product used in very small amounts should be purchased in small units, not large ones. For instance, purchase very small amounts at a local grocery store only when needed.
- Streamline the list of products carried. For example, streamline three sizes of ground beef patties. Through critical analysis, reduce this down to one or two sizes of ground beef patties.
- Manage the menu to use each item in the inventory at least two to three times during the menu cycle.
- Examine special dietary products for possible consolidation with regular products. In facilities serving a number of special diets, there may be a tendency to carry two types of each fruit, vegetable, bread, frozen entrée, baked product, and so forth. One product may be for clients requiring modification of salt, sugar, or fat. Another may be for clients with no dietary restrictions. By reviewing dietary needs and product options, you may be able to select one product to serve both needs. Examples are: a juice-packed canned fruit or a healthy convenience food.
- Avoid minimum purchases from specialty or secondary vendors. If a $500 minimum order is required to get the $30 specialty cookie, then skip the cookie.

Food Issuing Practices

A controlled process for withdrawing products from storage for use is called **issuing**. Here, the idea is that not just anyone can go take what is needed. Instead, someone has to issue a product. The active process of issuing denotes control, responsibility, and accountability. An effective food issuing system does three things:

- Matches items removed from storage with those required for actual food production.
- Supports security procedures.
- Documents the quantities of items issued for record-keeping and accounting.

Clearly, these objectives require basic controls and documentation. Many facilities use a **food requisition**. This form organizes requests for food and non-food items to be dispensed from inventory. The form documents the transactions and assigns responsibility for the cost when items are requisitioned by outside departments. An example appears in Figure 24.11, found in the Supplemental Material for this chapter. Unit price and food cost may or may not appear on the form, depending on how the accounting system is structured.

The issuing process is managing the movement of ingredients to production and service areas. Each facility should establish policies about inventory issues. For example, who may complete the requisition and authorize inventory withdrawal? When should

GLOSSARY

Issuing
Process for withdrawing products from storage

Food Requisition
A documented request for specific products and quantities

View the Supplemental Material for this chapter for Figure 24.11, Food Requisition Form.

products be issued? Are receiving areas charged for the items issued? What items can be requisitioned?

A basic plan may be that the cook completes a food requisition for recipes to be prepared for the next meal period. A standardized recipe will indicate the types and quantities of necessary ingredients. In a more comprehensive computerized food production system, a printout may show what withdrawals will be needed days in advance based on forecasted levels.

After the food requisition is completed, it goes to the storeroom for issuing. An employee assigned to storeroom management pulls the products needed, and delivers them to designated areas. The person who receives the items verifies the delivery and signs off that everything has been received.

In another example, a service employee requisitions ready-to-use products from inventory. For example, a cafeteria employee stocking the cold service area may request cartons of milk, fresh fruit, and other items. The same steps hold—the cafeteria employee completes a requisition, the assigned storeroom employee fills it, and the cafeteria employee checks and signs off on it. In many ways, this process is similar to the initial receiving process. Each person involved in the transaction is responsible for accuracy and verification, and is accountable for the products.

Controlling access to storage areas is a prime concern in security at the time of food distribution. After items are issued and transferred to food production or service areas, the issuing process is complete.

In a very large facility, some food may be stored off-site in a warehouse. Again, the process follows the same principles. However, the requisitions must be organized and communicated well in advance of need. Assigned employees pull products for use and deliver them to the requesting location.

In another scenario, some food production and dining service facilities accommodate issuing systems for areas that maintain par inventory levels. Consider items on nourishment carts in nursing stations or supplies in a decentralized pantry where rethermalization of trays takes place just before meal service. As items in these areas are reduced to a predetermined level, a specified quantity of additional products is issued to build the inventory levels to a predetermined par level.

A modification of this system is the exchange cart process. In this model, an employee stocks a cart with required supplies (following a predetermined list), and wheels it to a pantry. Then, the employee exchanges this cart for an old cart. He takes the old cart back to the kitchen for restocking of remaining inventory.

Some food production and dining service facilities use computerized issuing systems while others use optical reading devices that read information from bar codes and enter it into computerized information systems. Software calculates the quantity of products leaving storage areas and maintains an ongoing count of products in inventory, supporting a perpetual inventory system.

A stockless inventory system works in some facilities. For example, a satellite unit may have little or no inventory on hand. Products to be prepared/served are brought to the facility daily. Any remaining products are taken back to the central preparation area at the end of the serving period. While not practical in many facilities, this system is useful when satellite facilities have very minimal food storage areas. In this system, very frequent deliveries of necessary products are essential.

Even small facilities can implement the basic principles of issuing control. Perhaps expensive and/or theft-prone items are kept in locked storage. Management staff can be present for issuing these relatively few items at specific times preceding production. Other items can remain available in storage areas for request on an as-needed basis by production personnel.

Small food production and dining service operations may not find it practical to use a formal food requisition system. However, these facilities might require that a CDM, CFPP be physically present at the time withdrawals are made from inventory. Some facilities may use a requisition taped to the wall or door of each storage area. Staff members authorized to withdraw products from storage can then enter information onto the form. Consistently enforced policies regarding storage areas being off-limits to unauthorized personnel can reduce the number of employees who issue products to themselves. Close supervision is necessary to assure that personnel adhere to this procedure.

Requisitions can be used by the CDM, CFPP to match the quantity of items withdrawn from inventory with that used in actual food production as a method of monitoring product movement and control. The objective in issuing is to distribute needed items for production efficiently, safely, and economically. Related to this objective is to keep food stocks secure from theft and pilferage. Record-keeping is a supportive service, but not an objective unto itself. The end result is effective food distribution throughout the operation.

Purchase Orders

Once inventory needs have been determined and vendors selected, it is time to place a purchase order. A **purchase order** is a business document that specifies what is being purchased, in what quantity, from whom, for whom, and under what terms. In most facilities, a predetermined purchase order format and set of related procedures already exist. Additional information that may appear in a purchase order includes: the vendor's item number, an internal inventory number, and the purchase unit (e.g., case).

Typically, a purchasing agent (Storeroom or Purchasing Supervisor) bears responsibility for making purchases. In smaller facilities, the CDM, CFPP or designated cook may place the order. In large multi-site facilities, purchasing may be handled by a purchasing department, or a buyer serving a number of food production and dining service operations. Note that it is important to clarify who is authorized to make a purchase order. If the CDM, CFPP ordinarily holds the authorization, others should be designated to place an order when the manager is not available, such as during a vacation or an emergency

Managers use web-based ordering systems to connect with a vendor's online order entry process directly. Most software and web-based options provide detailed reporting of purchasing history. This is valuable for cost analysis, as well as for determining usage history.

> **GLOSSARY**
>
> **Purchase Order**
> A business document that specifies what is being purchased

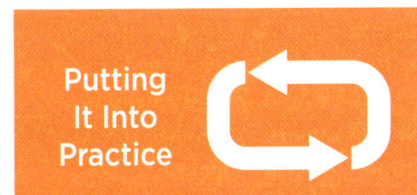

7. Your facility has an open storeroom where the cooks and other employees walk in to get what is needed. As a result, there are variances in the physical and perpetual inventory. How would you implement a requisition form and system of issuing food and supplies?

Purchasing Ethics

With the authority of purchasing comes the responsibility of ethical practices. Business ethics identify purchasing decisions based on objectives of the facility and not influenced by personal factors. This is essential to the sound fiscal operation of a facility, as well as professional standing. Most facilities have a policy addressing ethical practices. Become familiar with this policy and follow it.

Broadly recognized ethical practices dictate that a purchasing agent not accept meals, gifts, or favors from suppliers. In addition, treat all suppliers and potential suppliers fairly and equally. For example, in a competitive bid process, include all possible candidates. Final selections of vendors are based on the criteria described above, including price, value, and service. An ethical CDM, CFPP continuously evaluates purchasing choices on an objective basis and remains open to new opportunities. Sometimes, the most appropriate business decision is not the personally preferred decision.

From forecast to specification to purchase order, it is clear that there is a great deal of planning, attention to detail, and sound management required to perform effective purchasing.

Security and Controls

Throughout the process of purchasing, receiving, storing, and issuing food, there are ongoing security concerns. Many relate to the flow of products from one task to the next. The first concerns come into play in the purchasing process, where a form of theft or error can occur. Here are some of the issues:

- **Kickbacks.** Kickbacks involve the purchaser working in collusion with someone from the supplier's company. In one type of kickback scheme, products are purchased at higher than necessary prices; the two thieves split the difference between the real and inflated price. The payment can be in money or gifts. Either way, the food production and dining service operation is the loser. Routine review of invoices and competitive bids can identify this unethical practice.

- **Padding the invoice.** This means adding items that were not received, and/or increasing the invoice by adding unreasonable "handling" or other charges. This scheme works well when the employee who purchases also does the receiving. The recommended accounting practice encourages separated purchasing and receiving tasks.

- **Fictitious companies.** Personnel who purchase can steal by setting up a "dummy" company to submit invoices for products that were never received. To identify this, periodically review the distribution summary generated by the Finance Department that lists every check cut for the department with the payees' names to ensure that all vendors listed are valid.

- **Duplicate invoices.** Suppliers may send an invoice through twice if the facility does not have an internal system to verify which invoices have not been paid and cancel invoices that have been paid. This type of problem may happen unintentionally and is not necessarily a sign of bad faith or malicious intent. Reconciling the invoice number against the monthly billing statement from the vendor with the distribution summary of checks cut helps identify duplicate invoices and adjustments to the delivery statements caused by credit memos. What's important is to have basic accounting practices in place to address any failures, omissions, or errors.

- **Credit memo problems.** Financial loss can occur when products are not delivered and no credit memo is issued to reduce the original delivery invoice accordingly. A similar problem can occur if a product is rejected and the supplier fails to process a credit memo. CDM, CFPPs can require that a credit memo be issued and attach it to the delivery invoice whenever shortages or related problems occur.
- **Delivery invoice errors.** Intentional or unintentional arithmetic errors, short weight or count, quality deviations, and similar mistakes can cost food production and dining services money. It is important to check the arithmetic on invoices. Regardless of whether these are innocent errors or intentional frauds, the bottom line is the same. The facility loses money.
- **Quality substitutions.** Downgrading a product with the hope that it won't be noticed is a type of theft that can sometimes occur. Paying more for a lower-quality product can be prevented by proper receiving practices.

> Note: In most organizations the Accounts Payable staff do not know or understand what is appropriate or consistent billing for the operation. They see an invoice from an approved vendor for food items with what appears to be the manager's signature of approval, so they pay it. If someone has figured out how to get around the system and is buying food not delivered to the facility, but hiding the invoice in with legitimate invoices, Accounts Payable will pay it.
>
> Review the invoices carefully before approving for payment. Review the "Distribution Summary" of checks issued to verify that all invoices were valid. Restrict "will call" picks-ups to Manager Approval Required. Invoice fraud is easier than you think because we do not review our own records.

Security concerns become important at time of receiving, too. There are many opportunities for employee and supplier theft. Consider the following examples:

- The facility receives the wrong item, such as ground beef at 30% fat instead of 20% fat. If the employee does not catch this error, the higher price for a lower-quality product is now in the system.
- The facility receives a short weight or count and fails to notice. Now, the food production and dining service operation pays for a product it does not even have (and may not have enough food for scheduled production).
- Delivery of a product containing a filler, such as ground meat to which ground ice has been added.
- A similar scenario is meat that has not been trimmed to specifications. In this case, weight of the product may match the invoice, but edible yield factor is lower; you are paying more per ounce of Edible Portion.

To help guard against loss at the time products are received, focus on some basic principles. First of all, schedule deliveries to allow adequate time for careful check-in of products. Next, make the investment in training for receiving staff. Recognize staff for their role as gatekeepers, and assure they understand the details and mechanics of how to accomplish their mission.

While direct access to the receiving dock is efficient, the receiving doors should not be left open or unsecured. An audio signal can be installed to permit delivery staff to signal when they have arrived. Delivery persons should be under visual supervision of receiving staff during the entire time they are in the facility and access to possible deliveries is controlled.

In storage, yet additional problems can arise. The most common is theft (also called pilferage), either by food production and dining service employees, house staff, or outsiders to the facility. Several practices can help reduce pilferage:

- Move deliveries to their storage locations as quickly as possible.
- As an additional control, prohibit access to storage areas.
  > Locking all storage areas and controlling access to keys is a generally accepted practice.
- Have a clear policy about who may or may not enter the storage areas.
  > Post signs on storage areas to reinforce the policy.
  > Enforce the policy and escort non-departmental or outsiders out of any storage areas.
- Manage personal items and access in storage areas, for example, employee lunches or a client's birthday cake.
  > If allowed by the facility, have a policy that designates a special reach-in cooler away from the general storage areas for outside items.
- Develop policies that prohibit staff from taking "leftovers" from the facility without the manager's signed approval stating that the employee is authorized to remove this item from the building. It names the item(s), and contains a date and authorized signature.
  > If leftovers are available for employee use, at no charge, there will always be "leftovers" of the most popular items.
  > In some facilities, all employees leaving the building are asked to show their property to a security guard on the way out the door.
- Secure storage during off-hours access.
  > There may be only one or two employees working, such as a late night clean-up employee or an early morning storeroom employee. When possible, secure areas that do not require access during these times.
  > In addition, coordinate with a security manager, an evening administrator, or someone else to provide monitored access to the department after hours.

Security of the department is a concern beyond the potential theft of product. It also relates to the safety and wholesomeness of the food items. Intentional or inadvertent contamination of the food supply can affect every client in the dining room. Coolers left slightly open overnight by a distracted aide can result in thousands of dollars in lost food products. The safety of the food supply is the goal.

Paying for Purchased Products

The role of the accounting department deserves special attention in this discussion because all products received must be paid for accordingly. Designing a system that incorporates the accounting function as an integral part of the purchasing task is very important.

Putting It Into Practice

8. There are many ways in which purchases can be mishandled resulting in unethical practices. What are some principles that can be put into place to safeguard against this?

In small food production and dining service operations, the owner or CDM, CFPP may be both the purchaser and the bill-payer. As facilities become larger, these tasks are split between operations and accounting or office personnel. As food production and dining service operations grow bigger still, purchasing responsibilities may be assumed by the Procurement or Purchasing Department in an increased effort to separate duties. Typically, a flow of documentation is used to help the manager, accountant, and supplier communicate with each other. This documentation may be paper-based, or it may be maintained in a computer system.

One type of document is a source document. This means it is a source of original entry for financial information into the accounting system. For example, a time card may be a source document for payroll. A purchase order is a source document, as is a signed invoice. Figure 24.12 identifies the source documents and flow of accounting information in a small facility, from the time that an order is placed until the supplier is paid.

At the end of the day or shift, purchase orders and delivery invoices are forwarded to the designated manager or bookkeeper. This person is responsible for:

- Ensuring that there are no differences in quantity and/or price between items ordered (purchase order) and received (delivery invoice).
- Verifying that arithmetic extensions on the delivery invoice are correct.
- Submitting and filing the invoice for payment by accounting.

Procedures may be modified by larger food production and dining service facilities.

Although responsibility for purchasing tasks may vary from one facility to another, it is most common for a food production staff member to bear responsibility for purchasing food. This is because the specification and selection process requires an in-depth knowledge of food and the needs of dining services.

There are generally two methods used to pay suppliers for purchased products. One is managed by invoice, while another is managed by statement. An **invoice** is a document designating what has been purchased, accepted, and at what price. The purchases are totaled as the amount due. A **statement** is an accounting document that summarizes all invoices, credits, and payments for a given time period and provides the bottom line, as the amount due.

> **GLOSSARY**
>
> **Invoice**
> A document designating what has been purchased and accepted
>
> **Statement**
> A document that summarizes all invoices, credits, and payments for a given time period

Figure 24.12
Source Document Flow in a Small Facility

With the by-invoice plan, the CDM, CFPP takes the following steps:

- Review invoices received daily. Question and correct any matters of concern. Be sure that the final figure on each invoice reflects all discrepancies, credits, or adjustments noted by the receiving clerk.
- Assign dollar amounts to appropriate accounting department codes (food, paper goods, chemicals, etc.), mark the invoice "approved for payment," sign and date them.
- File invoice by due date.
- On a scheduled basis (such as once per week), forward invoices for payment to accounting:
  > Typically, accounting cuts checks for vendors one day a week so all invoices should be submitted at least one day prior for prompt payment.

With the less common by-statement plan, the CDM, CFPP begins as above, but then follows a slightly different process. Here are the steps:

- Review invoices from receiving daily. Question and correct any matters of concern. Be sure that the final figure on each invoice reflects all discrepancies, credits, or adjustments noted by the receiving clerk.
- Assign dollar amounts to appropriate accounting department codes (food, paper goods, chemicals, etc.), mark each invoice "approved for payment," sign and date them.
- File invoice by supplier, in an organized date sequence. For example, all invoices from Axl Distributors go into the "Axl" file, with oldest invoices in the front, and newest in the back.
- Wait for a statement from each supplier to arrive.
- When the statement arrives, pull all invoices from this supplier's file. Verify the statement against the invoices. If there are any discrepancies, contact the supplier for clarification or adjustment. Then, process the statement for payment.

In most facilities, documents approved for payment then go to a business office or accounting office, where designated personnel actually cut the checks and mail them. Regardless of whether payments are managed by-invoice or by-statement, similar procedures are necessary to prepare the documents for payment.

Monthly Spend Down Tracker

Managing the purchasing process to stay within budget is often a difficult task. A number of systems have been designed from simple paper and pencil to formal computer systems that control costs to the penny.

The simplest system is to invest in a steno notepad and a calculator.

- Start with the annual budget for all food and for all non-food items.
- Divide the total by 12 for a monthly target or by 52 for a weekly target.
- Enter that amount at the top of the page.
- Write down every invoice received by date, invoice number, vendor, amount, and the date the invoice was sent to accounting.
- Subtract that amount from the total and keep track of how much money is left for the week or month.

- If at the end of the month and there is not much left, adjust the purchases.
  > Or, if it looks like you have a generous amount left in a 30-day month, buy a little extra (insurance) quantity for the 31-day month coming.

A more structured program or computer spreadsheet may be available from the vendor, online, or set one up to meet the facility's needs on the computer. Figure 24.13 is an example of a simple Spend Down Spreadsheet, and can be found in the Supplemental Materials for this chapter.

The Spend Down Tracker closes the purchasing cycle by documenting the approval for payment of products specified, ordered, received, inventoried, and used. Purchasing is a major element of the CDM, CFPPs responsibilities impacting budget, food quality, menus, and client satisfaction.

View the Supplemental Material for this chapter for Figure 24.13, Spend Down Spreadsheet.

Figure 24.14
Sample Monthly Spend Down Tracker
Purchases for the Month August 2020

		FOOD	NON-FOOD	TOTAL
	Annual Budget	$ 365,000	$ 36,500	$ 401,500
	YTD Spend	$ 192,142	$ 16,660	$ 208,803
	Monthly Budget	$ 31,000	$ 3,100	$ 34,100
	MTD Spend	$ 6,831	$ 1,517	$ 8,349
	Remaining	$ 24,169	$ 1,583	$ 25,751

DATE	INVOICE NUMBER	TO ACCT.	VENDOR	FOOD	NON-FOOD	TOTAL PURCHASES
8/2/2020	1259543	8/6/2020	Good Food Del	$ 3,512.33	$ 251.00	$ 3,763.33
8/4/2020	826543	8/6/2020	Bread	$ 393.25	$ —	$ 393.25
8/4/2020	62582	8/6/2020	Dairyman	$ 563.11	$ —	$ 563.11
8/6/2020	1259677	8/6/2020	Good Food Del	$ 2,362.80	$ 1,266.03	$ 3,628.83
						$ —
						$ —
						$ —

Chapter References

RESOURCES	
Ethics in Procurement	https://www.procurement-academy.com/ethics-procurement/
Group Purchasing	https://en.wikipedia.org/wiki/Group_purchasing_organization
School Food Service Purchasing	https://www.canr.msu.edu/michiganfood/uploads/files/Inst_Food_Purchasing_Report.pdf
USDA Commodity Procurement	https://www.ams.usda.gov/selling-food

Revenue and Cash Handling

Overview and Objectives

Revenue generation and cash transactions are an integral part of foodservice operations. Cafeterias and retail operations in most facilities are expected to break-even, or bring in a profit. In this chapter, we will explore ideas for generating and managing revenue and examine protocols for cash handling. After completing this chapter, you should be able to:

- Research and analyze revenue-generating opportunities
- Supervise cash activities and reports
- Calculate cost and set prices for catered events
- Plan food service and menus for catered events
- Estimate price-per-unit serving for catered events
- Use cost-control techniques to balance revenue budget
- Prepare business plan and justification for new revenue-generating programs
- Promote existing and new revenue-generating programs

It is not enough to merely provide outstanding products and services in the foodservice industry. Managers must also create and maintain profitable foodservice operations. Simply put, driving revenue, while controlling expenses.

In the most basic terms, revenue is money or dollars brought into the operation, also known as sales. All foodservice operations have expenses, but not all have "sales." Some non-profit onsite foodservice operations provide their products to guests as part of a larger operation. For example, patients in the hospital do not pay for each of their meals individually, prisoners don't pay for their meals, and a few businesses provide an employee cafeteria where the food and beverage are free to the employee. In these situations, the revenue comes from some overall organization budget and participation may be measured instead of revenue. Even in these kinds of operations, managers typically must still work within their revenue budgets.

The selling of food and beverages is obviously the main source of revenue. Proper marketing of the foodservice operation is also vital. Simply put, there are four different ways to make more money in the foodservice industry. 1) Bring in more customers. 2) Get them to come back or purchase more often. 3) Get them to bring others with them. 4) Get them to spend more while they are there (increase the average check).

Revenue-Generating Services

The key objective of implementing revenue-generating services is to increase gross revenue in the operating statement. Depending on the overall financial plan of the facility, this money may increase profits or fund other activities. Opportunities for generating revenue in any foodservice department are abundant and generally draw upon the resources in place, such as physical facilities for producing food, a ready client base, culinary talent, and business support services within the facility. Thus, the possibilities are limited only by the imagination and resourcefulness of the Certified Dietary Manager®, Certified Food Protection Professional® (CDM®, CFPP®).

Some options may employ special merchandising techniques in a cafeteria, while others may require creating new systems and services. Some may use the existing client base, such as employees of the organization, while others may extend the client reach further into the community.

The CDM, CFPP can use a variety of techniques to manage revenue-generating services such as: supervising cash activities and reports, business planning including a profitability analysis, calculating costs for services, and promoting revenue-generating services.

If done and thought out correctly, catering represents a potentially lucrative revenue stream for restaurants looking to expand and diversify as well as onsite food service operations looking for other avenues to attract customers and add to the bottom line.

1. Your hospital foodservice department is looking at ways to generate revenue. Brainstorm and identify five different opportunities for revenue generation.

Figure 25.1
Increasing Your Revenue Through Catering

- Choose your catering format
- Develop your menu
- Designate and communicate with catering staff
- Establish your kitchen design and equipment
- Master costs and finances
- Be diligent with marketing
- Utilize supporting resources

Source: https://www.restaurant.org/articles/operations/increase-your-revenue-through-catering

Business Planning

While it is not practical to implement a long list of revenue-generating services all at once, a CDM, CFPP should carefully weigh the strengths of in-house resources along with the various opportunities. It is important to conduct some financial analysis to decide which option is most likely to meet the revenue objectives.

Some revenue-generating options pinpoint high-profit menu items. Specialty coffee is an excellent example. Taking the cue from the foodservice marketplace, specialty coffees are very popular, and clients are willing to pay extra for a cup of premium latte, cappuccino, or iced coffee. The added revenue comes from quality ingredients, along with creative merchandising, while the raw food costs are relatively low. Some revenue concepts may require extra labor time along with an increase in raw food expenses. Providing take-out holiday foods is an example. For this idea, some additional staff time may be needed, as well as purchasing additional ingredients.

Any time your idea begins to incur extra costs, a profitability analysis is warranted. A **profitability analysis** is a financial calculation that compares costs with revenues to determine whether an idea is profitable. To create one, detail the costs, set a selling price, project a sales volume, and then calculate the bottom line. Figure 25.2 provides an example for take-out deli trays. Another type of financial calculation is a **break-even analysis**.

For some ideas, an investment may be required, e.g., purchasing new equipment or building a snack shop or purchasing a kiosk for mobile food sales. If there is a significant budget cost to an idea, the next step is to create a **business plan**.

A business plan is a formal document that includes the following:
- Goal.
- Overall description of the revenue-generating service, including the proposed products and/or other services.
- Description of the target market (who will purchase the products and/or services).
- Pricing strategy that includes a review of the competition for the products and/or services.
- Detailed timeline, including the management team responsible for each task.
- Financial projections with pricing, sales volume, costs, labor, expenses, payback period, and net revenues.

View the Supplemental Material for this chapter for the Focus on Formula video to Calculate Profitability Analysis.

GLOSSARY

Profitability Analysis
Financial calculation that compares costs with revenues to determine whether an idea is profitable

Break-Even Analysis
Financial calculation that compares costs with revenues to determine if a profit is possible

Business Plan
A formal document that provides details for a proposed revenue-generating service

Figure 25.2
Profitability Analysis: Take-Out Deli Trays

COSTS:		REVENUE:			
1. Food		Selling Price per Tray	$21.95		
Ham	$0.60	Total Production Cost per Tray	$11.01		
Turkey	1.20	Gross Profit per Tray	$10.94		
Soft Cheese	0.72				
Gouda Cheese	0.51	# Trays Sold		Gross Profit	Net Revenue
Jack Cheese	0.37				
Crackers	0.93	5	X $10.94 =	$ 54.70 -$120 =	($65.30)
Garnish	0.14	10	X $10.94 =	109.40 -$120 =	(10.60)
Food Total	$4.47 per tray	11	X $10.94 =	120.34 -$120 =	0.34
2. Packaging		15	X $10.94 =	164.10 -$120 =	44.10
Packaging Materials	0.19 per tray	20	X $10.94 =	218.80 -$120 =	98.80
3. Labor		25	X $10.94 =	273.50 -$120 =	153.50
30 minutes—1 employee@ $12.70/hr., including benefits	$6.35 per tray	50	X $10.94 =	547.00 -$120 =	427.00
	$11.01 per tray	75	X $10.94 =	820.50 -$120 =	700.50
4. Advertising		100	X $10.94 =	$ 1094.00 -$120 =	$974.00
Advertising Cost	$120.00 total				

In essence, a business plan is a blueprint for all aspects of the new business. Thus, the profitability analysis needs to expand to include a more detailed accounting of:

- Capital expenditures.
- Building or renovation costs, equipment cost, initial supply acquisitions.
- Advertising costs.
- A timeline of projected sales volumes, pricing, and profit or loss.

Promoting Revenue-Generating Services

Let's say that you have chosen to expand catering as a revenue-generating service. How will clients, either internal or external, know about the expanded service? **Marketing** is part of doing business today, especially in the foodservice industry.

Marketing and Image

Have you ever been responsible for selecting a nursing home for someone? Many healthcare consumers today follow advice from a number of organizations, such as the AARP, the National Council of Senior Citizens, and others when they look for a facility. A specific tip offered by these organizations is simple and consistent: visit the facility during meal time.

This is powerful information. What it tells us is that in a healthcare environment, the dining services department may have significant impact on the decisions of others to use the facility's services. This is just one example of why marketing is important in a dining services operation.

GLOSSARY

Marketing
Presenting products or services to clients (and potential clients) in a way that persuades them to buy

More specifically, marketing activities can have great impact on the immediate sales within an operation, such as sales of the lunch special in an employee cafeteria, or sales of products in a convenience store. Thus, a CDM, CFPP needs to consider marketing on two levels: the role of dining services marketing in fulfilling facility objectives, and the role of marketing in fulfilling the objectives of the dining services operation.

Let's take a closer look at the process of marketing. At the highest level, we know that marketing has to do with presenting products or services to persuade people to buy them. There are several components to a marketing plan: advertising, promotion, and direct communications with clients or potential customers.

The basis of marketing relies on the image, which is the view or perception of products and services, as presented in the marketplace. A successful business creates an image of what its products or services represent. Often, this comes directly from the corporate vision. It relates to the idea of identifying (or creating) the client's needs and defining how the business will meet that expectation.

Here is an example: Axl Hospital has a vision to provide state-of-the-art health care, blending technology with human compassion to meet clients health needs. From this vision, Axl Hospital would want to build an image in the marketplace that:

- Focuses on caring for people.
- Relates the technical excellence of the hospital's resources.
- Explains the benefits of this combination to potential clients.

Now, any marketing activities Axl conducts are likely to revolve around these ideas. When Axl Hospital produces a billboard for local highways or places a radio advertisement, at least one of the themes listed above will be reflected. Figure 25.3 lists some examples of specific images that might be defined by a dining services operation.

The image is somewhat specific to each facility, and becomes part of its corporate personality. The more consistently a facility uses and supports a cohesive image, the more various campaigns and communications will work together in synergy to generate powerful results. Hence, the CDM, CFPP should define the departmental marketing efforts around the facility's mission and image.

Advertising and Promotion

Once image is established, a facility can begin conducting effective advertising and promotion. What do these terms mean? Advertising means placing persuasive announcements in the marketplace to generate sales. These announcements may take the form of newspaper ads, radio ads, television commercials, or even banner ads on

Figure 25.3
Images a Dining Services Department Might Convey in Marketing Efforts

SETTING	EXAMPLE OF AN IMAGE
Employee Dining	Provides the freshest food with quickest service
Hospital	Provides highly personalized meal service with respect for individual needs
Nursing Home	Offers home-style food in a home-like environment
School	Provides the most nutritious meals with a commitment to the well-being of students

the internet. Advertising is also done through direct mail campaigns, email campaigns, and other techniques.

Promotion

Promotion is a little more general, referring to any activity that is designed to publicize a product or service. It may take the form of press releases sent to a local newspaper or even menus posted in a dining area.

Interestingly, promotion can have a secondary effect beyond support for sales. For example, in a healthcare facility where the mission is to promote the nutritional well-being of clients, part of the task may simply be to persuade clients to eat. How the menu and the food are presented may make a big difference. The dining environment and the service provided have an impact too. Hence, the ability to promote food becomes a clinical care concern as well as one of business development.

Following are some examples of advertising and promotion activities a foodservice operation might use.

Posted Menu

One of the most basic tools for promotion in any dining services operation is the menu. This simple document offers a superb opportunity to call attention to the food, to reinforce a defined image, and to build sales and/or acceptance. A menu is always of interest to dining clients. When available, it may be studied far in advance of meal service times.

What makes a menu an effective promotional tool? First of all, it must be easy to read. A clear layout groups offerings by days and meals that are readily identified. It uses a font that is easy to read and adequately sized. Often, it uses clip art, borders, or images to draw attention to its contents.

Here are a few specific tips used by graphic designers:

- Use consistent alignment, generally to the left. Do not center everything, as this is difficult to read.
- Use a consistent design for menu headings that is larger type, bold type, and/or a unique font. Often, a good choice is a sans serif font (one in which the strokes contain no decoration).
- Select and use one font for the remaining contents of the menu.
- Use ALL CAPS sparingly, as it is difficult to read. Generally, it works best only for brief headings.
- Use little or no clip art. It draws attention away from menu contents. Do not let it compete with the words on the menu.
- When used, select pieces of clip art that are compatible with each other in style. They should look like they were all drawn by the same artist, even if they weren't.
- Use colors carefully. Generally, dark type is easiest to read. It should have good contrast. For example, black type printed on dark blue paper will not be very readable. Dark blue type on white paper will.
- Use each design element for a purpose, such as to highlight an important idea. Do not overdecorate, as this actually impairs readability and makes the menu difficult to understand.

> **GLOSSARY**
>
> **Promotion**
> Activities designed to publicize a product or service

Many facilities now offer their menu digitally to their customers through their website or QR codes posted around the dining facilities. It is important to ensure that the menu is updated regularly online and includes information about the facility, hours of service, payment options, and a phone number for take-out or catering.

In a healthcare facility where clients complete a selective menu, the promotional opportunity is on the menu form distributed to clients. Once again, readability issues are very important. The type should be large, clear, and dark, with good contrast to the paper on which it is printed.

Naming Products

What to call the items offered on a menu? This is a subtle but forceful choice. For instance, which of these products is more tempting to select from a menu—coffee cake or fresh-baked coffee cake? Tossed salad or garden green salad? Vegetable soup or autumn minestrone?

The name is a promotional activity. Furthermore, the name can go a long way in conveying the image defined for the dining venue. Figure 25.4 lists some examples of product names that relate directly to the appearance a foodservice department might wish to convey.

Definitely, the choice of a name builds an image about the food. There is a caution here, however. A name should still be clear and as descriptive as possible. The challenge is to communicate clearly and creatively at the same time. For example, the name double fudge delight sounds interesting, but we don't know what it is—a drink? A cake? A cookie? An ice cream sundae? So, a name should convey enough information to avoid confusion or surprises, which can backfire and disappoint a client. This is especially important in a setting where clients order their food without seeing it, e.g., from a hospital bed. Many CDM, CFPPs also add brief descriptions to menu listings to tell more about the food.

Figure 25.4
Naming Products to Convey an Image

IMAGE	PRODUCT NAMES
Fresh Food	• Garden Green Salad • Fresh Diced Apples • Harvest Frittata • Wholesome Cornbread
Home-Style Foods	• Down-Home Biscuits • Home-Style Beef Stew • Martha's Apple Pie • Robust Bean Soup
Upscale Food	• Portabella Pastry Puff • Authentic Bruschetta • Spinach Roulade • Blackened Salmon

Where can you go to obtain inspiration for naming products? Cookbooks, restaurant menus, trade magazines, and recipe websites can all be good sources for ideas. Of course, customize the names to the organization, and clearly avoid using the unique product names of other commercial establishments. Avoid overly flowery descriptions that confuse or mislead the client (and may commit you to purchasing product specified by name but not always available):

> **Sally's Homemade Chicken Pot Pie**—A delectable blend of petite peas with garden fresh carrots and Blue Lake green beans, simmered with aromatic garlic and new season pearl onions that complement the diced red potatoes.
>
> **Sally's Homemade Chicken Pot Pie**—A blend of fresh vegetables simmered with diced white chicken meat in a light cream sauce, topped with flakey pastry dough browned to perfection.

Meal Deals

Special deals or meal packages often constitute a way of promoting food. Lunch specials or Prix Fixe meals are examples of meal deals. Prix fixe is French for "fixed price" and is pronounced "pree fiks." Fixed price menus are typically full course meals consisting of an appetizer, entree, and dessert, though they may feature less or more courses than the typical 3-course meal. The price tag usually reflects a cost savings than if the items were ordered individually. In marketing, this approach is called bundling. Bundling can increase sales. At the same time, it can often speed up the service in a restaurant or cafeteria, as clients make their choices more quickly.

Discounts and Coupons

Discounts can be a way of encouraging greater sales volume. An example of a discount in a convenience store might be an offer to purchase one deli sandwich and receive the second one at half price. This type of offer is often short-term, and of course pricing must be calculated to be cost effective for the operation.

For a new product or service, a promotional special or coupon can be a valuable marketing tool. A promotional special at a low price, or a coupon for a free introductory trial, can motivate clients to try something new without feeling that they are taking risks. For example, to advertise a new meal delivery service for clients of an independent living community, you might offer a coupon good for one free home-delivered meal.

Loyalty Programs

Another approach is to reward clients for loyalty or repeat business. Most facilities have apps that can be downloaded and the customer scans and earns points for every purchase. After a certain number of points, the customer can get a free item.

In debit card systems, a client may earn so many points for every $100 placed on the card. The value is added to the debit balance. There are many possibilities, but the objective is always to encourage a client to continue using the service. Continued business is valuable and can contribute significantly to revenues.

Special Signage

As food is displayed, special signs can draw attention to products and advertise them. A cafeteria offering healthy fare items may develop a special graphic to identify these products throughout the service area. A sign may also be used to highlight a featured item or a special price. A sign should be simple, clear, and easy to read. It should be attractive but should not detract from the visual impact of the food itself. It should not block view of the food products.

Newsletter

Getting a customer database in place and sending them an e-news can be a simple tool for telling clients more about the operation. You may also get information and reach people who are closely involved with customers, such as family members of nursing home clients, or visitors to a hospital, or parents of students in a public school. Quite often, the most effective newsletters are very short. A set of two or three brief articles can address new offerings, new services, the mechanics of interacting with the foodservice department, the ways in which foodservice staff can be reached to discuss clients' needs, and much more. Here again is an opportunity to support the defined image by including content that tells more about what you do, how you do it, and why you do it.

Some dining services operations offer nutrition tips in a newsletter, too. They may also include a signature recipe from an in-house culinary expert. Ultimately, the emphasis of a newsletter designed for marketing purposes should be to build image, to help clients, and to advertise products or services through editorial content.

Specific Product Promotions

On a rotating basis, a CDM, CFPP may promote specific items on the menu. This can encourage clients to try new fare, and may thus expand sales and establish new loyalties. Branded food items create a ready opportunity for promotion. Brand names should be featured prominently in menus and on signs.

Some operations use self-branding concepts. This means they create their own special product line based on a theme or identity, and create a unique name for this line of products. This can be an excellent way to hone an image and to promote food items.

An operation that offers home meal replacements or take-out items or gift baskets can most certainly promote these products uniquely, too. Signage, fliers, community advertising, and public announcements can all support this effort.

Theme Meals and Events

Particularly in situations in which a client group represents repeat business over extended time periods, there is a genuine need to break up the monotony of cycle menus, and produce renewed excitement in meal service. One way to do this is to present theme meals. Theme meals are built around a theme, such as a holiday, a season, an event, a type of food, a destination, an ethnic cuisine, a cultural custom, a famous character, a cooking style, or almost any idea. Figures 25.5 and 25.6 present ideas for theme celebrations.

Figure 25.5
Theme Example: Halloween Special Menu

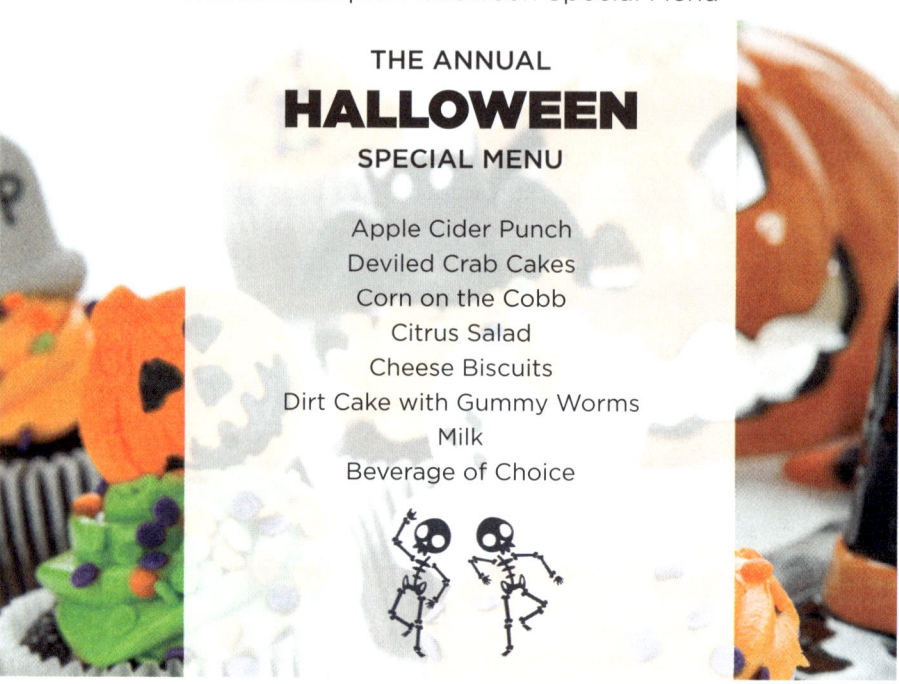

Figure 25.6
Theme Example: Luau Entrée

The success of a theme meal is more than food alone. Dining is a sensory experience that encompasses not just flavor, but ambiance, sounds, and sights, too. In a skilled nursing facility, a theme meal is often a full-blown event, and it becomes an interdisciplinary project. Recreation therapists often become very involved and help to plan the themes, the decor, and the activities that will turn a meal into an experience. Some of the details that can make a theme meal successful include:

- Decoration of the dining area.
- Special entertainment.
- Games and activities.

- Background sound or music.
- Theme-related serviceware and napkins.
- Characters/servers dressed in special costumes.

Theme Weeks

A related idea is a theme week, in which a special theme may work its way through an entire week. For example, a holiday season theme may include specialties each day of the week, such as eggnog, holiday cookies, and more. Ideas for full weeks can also piggyback on publicized recognition weeks/months, such as National Nutrition Month, Pride in Food Service Week, or many of the health-related promotional weeks that occur throughout the year.

Needless to say, theme dining ideas require menu creation and advance planning. Some CDM, CFPPs save their holiday menus, theme menus, and other materials for re-use in the future. Search online for theme day or party ideas. Contact the vendors and food distributors for marketing support and concept meals.

Open Houses

An open house is often a way to help the families and significant others of the clients become more familiar with the service and try the food themselves. In addition, an open house can bring in potential clients.

Press Releases

An inexpensive way to promote products and services is through the use of press releases. For example, an open house may be announced in a press release issued to local newspapers, radio stations, and television stations. A press release is a brief document developed specifically for the media. When writing a release, keep these tips in mind:

- Write a clear headline that tells what this is about.
- Write a lead sentence that gives the key point.
- Add further description about the announcement, followed by more information about the facility.
- Provide contact details for more information, and invite inquiries.
- When possible, provide a photo for print media.
- Clear the announcement with in-house marketing or media relations department, or senior leadership.

Media representatives do not always use a press release as is. They may call to obtain more information or conduct interviews, and write the story according to their own editorial guidelines and needs.

Website and Social Media

Many dining services operations use a website and social media avenues (Facebook, Twitter, Google Alerts, etc.) to communicate with clients and promote products and services. A website may include upcoming menus, a few featured recipes, profiles of the culinary experts, contact information (address, phone, fax, and email), and descriptions of special offerings. Some dining services websites offer online ordering, too.

To make use of this medium, always keep the site fresh and up-to-date. Menus, for example, should always be current. In some facilities, it is appropriate to offer special coupons on a website and via social media to promote sales and for effective marketing.

Brochure and Fliers

A printed piece can be available to promote special products and services. A flier may also be used to promote catering, home meal delivery, nutritional counseling, or other features. As with printed menus, a promotional brochure should also be neatly designed without excessive decoration. It should be easy to understand, and should always include identity and contact information.

With a desktop publishing program and a color printer, a CDM, CFPP may produce many pieces in small runs from a simple computer system. Some managers use pre-printed, specialty papers to make design a little easier.

A basic approach for writing a promotional piece is to follow these steps:

- Identify the audience. Who will read this piece? Make sure that everything written is directed to this group.
- Write a brief sentence describing the concerns or needs the product or service will meet.
- Then tell how the product or service will help.
- Briefly describe the features of the product or service. Bullet points are often effective for this part.
- Summarize the benefits the client will enjoy as a result of using the product or service.

Catering Services

While catering is a service mechanism, it also doubles as a promotional vehicle for many operations. Every time catered food is provided, the food and service is placed in front of potential clients. If the facility caters within the community, there is an ongoing chance to build the image and generate interest in the facility. This can be a superb way to support the broader marketing efforts of the facility, while also generating revenue.

Informal Promotion

This is one of the most effective marketing techniques of all time. It is better known as "word of mouth." A client who enjoys a positive experience tells others about it. This is inexpensive, honest marketing, and it is a natural byproduct of simple, ongoing attention to clients' needs. A personal recommendation for the products or services will likely have a profound impact.

Calculating Costs for Services

Costing and Pricing

Any retail operation has the potential to be a significant revenue generating service or a source of additional cost to the organization. It is important to plan pricing to ensure the retail operation meets the facility's financial objectives. Often, the guideline stated by senior leadership is to break even or make at least a little profit. However, the expectations of menu offerings and the customer willingness to pay rarely result in a profit for the facility.

Pricing a menu item should reflect the cost of the food needed to make the item, the labor to prepare it, serve it and clean up at the end of the meal, plus the supplies like china, detergent, and serving pans. In a true profit environment, the cost of overhead expenses, such as utilities, rent, insurance, and property taxes also needs to be included in the calculation. Without a magic wand to make food appear, every expense and minute of labor, down to the cost of the individual foil wrap for baked potatoes, is part of the cost.

There are a number of different ways to calculate the cost and determine the price point for each item on the menu.

Detail Cost Analysis

Add up all expenses and set the sell price to cover the cost.

- Based on the cost calculation of a standardized recipe, determine the food cost of the portion being sold (refer back to Chapter 3 for information on the costing of a standardized recipe).
- Add to the food cost the cost of every minute of labor associated with the portion being sold.
  > Remember to include the labor time of the person who took the inventory and added the ingredients to the order from the vendor.
  > And the labor of the dishroom crew to wash the pots.
  > And the Accounts Payable person who wrote the check to the vendor for the food delivery.
  > And the finance person who reconciled the bank statement of checks paid against checks written.
  > And every minute of other labor related to the menu item.
- Add to the food and labor cost the supply expenses related to the menu item:
  > Dishmachine detergent
  > China, silverware, glassware
  > Disposables
  > Office supplies
- Total the expenses (assuming building and overhead expenses are not included) and set the price for the menu.
- If Food Cost is $1.70, Supply Cost is $0.22, and Labor Cost is $3.04, then the total cost is $4.96.
  > $4.96 would be an odd price, so round it to $4.99.
  > Notice there is no profit in this sell price.

Food Cost as a Percent of Sell Price

Using the recipe food cost and a predetermined target food cost percentage, calculate the menu selling price.

- Often, a dining service will set their food cost target at 33-40%.
- Based on the cost calculation of a standardized recipe, determine the food cost of the portion being sold (refer back to Chapter 3 for information on the costing of a standardized recipe).
- If the food cost is $1.70 per portion and the target food cost percent is 35%, then (here comes the math):

$1.70 \quad\quad \$?.??$
$35\% \quad\quad 100\%$ = Calculated Sell Price

Cross multiply and divide
1.70 times 100 = 170
170 divided by 35 = $4.86
$4.86 would be an odd price, so round it to $4.85 or $4.89

Food Cost Times a "Factor"

Many menus use a food cost times a factor of 2.5 to 3, as a quick estimate of the food cost percentage. A factor of 2.5 is equal to a 40% food cost, while a factor of 3 is equal to a 33% food cost.

- If the food cost is $1.70 per portion and the factor is 3, then the sell price is 3 times $1.70 or $5.10.
  > $5.10 would be an odd price, so round it down to $4.99 or up to $5.29.
  > Notice there is some profit in this sell price.

Pricing Buckets

Operators and guests do not want to see 50 items with 50 different prices. Streamlining the menu pricing into some similar price points makes the menu easier to read.

- For example, in a cafeteria items may be grouped into three or four price point buckets: $3.29, $3.99, $4.79, and $5.29.
- Using the preferred method to estimate the price point, assign the menu item to the appropriate bucket.
- The level of profit or loss is an estimate.
  > Some items may even be underpriced because they fit a lower bucket better than the "profitable" bucket.

In general, customers have become accustomed to pricing that is set at five cent or nine cent increments. Products are rarely priced as $4.37. Operators and guests alike would expect that price to be $4.39 or even $4.49. Rounding of the pricing to the five or nine cent points makes the menu more consistent with what the customer expects to see.

Non-Cash Revenue

Catering represents a specialty service provided based on demand and it can be a revenue generating service. However, often the target market is the clients internal to the facility. A catering service within the community may generate cash revenue for the department, but it may be a loss if the pricing does not cover the expenses.

For in-house clients, the catering transaction typically occurs within the organization's bookkeeping, indicating an expense on one department's budget that becomes a credit in the dining services department's budget. Generally the cost of the catering services

Putting It Into Practice

2. Your food cost for a Thanksgiving prix fixe meal is $8.40. Using the food cost of 35% as a percent of sell price, determine the price on your menu.

that are transferred to another department reflect food cost only and even then are under-valued relative to true cost. Labor and supply costs are often not included so the function is provided at a loss to the department.

Catering charges should not be taken as a reduction in cost to the food expense sub-account on the budget. Food cost is food cost. The only credits that should be taken against the food cost sub-account are vendor credit memos, manufacturer's rebates applied to the food cost account, and GPO or prime vendor incentives assigned as a reduction in cost. Interdepartment charges for catering should be entered as a credit for dining services in a separate sub-account in the expense section of the budget. Any cash revenue generated by catering should be recorded as income in the revenue section of the budget.

As with the cafeteria, there are different pricing options for catering services; what is used may depend upon the type of services being offered.

Fixed Pricing

If catering activities consist of in-house catering, such as meals for staff, board meetings, and training sessions, fixed pricing may be preferred. Fixed pricing is where a defined cost for a variety of menu items is established in advance. Figure 25.7 is an example of a requisition to be completed by those requesting in-house catering services, followed by a fixed menu for catering items in Figure 25.8.

Custom Pricing

Custom pricing is mainly used for external events where the cost of the catering is determined after all of the details about the event have been defined. Once the basic expenses are tallied, price the event by using a percentage that meets the financial objectives. Some facilities use a food cost percentage method, some use a total cost percentage method, and others use the factor method. Today, many software packages can help determine the menu prices by just entering the menu item and the portion size. The software is set up to calculate cost percentage and determine the selling price.

View the Supplemental Material for this chapter for Figure 25.7, Sample Catering Requisition; and Figure 25.8, ABC HealthCenter Sample Catering Menu.

Planning a Catered Event

First, confirm that the date, time, and location are available. Consider the size and style of service being requested. Select the menu. Most dining services departments develop a set of catering menus to suit various occasions. For example:

- Breakfast
  > A simple coffee and breakfast pastry bar
  > A continental self-serve breakfast
  > A full service buffet breakfast
- Luncheons
  > A casual soup and sandwich
  > A more elegant luncheon
- Dinner
  > A quick pizza and salad buffet
  > A formal annual Board of Directors white linen dinner

The CDM, CFPP or catering coordinator should meet with the client to review menu choices and select a specific menu or design a custom meal for the event.

The advantage of working with pre-defined catering menus is that the planning process is significantly streamlined. Using catering menus (with minor adjustments and customization) will minimize managerial time in working out pricing, recipes, purchasing needs, production plans, and service needs. A specialty menu for high-end events takes considerably more resources, as each step has to be planned and tested down to the point of placing special orders for food items not normally purchased.

All catering events should be documented either as an in-house catering request or as a formal business contract for external clients. A written document is important for confirming the order and related details. Later, it is also used for invoicing or accounting.

- Confirm date, time, and location of the event.
- Determine the number of people to be served.
- Define service expectations. Is this for a fine dining event or a casual snack? Is this for a buffet or tabled-waited service?
- Plan the work schedule, responsibilities, supervision, and staffing to include adequate time before, after, and during the event to cover setup, preparation, service, and clean-up.
- Plan and request the physical support required, such as room setup.
- Plan the ambiance, food presentation, and table setting (if applicable).
- As relevant, plan and order flowers, linens, uniforms, special equipment rental, and any other needs.
- Forecast food and any special beverage needs; place orders.
- If alcohol is to be served, check on the local ordinances regarding age of the servers, licensing, and insurance requirements.
- Train employees, as needed, to carry out setup and service expectations.

These steps need to be taken in some form for all catering, even if it is just delivering coffee to a meeting.

Supervising Cash Activities and Reports

The operation needs to have specific operating procedures for the cash register or POS (point of sale system). At the beginning of the work shift, the cashier should count the cash bank assigned to the register and verify the cash amount. During all cash counting operations, two people should be present: a cashier and a supervisor or CDM, CFPP. These two verify each other's work.

At the end of the shift, the cashier should complete applicable cashier records. A cashier and supervisor or manager count the cash, record the sum, and sign or initial the cash record. During the cafeteria operation, there may be times when the cashier must void a transaction or make other corrections. A manager or supervisor should authorize this. Standard operating procedures should be developed for handling issues such as these.

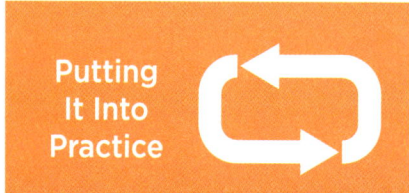

3. You have been asked to cater the senior graduation breakfast at a high school. What are the steps you would take to plan the event?

While cash-handling procedures vary by operation, some basic procedures generally apply.
- Keep the cash drawer closed when not in use.
- Give each new cashier his or her own bank (the base amount of change in the "till" used to open the cash register).
  > The size of the bank should reflect the level of business that typically goes through the register during the cashier's shift.
  > Cashiers should count and sign the cashier's log for receipt of the bank at the beginning of their shift.
- At the end of a shift, check out the cashier.
  > Count the cash in the drawer.
  > Set aside the defined bank amount.
    - The bank is the bank – do not short it to make the deposit whole.
    - The cashier should NOT know what the cash register records as the correct amount for the deposit.
  > All remaining cash is the deposit.
  > Document the checkout for cash, credit cards and department charges.
  > Both the supervisor and cashier sign the cashier's log at the end of the shift.

If credit cards or debit cards are accepted, ensure that the policies regarding data security are in place.
- Reconcile the cash deposits, credit card receipts, and department charges to the cash register Z reading.
  > Record any amount over or under on the cashier's log.
- Have policies and procedures in place for addressing discrepancies between cash in the drawer and actual sales.
  > Address the steps if the amount is significant.
  > Address the steps if the cashier consistently makes errors in cash handling.
- Train each cashier on use of the system and keep a reference or manual available.
- In a POS system, be sure that register buttons that are keyed to specific items match the menu, and that cashiers know on which key to enter each item.
- Be sure that pricing is up-to-date in the system.

4. How would you address any variance in cash handling?

Chapter References

RESOURCES	
Increase Your Revenue Through Catering	https://www.restaurant.org/articles/operations/increase-your-revenue-through-catering
Meridian Public Schools: What's on the Menu	https://www.merps.org/o/meridian-public-schools/page/food-nutrition--2
UCLA Health Catering Menus	https://www.uclahealth.org/catering/menus

Financial Reports and Cost Control

Overview and Objectives

The management of financial resources involves financial accountability on the part of the department manager. While this includes cost control, it also involves the reporting of transactions and the periodic preparation of various reports based on those transactions. An analysis of these reports is crucial to reviewing cost-saving principles, recommending efficient purchasing practices, and analyzing program changes in planning future operations. After completing this chapter, you should be able to:

- Determine accounting periods and prepare an operating report
- Develop a variance report addressing actual costs versus budget
- Use food cost, sales reports, and census counts in financial management
- Identify techniques to control costs

Financial Tools

Throughout the Business Operations unit, we have discussed how to prepare purchasing specifications, manage revenue generating services, and monitor the cost of food and labor. The information presented earlier in the textbook identified the financial control process by setting standards and measuring performance. Now it is time to complete the cycle by comparing performance with standards and taking corrective action. Let's examine some of the financial reporting tools available. See Figure 26.1 for an overview of common financial documents.

Balance Sheet

The balance sheet for a not-for-profit organization is a statement of the facility's **assets**, **liabilities**, and net assets (what is left after all bills are paid). A balance sheet showing for-profit financial activities would include investor or stockholder information. This financial statement presents a snapshot in time (on the day it was generated, usually the last day of the accounting period). Different facilities have different accounting or financial periods; the most common are monthly, quarterly, semi-annually, and annually.

Operating Statement

The income statement or operating statement (also known as the profit and loss statement) is an important managerial tool for reporting the revenues, expenses, and profit or loss of an operation over an accounting period. Sales or revenue include the cash receipts, or the funds allocated to the foodservice department for the period. For example, in school food service, revenue would include government reimbursement for school breakfast and lunch as well as student cash receipts. Expenses would include the cost of goods sold, the payroll costs, direct and indirect costs. Net profit or loss is determined by subtracting expenses from revenue. In a not-for-profit organization, net profit is referred to as excess revenues over expenditures.

The operating statement is often generated at the end of each month. So, on January 5, the department manager may receive an operating statement that is current through December. The operating statement then shows the financial performance (revenues and expenses), as compared with the budget that was developed for the same period. This becomes a good tool for comparison and analysis. A report that reflects Year to Date numbers (which means a cumulative total of revenues and expenses in each budget category for the portion of the fiscal year that has been completed so far) is also generated to review current performance to the forecasted one in the budget. Figure 26.2 provides an example of a monthly operating report and a Year to Date report as well.

> **GLOSSARY**
>
> **Assets**
> Resources of a company. This includes cash on hand, accounts receivable, inventory, prepaid expenses, and fixed assets such as buildings and equipment
>
> **Liabilities**
> Debts of a company. This includes accounts payable, and accrued expenses such as annual mortgage payment

Figure 26.1
Comparisons of Financial Documents

BUDGET	BALANCE SHEET	OPERATING STATEMENT
A financial planning document that predicts where you want to be in the next year.	A snapshot showing assets, liabilities, and net assets on a given day in time—usually the last day of the financial period.	A financial report presents the net income or profit of an organization for the accounting period (which can be monthly, quarterly, annually, or a period decided by the organization).

As mentioned in the previous chapter, the preparation and approval of a budget is an important activity for the organization as it is used for tracking performance, and as a tool to manage revenues and expenses in the department.

On this sample report, the current period is identified in the report header as PERIOD ENDING MARCH 31, 2020. Under the current period heading are three columns: ACTUAL, BUDGET, and VAR for Variance.

Actual: Identifies what revenues were received in each of these budget categories, and what expenses were actually paid out during the current period of March.

Note: The term Actual is a little misleading as it refers to the amount Accounts Payable paid out during the month which does not exactly match the amount spent. Consider that the invoices for the 30th of the month are usually paid in the next month. Some finance departments estimate (accrue) the amount carried over from month to month.

Budget: Shows what the monthly budget was for these accounting sub-categories for the reporting period. This budget was established in advance for this fiscal year. In this example, a one-month budget for any category is the annual budget divided by 12, in other settings the budget number may be based on the number of days in the month (Total divided by 365 days in the year times 31 days in the month of March).

Variance: Shows how the actual figures compare with the budget as planned. A variance of zero means that the budget is precisely on target; there is no variance. For example, in the Revenue section for the current period in Figure 26.2, the total revenue is under budget by $518. This shows that the department received $518 less in revenue than anticipated for the month. Parentheses ( ) are used to show places where the actual values represent an operating loss for this budget category. The detail shows that the cafeteria revenue was underperforming for the month.

Now, look at the Expenses section. Notice that the wages paid to employees during March exceeded the budget. Thus, the report shows a variance of $3,596.

- In the section related to Supplies, some sub-accounts are under budget and some are over budget. Overall, the cost of Supplies was under budget by ($1,853).
- Finally, looking at NET REVENUE OVER EXPENSES shows that the bottom line totals for the month were over budget by $2,387. Between less than budgeted revenue and higher than planned labor costs, the savings in supplies was not able to make up for the losses.

Year to Date

In the right-hand section of this report, we see a major heading called Year to Date. Beyond March, this section of the report is identifying how the revenue and expense categories of the budget total from the beginning of the fiscal year until now. It is showing cumulative figures. Under the Year to Date heading are three more columns, ACTUAL, BUDGET, and VAR. These are identical with the three labels explained

> **GLOSSARY**
>
> **Budget Variance**
> A budget variance is the difference between the budgeted or baseline amount of expense or revenue, and the actual amount. The budget variance is favorable when the actual revenue is higher than the budget, or when the actual expense is less than the budget

1. Using Figure 26.2, prepare a monthly operating report for a campus dining service. List three possible sources of revenue and four expenses for that operation. Is the operation in the black or red (profit or loss)?

Figure 26.2
Sample Operating Statement (Monthly Budget Report)

RUN DATE: 040220
RUN TIME: 12:59 PM
Dept Code:510

A MEDICAL CENTER
OPERATING STATEMENT
ACTUAL TO BUDGET COMPARISON
PERIOD ENDING: MARCH 31, 2020

510 Food Operations

Data for the Month				Year to Date			
ACTUAL	BUDGET	VAR	DESCRIPTION	YTD ACTUAL	YTD BUDGET	VAR	BUDGET REMAINING
37	-	37	OUTPATIENT	150	-	150	-
37	-	37	TOTAL PATIENT REVENUE	150	-	150	-
31,407	31,962	(555)	CAFETERIA REVENUE	103,644	102,129	1,515	381,455
31,444	31,962	(518)	**TOTAL OPERATING REVENUE**	103,793	102,129	1,664	381,455
			OPERATING EXPENSE				
39,800	37,119	(2,681)	SALARIES	127,359	126,425	(935)	551,711
325	-	(325)	STAFF SERVICES	974	-	(974)	-
8,756	8,166	(590)	EMPLOYEE BENEFITS	28,019	27,266	(753)	121,376
48,881	45,285	3,596	**LABOR**	156,353	153,691	2,662	673,088
15,190	6,806	8,384	SUPPLIES-MEAT, FISH, POULTRY	47,091	20,750	26,341	74,700
15,394	25,091	(9,697)	SUPPLIES-OTHER FOOD	63,657	74,700	(11,043)	371,840
2,335	2,774	(439)	SUPPLIES-SUPPLEMENTS	7,471	7,968	(497)	33,200
(4,499)	(4,339)	(159)	SUPPLIES-FOOD TRANSFERS	(14,396)	(12,948)	(1,448)	(51,460)
(37)	35	(72)	SUPPLIES-OTHER MEDICAL	(117)	100	(217)	534
437	348	89	SUPPLIES-CLEANING PRODUCTS	1,398	1,029	368	3,637
363	429	(65)	SUPPLIES-MINOR NON-MEDICAL EQ	1,017	1,245	(228)	6,737
83	131	(48)	SUPPLIES-OFFICE & ADMIN	283	398	(116)	1,853
1,358	1,371	(13)	SUPPLIES-OTHER NON-MEDICAL	3,396	4,150	(754)	21,719
1,358	1,371	(13)	SUPPLIES-UNIFORMS	232	83	149	396
30,864	32,717	(1,853)	**SUPPLIES**	110,539	97,571	12,968	463,618
3,497	2,771	726	PURCHASED SERVICES	9,636	7,968	1,668	33,062
266	317	(51)	REPAIRS & MAINTENANCE	851	955	(104)	3,864
26	124	(97)	OTHER	87	365	(278)	1,479
1,379	1,831	(452)	DEPRECIATION/AMORTIZATION	4,412	4,980	(568)	22,581
18	17	1	RENTAL/LEASE	47	47	(1)	208
84,931	83,062	1,868	**TOTAL OPERATING EXPENSE**	281,923	265,577	16,347	1,164,837
(53,487)	(51,100)	(2,387)	**NET REVENUE OVER EXPENSES**	(178,130)	(163,448)	(14,682)	(783,382)
			STATISTICS				
2,517	2,807	290	TOTAL HOURS	7,298	8,128	(830)	33,003
2,061	2,188	(127)	PATIENT DAYS	6,596	6,784	(188)	25,783
8,621	9,257	(636)	MEALS	26,431	26,956	(525)	109,196

above, except that they cover a different time period, giving a cumulative report on financial performance for the year to date. Many organizations also include a column for BUDGET REMAINING that helps the department manager know how much money is planned for the remaining months.

The example in Figure 26.2 shows that so far, the revenue has been $103,793, and this is $1,664 more than expected in the budget planning. This report also shows that even though the operation was over budget for expenses for March, in the cumulative year to date, the operation is over budget for expenses by an even larger amount: $14,682. In reality, the $2,387 is below the average of the first two months of the year and demonstrates that efforts on the part of the manager are bringing costs into better budget compliance.

Net Revenue Over Expense

The bottom line at the end of the report shows a profit (when revenues exceed expenses) or a loss (when expenses exceed revenues). For example, the month shows a net loss of $2,387. With continued effort and financial control, the manager may be able to be at or below budget by the end of the fiscal year.

Preparing and Using an Operating Systems Statement

Responsibility statements (monthly financial report, or operating statement, or profit & loss) are prepared by the finance department. As noted above, typically the Supplies cost figures reflect the amount paid during the month by Accounts Payable and may not be consistent with what was purchased during that month. Bill payments are often 15-45 days out from the time the product is delivered and invoiced.

The Finance Department looks for variances and may provide a guideline of what areas need to be addressed. Often, they are not concerned that small amounts over or under be explained, so they may specify that items with a variance more than $500 or 5% need to be explained in a variance report.

The variance report is the opportunity to educate the senior leadership team on what the drivers are for the dining services department. An explanation might indicate that December's food expense is up because of holiday special meals and catering, or that the freeze alert in California will impact the availability and prices of vegetables and consequently the menu in the dining room.

The variance report is also something to share with department staff. By including staff in the financial information, they become invested in the corrective actions that need to be taken and share the positive impacts of changes made.

Steps in Variance Analysis

Review

First, review the performance in each category and keep notes.
- Is it over or under budget? Do you know why (like the changing price of chicken)?
- Was there a new service started during the month?
- Was a unit closed for renovation?
- Was there a major holiday with increased catering?
- Was there a large dishware delivery during the month?

Compare
- Has the performance improved since the prior month or over the course of the last six months?
- Do the numbers match the expectations?
- Is the variance related to seasonal fluctuations?
- Or, are the numbers a surprise?

Ask Why
- Is there a clear reason for the variance?
- Do you know what is driving the costs?
- Sometimes unexpected jumps in business, such as increased catering or snack shop sales, can also generate increased expenses (to purchase more food and pay for more employee hours in order to honor increased service demands). This is not a bad thing. It can be a sign of business growth.
- The important figure to monitor in this situation is the net gain or loss.

Recommend Cost Saving Practices
- Is labor expense too high?
- Are overtime hours excessive?
  > Look carefully at the schedules and find a way to cut back.
- Is the cafeteria showing a drop in revenue?
  > Check the sales records, identify specific items on the menu for change.
  > Update the menu mix, pricing, or other areas.

If you are over budget for expenses—or under budget for revenues—this can contribute to a cash flow issue for the facility. Either of these situations is potentially troublesome and represents an opportunity to analyze and change as quickly as possible. The primary responsibility in managing a budget is to help meet the financial objectives of the facility and maintain financial viability.

Food Cost Report

Calculating food cost for a financial period is tricky as purchases during that period do not equal food cost. There may have been past inventory that was used for food preparation and/or purchased product that has only been partially used during the period. A food cost report is an important tool as it calculates the actual expense and represents a large portion of the budget. When a computer order/entry system is available, this report may be accessible by the manager through the same software used for purchasing. Figure 26.3 in the Supplemental Material shows a form that can be used for calculating food cost and food cost percentage.

View the Supplemental Material for this chapter for Figure 26.3, Food Cost Report.

2. The operating budget for May shows a much higher actual food cost than the budget. What steps would you take to address this variance?

Cost-Saving Purchasing Practices

In addition to reviewing food cost reports, the manager should be staying current with market trends. If there has been a freeze in Florida and orange juice is a daily menu item, review the product specifications to ensure that Florida is not specified as the only source for orange juice. Often, the vendors provide Weekly Product Updates that cover produce, fresh meats, seafood, and the status of staples such as the upcoming peach pack for the next year. There are websites that can track market trends such as http://www.americanrestaurantassociation.com/market-center. When food costs are increasing, start monitoring the market trends for the most expensive items such as meat and produce, work with the vendors, and adjust the menu, the purchases, and the individual products to get the best prices.

Sales Report

Another report that can be extremely useful to a Certified Dietary Manager®, Certified Food Protection Professional® (CDM®, CFPP®) is a sales report for cash operations such as a cafeteria, a restaurant, a C-store (convenience store), or others. A sales report provides a pulse on daily revenues. In addition, it can provide a basis for comparison of food sold with food prepared.

A common way to receive a sales report is through the reporting feature of a point of sale (POS) system. This is a computer-based cash register system. It records transactions and maintains very detailed records of sales. Information may be reported by location, date, meal period, menu item, and much more. Most POS systems provide a broad range of reporting options. It is worthwhile to become familiar with the POS system in the facility, examine options, and specify the reports needed for review.

The CDM, CFPP has an important role in the control of sales generated from cash operations. For effective control, the manager needs to know what the amount of sales should be and needs to know what sales actually were. Any discrepancies need to be investigated and corrective action promptly taken.

Let's take a look at each of these control points.

1. **Know what the amount of sales should be:** In a cafeteria or dining room situation, there can be errors in portioning, errors in ringing up food, and other situations that lead to poor control. Regardless of whether mistakes are intentional or accidental, the impact on the dining services operation will be the same: sales revenues that should be collected will not be collected. To control cash in a dining services operation, a CDM, CFPP has to examine some basic information, and reconcile accordingly. Using a food usage record, as shown in Figure 26.4, provides a control mechanism because it shows what food has been issued to the serving area, what is left over, and what has actually been used.

   In this example, mashed potatoes is a menu item featured on the cafeteria line. As the line opened, one pan of potatoes was issued to the line. During the meal period, two additional pans were sent to the line. A total of three pans were issued. At the end of the meal period, only half of one pan remained. Therefore, two and a half pans have been used.

If each pan contained 30 servings, then the total number of servings that should have been sold is:

- 2.5 pans x 30 servings per pan = 75 servings

    If each serving should have sold for $0.60, then total revenue that should have been collected for mashed potatoes is: 75 servings x $0.60 per serving = $45.00

    So now, both an item count and a dollar figure have been calculated for the amount of mashed potatoes sent to the cafeteria for service.

2. **Know what actual sales were:** At the end of the serving period, the POS report lists what the real item count and dollar figures were for mashed potatoes for the same time period.

3. **Compare expected with actual:** For example:

Sales for Mashed Potatoes	Projected	Actual
# of Servings	75	68
Total Revenue @ $0.60	$45.00	$40.80
To Calculate the Over or Short of Actual Sales:		
Percentage $45.00 - $40.80 = $4.20 divided by $45.00 = .093 or 9%		

There is a 10% discrepancy. What might cause this?

- Perhaps the cook did not produce or obtain the intended yield from a recipe, and/or did not properly fill the pans before service.
- Perhaps the servers over-portioned the potatoes, giving a little too much to each person.
- Perhaps several servings were dropped and discarded.
- Perhaps, at checkout, a cashier neglected to notice potatoes on several plates and did not ring them up.

These are just a few examples of how discrepancies can occur in sales. To manage costs in the operation, investigate causes of discrepancies such as these and implement finer controls. To exert the greatest impact, focus on menu items with the highest costs, prices, and volume.

Realistically, these figures will not be perfect matches all the time. However, a CDM, CFPP needs to manage the service by:

- Establishing a standard for the variance that will be permitted (e.g., 2-3%)
- Making the routine comparisons.
- Investigating discrepancies.
- Making corrections as warranted.

Census Variations

Monitoring the census or client count is part of the key to sound financial management. Many of the operating costs are based on projected census or client figures. Revenues are often tied to the expected activity represented by census counts. As the census or client count changes, adjust the expenditures accordingly in order to keep the budget on track.

Figure 26.4
Food Usage Record—Cafeteria

Date: _____ Serving Period: _____

Item	Quantity Issued				Amount Left	Total Used	Sales Income Per Pan	Total Income
	#1	#2	#3	Total				
Mashed Potatoes	.50 pan	.50 pan	.50 pan	1.50 pan	.25 pan	1.25 pan	$18.00	$22.50

Projected Income: _____ Actual Income: _____

Consider this example:
- You work in a facility where the census may vary and has dropped from 200 to 160 (that is a 20% drop).
- The budget for both food and labor is based on a census of 200.
- Understand that with a lower census, the facility will be experiencing a decrease in revenues, because it will receive less reimbursement for services.
- Because the census dropped, so did the traffic in the cafeteria, therefore, cash revenues have decreased as well.
- To maintain a balanced bottom line, the cost factors related to food and labor need to be adjusted downward, either through budget control, cuts in services, or system reductions, such as layoffs.

In many dining services arenas, reimbursement is limited and even unpredictable. Expenses are managed with tight control. It is not uncommon for a facility that depends upon a census to experience budget cuts, even during a fiscal year whose budget has already been approved. For example, there may be push to reduce labor by eliminating overtime, leaving an open position unfilled, or cutting back hours for employees. A reduction-in-force (RIF) may be the final step.

A CDM, CFPP can keep control of the budget, and support the facility's financial goals at the same time, by working proactively to respond to changes in census. Figure 26.5 outlines a process for doing this.

Techniques to Control Costs

A census variation may require small adjustments to the labor force such as having each employee work a little less, maybe letting a breakfast cook leave early. However, food services is dynamic and sees monthly fluctuations in revenue. Hence, a number of specific cost containment techniques can help to minimize costs. Here are some examples that were discussed earlier in greater detail within their respective chapters:

Menu

- Adjust menus seasonally to take advantage of food prices that fluctuate by time of year. For example, strawberries may be inexpensive in June, but very expensive in February.
- Cost each menu. Know the specifics and the averages.
- If serving multiple diets, consolidate menu offerings when appropriate to reduce the number of different items for production. Be careful of using one-pot recipe cooking as it becomes so restrictive, it compromises taste and quality for the liberal diets.
- Examine ways to consolidate items produced at any one meal for multiple service areas. For example, consider whether a soup produced for the dining room meal service may also be used for client service or a catered event at the same time.
- Perform a cost comparison of condiments that arrive pre-packaged in individual service units with condiments that are pre-portioned by employees. Also consider the portion size of each condiment that is pre-packaged in individual service units.
- Carefully evaluate make-versus-buy decisions, and determine the cost effectiveness of using convenience foods.

Figure 26.5
Proactive Labor Adjustment

STEP	PROCEDURE	EXAMPLE
1	Determine the usual number of labor hours required in one work day. This is a total of all hours worked by all employees in one day.	You operate with 50 hours.
2	Determine your usual census.	Your census is 200.
3	Calculate a ratio of daily labor hours to census.	Your ratio is: 50 ÷ 200 = 0.25
4	Monitor census. When it changes significantly, determine an adjusted number of labor hours that will keep the ratio stable.	Your census has dropped to 150. To maintain a ratio of 0.25, multiply your new census by the ratio you established in Step 3: 0.25 x 150 = 37.5 hours.
5	Adjust labor	Now, adjust your daily schedules to use about 37.5 hours of labor per day, instead of your usual 50.

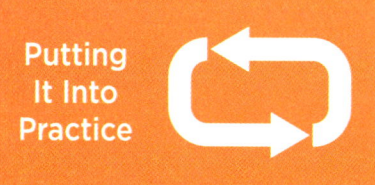

Putting It Into Practice

3. Your census has dropped significantly over the past month, increasing the labor costs. The administrator has just informed each department that they have to cut one FTE. What steps would you take?

Labor

- Match scheduled labor to staffing needs.
- Design daily assignment tasks to maximize workflow and reduce backtracking.
- Evaluate the labor cost of scratch-made menu items to convenience product items.
- Flex the daily staffing level to reflect the census or client count.

Food Purchasing

- Access a Group Purchasing Organization or obtain and use competitive bids for products.
- Examine opportunities for product rebates; track and obtain rebates.
- Ask a Registered Dietitian Nutritionist to help evaluate the use of nutritional supplements and tube feeding products. Determine whether supplementation is provided in the most cost effective manner.
- Research grade and quality for products carefully. Avoid specifying premium quality when it is not necessary for a particular recipe.

Receiving and Storage

- Verify that receiving procedures are being enforced so that deliveries match purchase orders.
- Check invoices to be sure they are correct.
- Monitor use of FIFO inventory rotation.
- Establish procedures for identifying inventory shrinkage.
- Practice security measures to protect inventory from theft.
- Ensure that perishable foods are put away quickly.
- Monitor storage conditions, such as temperature, to maximize product shelf life.
- Monitor food that is wasted due to spoilage, and intervene to prevent waste.
- Evaluate purchasing schedules for perishable foods such as fresh fruit. If needed, adjust the schedule or the quantities purchased.
- Evaluate the purchase unit of any product not fully used before part of it spoils.

Food Production and Service

- Cost each recipe.
- Take the time to calculate the labor element for each recipe to obtain a more refined analysis of cost.
- Monitor compliance with portion control guidelines.
- Examine ingredients in recipes. Ask whether a similar ingredient could also work. Compare costs. (Example: Which is less expensive for the recipe: ketchup or tomato paste?)

4. How would you minimize costs if you are noticing an increase in food waste?

- Forecast production quantities.
  - Monitor leftovers and make adjustments.
  - Use leftovers for other points of service when possible to avoid food waste.
- Scale standardized recipes to required needs on an ongoing basis.
- Monitor compliance with standardized recipes.
- Analyze time-intensive tasks in production and seek alternative methodologies.
- Evaluate the value and options for providing more self-service items to reduce labor requirements.
- Examine service and delivery systems for efficiency and streamline, if possible.
- Analyze ordering processes or individual menu systems for efficiency and streamline, if possible.

Non-Food Supplies

- Check to be sure all chemical products are being used in proper amounts and concentrations.
- Investigate use of alternative products; compare costs per usage unit.
- Cost the use of disposable products against the cost of reusable products.
- Ensure that disposable containers are not oversized for their intended uses.
- Check storage and display of disposable products.
- Train staff about when to use (or not use) disposable products.
- Examine dispensers for paper goods to make sure they easily distribute a single-use item without waste.

Using these cost containment techniques, a CDM, CFPP can positively contribute to the financial success of the facility.

Chapter References

RESOURCES	
Gregoire, Mary (2013). *Foodservice Organizations, A managerial and systems approach, 8th ed.* Upper Saddle River, NJ: Pearson Prentice Hall	
Tips for Managing Food Service Costs	https://cspinet.org/sites/default/files/attachment/tips%20food%20service.pdf

APPENDIX A
Focus On Formulas

CALCULATING AND CONTROLLING COSTS

FOOD COST AS A PERCENT OF SALE

Components	Formula	Example	Result
• Monthly Food Cost • Monthly Sales Total	• Monthly Food Cost / Sales	• Monthly Food Costs: $13,415 • Sales: $39,012	13,415/39,012 = .34 .34 x 100 = 34%

MAKE OR BUY

Questions to Ask

- What is the final quality if purchasing a convenience item?
- What is the labor requirement of a convenience food vs. made from scratch?
- What is the cost difference between a convenience item vs. labor and food cost from scratch?

Components	Formula	Example	Result
• Food Cost of the Convenience Item • From Scratch Food Cost • From Scratch Labor Cost	From Scratch Food Cost *See—Recipe Cost From Scratch Labor Cost *This should include benefit cost as well	You are making a soup recipe. • The from scratch recipe cost is $22.00 • It takes the cook 1.75 hours to prepare and cook makes $18/hour. Add 30% for the benefit cost. From Scratch Labor Cost = • $18/hour x 30% = $23.40/hour • Labor Cost = $23.40/hour x 1.75 = $40.95 • From Scratch Labor Cost + From Scratch Food Cost = $40.95 + $22.00 = $62.95	• To create this soup recipe from scratch would cost $62.95. • Compare the from scratch cost to already made purchase cost (make sure to include labor, which should be minor) • If the cost to purchase the item + labor is less than $62.95, consider purchasing the item already made. If the cost to purchase the item + labor is more than $62.95, consider creating the item from scratch.

PROFITABILITY ANALYSIS

Components	Formula	Example	Result
• Selling Price of Item (SP) • Cost to Produce (C) • Gross Profit (GP) • Projected Sell Amount (PS)	• Gross Profit = Selling Price of Item (SP) — Cost to Produce (C) • Profit Analysis = Gross Profit (GP) x Projected Sell Amount (PS)	New Speciality Dessert • Selling Price per Pan = $30 • Cost to Produce (including food and labor) = $20.15 • Projected Sell Amount = 50	Profit Analysis = • $30-$20.15 = $9.85 • $9.85 x 50 • Profit Analysis = $492.50

FOOD COST

RAW FOOD COST PER MEAL

Components	Formula	Example	Result
• Monthly Food Cost • Monthly Meals Served (# of patients x 3 meals a day x 30 days)	• Monthly Food Cost / Monthly Meals Served	• Monthly Food Costs: $18,425 • Monthly Meals Served: 11,250 (125 patients x 3 x 30)	$18,425 / 11,250 = $1.64 raw food cost per meal

MONTHLY FOOD COST

Components	Formula	Example	Result
• Food Inventory at Beginning of Month (BFI) • Total of Food Purchases (FP) • Ending Food Inventory (EFI)	Food Cost Monthly = Food Inventory at Beginning of Month (BFI) + Total Food Purchases (FP) — Ending Food Inventory (EFI)	• During the month of October your inventory on the first of the month was $14,565. • Your food purchase total at the end of the month was $16,200 • Your food inventory at the end of the month is $17,350 • What is your monthly food cost? Food Cost Monthly = • Food Inventory at Beginning of Month (BFI) + Total of Food Purchases (FP) - Ending Food Inventory (EFI) • Food Cost Monthly: $14,565 + $16,200 - $17,350	Food Cost Monthly • $14,565 + $16,200 - $17,350 • Food Cost Monthly = $13,415

RAW FOOD COST PER PATIENT DAY

Components	Formula	Example	Result
• Monthly Food Cost (FC) • Total Patients (P) • # of Days (D)	Food Cost Per Day = • Monthly Food Cost (FC) / BY Total Patients (P) x # of Days (D)	Monthly food cost for September is $18,425 • Facility has 125 patients • September has 30 days	Food Cost Per Day = • $18,425 / (125 x 30) • Food Cost Per Day = $4.91

LABOR

MEALS PER LABOR HOUR

Components	Formula	Example	Result
• Total Meals Served • Total Hours Worked	• Meals Served in a Month / Labor Hours per Month = Meals Per Labor Hour	Your facility served 7,842 meals in a month and calculates 526 labor hours per month. What are the meals per labor hour?	• The meals per labor hour is 14.9 • 7,842 / 526 = 14.9

LABOR COST PER MEAL

Components	Formula	Example	Result
• Total labor cost per month (includes benefits) • Total number of meals served per month	Labor Cost (per month) OVER/DIVIDED BY Number of Meals Served = Labor Cost Per Meal	Your facility's labor costs in July totaled $36,825 • The number of meals served was 12,400 • What is the labor cost per meal?	• The labor cost per meal is $2.97 • 36,825 / 12,400 = $2.97

COST OF LIVING ADJUSTMENT

Components	Formula	Example	Result
• Monthly labor costs • Cost of living adjustment	Monthly Labor Costs x Current Labor Costs	• Monthly Labor Costs: $98,720 • COLA Provided: 1.9%	• .019 x $98,720 = $1,876 • $98,720 + $1,876 = $100,596

TURNOVER RATE

Components	Formula	Example	Result
• Average number of employees over a given time • Number of employees who left during that same period of time	2020 Calendar Year (January 1 - December 31) • 26 total foodservice staff • 5 staff members left during 2020 calendar year	• Your facility operates on a calendar year from January 1 - December 31. • In 2020, you had 26 foodservice staff members. During that year, 5 staff members left the facility. • What is the turnover rate for 2020?	• 26 staff members total in 2020 • 5 staff left during 2020 • 5/26 = 19% Turnover Rate

FULL-TIME EQUIVALENTS

Components	Formula	Example	Result
• Total number of hours paid in week/year (HP) • Number of hours of FTE (NH)	FTEs = Total number of hours paid in week/year (HP) / Number of hours of FTE (NH)	Your facility paid out 772 hours last week. How many FTEs is that equivalent to? • FTEs = Total number of hours paid in week/ year (HP) / Number of hours of FTE (NH)	• Full-Time Equivalents = 19.3 • FTEs = 772 / 40

Foodservice Management—By Design Appendix • A | 445

LABOR (Continued)

TRAY ACCURACY

Components	Formula	Example	Result
• Total # of Items on the Menu Ticket (I) • Total # of Errors Found on One Tray (E)	**Step 1** • Tray Accuracy = # of Errors (E) / # of Items (I) **Step 2** • Tray Accuracy x 100 = X% **Step 3** • 100% - X% = Tray Accuracy Percentage	You find 1 error among 8 items on a tray • Tray Acuracy = 1 / 8	• Tray Accuracy = .125 • .125 x 100 = 12.5% • 100% - 12.5% = 87%

PRODUCTIVITY RATE

Components	Formula	Example	Result
• Number of Trays (NT) • Measure of Time (MoT)	Productivity Rate = • Number of Trays (NT) / Measure of Time (MoT)	Your team can assemble 13 trays in 8 minutes. • Productivity Rate = 13/8	Productivity Rate = 1.6 trays/minute

RECIPES & INVENTORY

DRAIN WEIGHT

Components	Formula	Example
• Drain Weight • Amount for edible food portion	Price / Drain Weight = Price Per Ounce	• Product 1: $3.19/58 oz = .055 per oz • Product 2: $3.29/66 oz = .0498 per oz If quality is the same, product two is the better value for canned peas

RECIPES & INVENTORY (Continued)

RECIPE COST

Components	Formula	Example	Result
- Total cost of food items (TC) - Number of clients served (CS)	Recipe Cost: - Total cost of food items (TC) OVER/DIVIDED BY Number of clients served (CS)	You have a recipe for a scrambled egg dish for 50 people. What is the cost for the recipe and for each client? The recipe calls for 50 eggs, 2-1/2 cups milk, and 1/2 lb. of butter. - Eggs: $1.99/dozen - Milk: $3.29/gallon - Butter: $3.00/pound Determine the total food costs: **Eggs:** $1.99/dozen - 5 dozen eggs, or 60 eggs. - 5 x $1.99 = $9.95 $9.95/60 eggs = $0.17/egg - 50 eggs - 50 x $0.17 = $8.50 for eggs **Milk:** $3.29/gallon - 16 cups in one gallon = $3.29/16 = $0.21/cup - 2.5 cups x $0.21 = $0.53 for milk **Butter:** $3.00/pound - 1/2 pound = $3.00 x .5 = $1.50 for butter Total Food Costs = $8.50 + $0.53 + $1.50 = $10.53	Recipe Cost = Total cost of food items (TC) / Number of clients served (CS) - Recipe Cost = $10.53 / 50 = $0.21

RECIPES & INVENTORY (Continued)

EDIBLE YIELD FACTOR

Components	Formula	Example	Result
- As Purchased Weight (AP) - Edible Portion Weight (EP)	Edible Yield Factor = - Edible Portion Weight (EP) / As Purchased Weight (AP)	- 15 lbs. of eggplant (AP) - 12 lbs. of eggplant (EP) after trimming Edible Yield Factor = 12 lbs./OVER DIVIDED BY 15 lbs.	- Edible Yield Factor = .8 - .8 x 100 = 80% Edible Yield

SCALING A RECIPE

Components	Formula	Example	Result
- Original Yield (Y) - New Yield (N)	Conversion Factor = - New Yield (N) / Original Yield (O)	- Recipe serves 25 people - Need to serve 80 people Conversion Factor = 80 people / 25 people	- Conversion Factor = 3.2 In Action: - Recipe calls for 2-1/2 cups of rice - 2.5 cups x 3.2 = 8 cups of rice

View all Focus on Formulas on www.anfponline.org/ANFPtv

APPENDIX B
Commonly Referenced Food Temperatures

Activity	Temperature
Cooking	
All whole cuts of meat such as pork, steaks, roasts, and chops	145°F (15 seconds). Allow the meat to rest for 3 minutes before consuming.
Poultry, game, stuffed fish, stuffed meat, stuffed pasta	165°F (<1 second, instantaneous)
Ground meats (beef, pork, lamb), comminuted (minced or ground) fish, and raw eggs (not prepared for immediate service)	155°F (17 seconds)
Fish, seafood, meats not listed above, raw eggs prepared for immedate service	145°F (15 seconds)
Fruits and vegetables	135°F
Food cooked in microwave	165°F (2 minutes) Hold time after cooking
Reheating leftovers	165°F (15 seconds)
Reheating Food	165°F (Within two hours)
Washing	
Handwashing, Water Temperature	100°F
Dishwashing, Manual—Wash Water	110°F - 120°F
Dishwashing, Mechanical—Wash Water • Stationary Rack, single temperature • Stationary Rack, dual temperature • Single Tank, conveyor, dual temperature • Multi-tank, conveyor, multi-temperature	 165°F 150°F 160°F 150°F
Sanitizing	
With Hot Water (If immersion in hot water is used for SANITIZING in a manual operation)	171°F (a minimum of 30 seconds)
Chemical Sanitizer, Water Temperature • Iodine • Chlorine • Quats	 75° - 120°F (30 seconds) 100°F - 115°F (30 seconds) 75°F minimum (30 seconds)
Dishwashing, Mechanical • Stationary Rack, single temperature • Stationary Rack, dual temperature • Single Tank, conveyor, dual temperature • Multi-tank, conveyor, multi-temperature	 165°F 180°F 180°F 180°F

* *Not recommended for highly susceptible populations. Needs to be at minimum of 150°F*

Holding	
Hot Holding	Above 135°F (Check local regulatory authority if different requirements and follow the most stringent.)
Cold Holding	Below 41°F

Continued...

Activity	Temperature
Cooling	
TCS Cooling from Hot	135°F to 70°F within two hours, then 70°F to 41°F in four hours or less, for a total of no more than six hours.
TCS Cooling from Room Temperature	70°F to 41°F in 4 hours
Thawing	
Under Refrigeration	41°F or below
Under Running Water	70°F or below
Receiving	
TCS (Refrigerated)	41°F or below
TCS (Frozen)	0°F or below
Ice Cream	6°F - 10°F
Storage	
Dry Storage	50°F - 70°F
Refrigerated	41°F or below
Deep Chill	26°F - 32°F
Frozen	0° or below
Utensil Storage Between Uses	135°F water
Hazard Zone	**41°F - 135°F**

Reviewed and updated 12-2020

Index

A

A la Carte, 27, 343–344
ABC Analysis, 400
Academy of Nutrition and Dietetics, 54, 56, 248
Accommodations, 148, 151, 258
Accounting, 338, 341, 356, 392, 395, 401, 404, 406–408, 414, 426, 429–431
Acquisitions, 31, 414
Action Plan, 193, 204, 215–218, 223, 232, 239, 260, 312
ADA (American with Disabilities Act), 147–148, 160, 198, 246, 258, 270, 370
Advance Preparation, 86, 88
Advertising, 206, 414–416, 419
Aerobic, 275, 283, 287
Agenda, 231–232, 234, 239
Air Gap, 311, 330
Al dente, 70, 119
Allergens, 54, 104, 289–290, 384
Allergies, 30, 32, 35, 54, 75, 103–105, 278, 289–290
Anaerobic, 277, 283, 285, 287
ANFP, 130, 209–210, 244–245, 353
    See also Association of Nutrition & Foodservice Professionals
Anti-Kickback Safe Harbors, 390
Antibacterial, 251
Applicants, 145, 147–149, 154–155, 157, 159, 258, 265, 270
As Purchased, 48–49
Association of Nutrition & Foodservice Professionals, 209, 244–245
    See also ANFP
Audit, 18, 91, 97–98, 113–114, 117, 122–123, 140, 155, 259, 263, 265, 267, 395
    See also Self-Audit

B

Back-Siphonage, 330
Bacteria, 59, 61, 64, 69, 282–287, 297–298, 320, 322, 370
Batch Cooking, 30, 77, 120
Benchmarking, 129, 134, 245, 347
BFOQ, 148, 157
Bid Process, 387–390, 404
Biological Hazards, 282, 293
Bona Fide Occupational Qualifications, 148, 157

Brainstorming, 232
Break-Even Analysis, 413
Budget, 3, 25–26, 37, 50, 64, 116, 127, 133–135, 177, 182–183, 186, 188, 224, 234, 238, 329, 337–353, 355–360, 362–363, 369–370, 372, 381–382, 386, 391, 408–409, 411–413, 424–425, 429–434, 436–437
Buffet Style Service, 8
Building Codes, 366
Business Plan, 411, 413–414

C

Cafeteria, 8, 12, 25, 28, 31, 53, 85–86, 88, 105–106, 112, 115, 122, 134, 137, 139, 142, 148, 177–179, 184, 216, 230, 260, 285, 338–340, 342, 345, 347, 350, 366–367, 386, 402, 412, 415, 418, 424–426, 431, 434–437
Calibration, 302, 320–321
Can Sizes, 384–385
Can-Cutting, 387
Capital Budget, 329, 337, 340–341, 355–360, 369–370, 372
Capital Equipment, 355–356, 369, 374, 378
Capital Expenses, 345, 356
Carrier, 286, 314, 333
Carts, 4–6, 82, 317, 328, 356–357, 366, 368, 370, 398–399, 402
Cash Activities, 411–412, 426
Catering, 85, 102, 106–107, 138, 213, 230, 342, 345, 347, 350, 362, 412–414, 417, 422, 424–426, 428, 433–434
CCP, 38, 41, 281, 300–305
    See also Critical Control Point
CDC (Centers for Disease Control), 170, 282, 284, 294, 306, 310, 314, 335
CDM, CFPP, 3, 9–10, 14, 23, 25, 28, 31–33, 37, 40, 43, 48, 52–53, 58, 61–62, 64, 75, 78, 83–86, 88–89, 94, 98, 106, 110, 113, 116–117, 122–123, 127–128, 130, 135–136, 148, 151, 153–154, 158, 167, 170–171, 173, 179, 186, 192–196, 198–204, 206–208, 213, 215–216, 218–222, 228–229, 235–241, 244–248, 250, 256, 258–260, 262–265, 273, 277, 287, 289, 291, 299, 302, 305, 309, 313, 315–316, 318, 322, 327–329, 334–335, 338, 340, 342, 347, 351, 353, 358–359, 362–363, 366, 368–369, 374, 376–377, 382, 388–389, 391, 394, 396–400, 403–405, 407–409, 412–413, 415, 417, 419, 421–422, 425–426, 435–437, 440
    See also Certified Dietary Manager, Certified Food Protection Professional

Census, 84–85, 133, 176–177, 209, 224, 238, 339, 342, 348, 429, 436–439
Centers for Medicare & Medicaid, 5, 9, 16, 23, 28, 33, 98, 105, 114, 122, 125, 130–131, 136, 238, 310, 335
    See also CMS
Chain of Command, 133, 141–143, 228
Change, 238
Chemical Safety, 331
Chemicals, 164–165, 250, 262, 277, 283, 289–292, 311, 315, 321–322, 324–325, 331–332, 334, 345, 358, 368, 378, 408
Cherry Picking, 388
Ciguatera, 288
Clean vs. Sanitary, 324
Cleanability, 321, 366, 371, 373
Cleaners, 324
Cleaning, 49, 139, 163, 249–252, 260, 278, 283, 289, 291–292, 299, 307, 311, 316–328, 330–331, 334, 340, 361, 365, 368, 373–374, 376–378
Closed Question, 109–110
Clostridium Botulinum, 277, 283
Clostridium Perfringens, 284
CMS, 2, 5, 9, 16, 20, 23, 28, 33, 59, 98–99, 105, 112, 114–115, 122–123, 125–131, 136, 143, 169, 214, 238, 272, 310, 314, 335
Coagulate, 67
Code of Ethics, 14, 245–248
Cold Holding, 297, 308
Collective Bargaining, 352
Commercial Supplements, 94
Communication, 3, 14, 32, 51–52, 87, 115, 124, 140, 191, 193, 195, 198, 208–209, 211–212, 214, 227–241, 314–315, 331–332, 335, 352, 388, 415
Competitive Bidding, 388
Compliance, 30, 32, 50–51, 53, 58, 66, 83, 91, 98, 122–123, 126–128, 130, 153, 164, 170, 186, 188, 191, 212–214, 249, 251, 254–255, 265, 267, 309, 312, 318, 347, 366, 369–371, 390, 433, 439–440
Conditional Employee, 254, 257
Consensus, 199, 232
Construction Material, 316–318, 370, 372
Contamination, 59–60, 250–253, 261, 271, 277, 281–283, 285, 290–292, 297, 304, 317, 319–321, 326, 332–334, 377, 406
Continuous Quality Improvement, 114
Contracts, 127, 146, 187, 351–352, 377, 388–390
Control Points, 272, 281, 300–301, 305–306, 435
    See also HACCP
Convenience Foods, 362, 368, 438
Convenience Store, 2, 8, 106, 109–111, 415, 418, 435
Conversion Factor, 46–47
Cook-Chill, 6, 24, 82, 299, 312, 362–363, 368
Cost Containment, 438, 440
Cost Percentage, 339, 346, 423–425, 434
CQI, 114

Crisis Management, 281, 313
Critical Control Point, 38, 40–41, 66, 115, 272, 274, 281, 299–301, 303, 305–306
Critical Limit, 300–304
Cross-Contamination, 250, 277, 281, 290, 292, 319–321, 377
Cross-Training, 135, 177–178, 210
Customer Satisfaction, 18, 21, 106, 108
Cycle Menu, 26, 85, 122, 419

Danger Zone, 4, 171, 287, 398
    See also Hazard Zone
Date Marking, 297–298, 305
Decentralized Meal Service, 4
Decision Tree, 94–95, 97, 254, 301, 303
Delegation, 133, 141, 222–223
Delivery Systems, 6, 94, 97, 116, 356, 440
Design and Layout, 361–379
Dietary Guidelines, 19–20, 33
Disability, 77, 103, 146–148, 150–151, 155, 160, 198, 254, 258, 270, 370
    See also ADA
Disciplinary Action, 151–152, 169, 183, 186, 189, 192–193, 200–202, 205–206, 245–246
Discrimination, 145–148, 150–151, 154, 160, 246, 258, 270
    See also ADA
Disher/Portion Scoop, 27, 53, 55, 75
Disposable Glove Usage, 252
Disposable Products, 440
Diversity, 20, 189, 198–199
Downward Communication, 228
Drain Weight, 385, 387
Dress Code, 146, 162, 264
Dry Lab, 303
Dry Storage, 278, 317, 326, 332, 366

EAP, 201
Edible Portion, 48–49, 405
EEOC (Equal Employment Opportunity Commission), 146–147, 149–151, 153–154, 156–157, 160, 246, 258, 270
Electrical Safety, 265, 318
Emergency, 54, 90, 168, 213, 263–264, 266, 281, 307, 310, 312–315, 323, 329, 332, 335, 394, 403
Employee Assistance Program, 201 Employee Satisfaction Survey, 209–210 Employee Selection, 153–154
Employment Law, 136, 145–146, 153, 179
Empowerment, 207, 221, 225
Endpoint Temperature, 293–294, 305
Energy Costs, 363, 376
Energy Efficiency, 363, 365, 371, 373
Energy Usage, 363
Enteral Nutrition, 92, 95, 97, 99
Equal Pay, 147

Equipment, 1, 3–4, 6, 9–10, 18, 25–26, 31, 36–38, 43–45, 52, 68, 71, 82–83, 86–87, 89, 116, 118–119, 123, 151, 162–165, 173, 217, 219, 224, 231, 238, 249–251, 253, 255–256, 259–262, 265, 267, 271, 286, 289–292, 296, 298, 300, 302–303, 307–308, 311, 316–325, 327–335, 338, 341, 343–345, 349, 355–363, 365–379, 382, 386, 388, 398, 413–414, 426, 430

Equipment Repair, 303, 327–328, 344, 356–357

Ergonomics, 266

Ethics, 14, 243–248, 404, 409

Ethnic, 20–23, 103–104, 419

Etiquette, 235

Exempt Employee, 152, 155, 339

Exit Interview, 189, 207

Expenses, 18, 37, 94, 97, 164, 182, 206, 224, 338–341, 343–345, 348–349, 356–359, 371, 391, 412–413, 423–425, 430–431, 433–434, 437

F

Facultative, 287

Fair Labor Standards Act, 152, 187–188
 See also FLSA

Family and Medical Leave Act, 147

FDA, 54, 56, 59, 64–65, 72, 79, 83, 90, 121, 131, 170, 174, 250–252, 254–257, 264, 270, 287, 289–294, 297–299, 301–302, 304–306, 308–311, 314–316, 324–325, 329, 331–332, 334–335

FDA Food Code, 65, 72, 79, 83, 90, 121, 131, 170, 174, 250, 252, 254–255, 264, 270, 287, 289–293, 297–299, 301, 306, 309, 311, 316, 324–325, 329, 331–332, 334–335

Federal Employment Compensation Act, 153

Federal Unemployment Tax Act, 153

Feedback, 31, 52, 55, 88, 106–110, 114, 118, 124, 167–168, 171, 173, 186, 189, 191–193, 195–197, 200, 205, 208–209, 215, 219–220, 229, 232, 234

FIFO, 261, 278, 311, 381, 396, 439

Financial Terminology, 337, 339

Fire Safety, 237, 262–263, 265, 371

First In, First Out, 261, 278
 See also FIFO

Fiscal Year, 338, 341, 343–345, 399, 430–431, 433, 437

Flow of Food, 4, 87, 272, 274, 281, 291–293, 299–301, 303–305, 312, 315, 362

FLSA, 152–153, 187–188

FMLA, 147

Food Acceptance Survey, 101, 121

Food Allergies, 35, 54, 75, 289–290

Food and Drug Administration, 171, 250–251, 291, 310

Food Code, 59, 65, 72, 79, 83, 90, 121, 131, 170, 174, 249–252, 254–258, 264, 270, 278, 287, 289–295, 297–299, 301, 306, 308–309, 311, 316, 320, 324–325, 329, 331–332, 334–335
 See also FDA Food Code

Food Costs, 25, 50, 75, 82, 94, 338–340, 342, 346–348, 350, 413, 435

Food Hazards, 251, 282–283

Food Preparation, 37, 41, 57, 82, 120, 138, 161, 251, 253, 281–306, 308, 311–313, 315–318, 322, 329–330, 334, 362–363, 365–366, 373

Food Production, 9, 25–26, 31, 35–56, 61, 75, 77, 81–90, 115–116, 118, 123, 138, 190, 195, 208, 213, 215, 256, 259–260, 262–263, 266–267, 272–274, 283, 291–292, 298–301, 303–305, 308–309, 311, 315, 327, 334, 348, 356–357, 362–363, 365, 367–368, 370, 372, 376, 378, 382, 386–387, 389, 391–392, 398–399, 402–407, 439

Food Requisition, 401–403

Food Safety, 4, 9, 14, 39–41, 59, 67, 71–72, 83, 89, 115, 120, 129, 162, 170–171, 174, 223, 250, 254, 261–262, 270–271, 274, 278–280, 282, 288–289, 291, 297, 299, 302, 305–310, 312, 314, 316, 320–322, 324, 327, 329, 332–333, 377, 383, 391, 397–398

Food Security, 315

Food Storage, 40, 311, 315, 332, 334, 368, 378, 402

Food Waste, 57, 75, 86, 88, 165, 304, 440

Foodborne Illness, 170, 250, 253–255, 258, 272, 278, 281–284, 287–288, 290–291, 293, 299, 301, 305, 307–308, 310, 312–314, 322

Foodborne Illness Outbreak, 255, 282, 287, 291, 312, 314

Foodborne Infection, 283

Foodborne Intoxication, 283

Foodborne Pathogens, 254, 285–286, 294, 314

Foodservice Equipment, 290, 371, 379

Forecasting, 84–86, 88, 135–136, 356, 394

FOTTWA, 284, 287

Full-Time Equivalent (FTE), 133–134

Fungi, 282–283, 288
 See also Biological Hazards

G

Garbage, 261, 277, 322, 328, 330–331, 334, 358

Garnish, 63, 77–78, 94, 115, 138, 383–384, 414

Gluten-Free, 62–63

Goal, 3, 19, 28, 33, 114, 129, 134, 136, 165, 169, 174, 176, 178, 191, 194, 200, 209–226, 230–232, 239–240, 244, 260, 263, 335, 406, 413, 437

Grading, 58, 64–66, 272, 280, 310, 385

Grievance, 206, 352

H

HACCP, 38–40, 66, 89, 114–115, 138, 174, 191, 250, 272, 274, 281, 299–305, 312, 314, 320, 373

Hand Antiseptics, 252

Handwashing, 114, 165, 170, 250–253, 255, 261, 286, 292, 311, 318, 329, 368

Hazard Analysis Critical Control Point, 40–41, 66, 115, 274, 299, 306
 See also HACCP

Hazards, 250–251, 260, 265, 267–268, 270–271, 277, 282–283, 287, 289, 291, 293, 299–302, 304–305, 331–332

Health Insurance Portability and Accountability Act, 129, 169, 246
See also HIPPA
Heat Exhaustion, 263–264
Heating, Ventilation, and Air Conditioning System, 317
Hepatitis, 254, 257–258, 272, 286
HIPAA, 129, 147, 161, 168–169, 172, 174, 213, 245–247
Hiring, 134–136, 143, 145–146, 150–151, 153, 159, 218, 258, 315, 338
Holding, 25, 31, 38, 51, 68, 77, 89, 106, 120, 138, 171, 244, 250, 261, 269, 278, 284, 288, 291, 295–301, 305, 308, 311, 320–321, 330, 357, 362, 368
Hospital Consumer Assessment of Healthcare Providers and Systems Survey, 105
Human Resource Department, 135
HVAC, 317, 328, 365
Hygiene, 170, 250, 285–286, 288, 291, 299, 302, 311

I

Ice, 53, 66, 73, 93–94, 275–276, 279, 285, 293, 297–298, 328–330, 357, 363, 398–399, 405, 417
IDT, 117, 128
    See also Interdisciplinary Team
Image, 105, 220, 256, 296, 320, 414–417, 419, 422
Individually Quick Frozen, 66
Ingredient Control, 81
Injury, 89, 153, 164, 201, 256, 260, 261, 265-269, 291, 365
Insects, 317, 333–334
Inservice, 174
Inspection, 59, 64–65, 115, 123, 130, 148, 250, 258–260, 265, 267, 271–275, 280, 307–312, 316, 320–322, 327, 334–335, 376, 384–385
Insubordination, 201
Integrated Pest Management, 307, 334
Interdisciplinary Team, 97, 117, 128, 130, 231
Interview Process, 108, 145, 154–155, 198, 218
Inventory, 18, 31, 37, 50, 53, 75, 84, 86, 136, 213, 247, 261, 273, 315, 332, 346, 362, 378, 381–382, 386–387, 390, 392–403, 423, 430, 434, 439
Inventory Valuation, 392
Invoice, 137, 271, 274, 345, 382, 389, 391, 398, 404–405, 407–409, 431, 439
IQF, 66

J

Jewelry, 146, 170, 252, 261
Job Analysis, 133, 136–140, 191
Job Description, 133–134, 136–140, 143, 154–155, 157, 162–163, 181, 183, 191
Job Sharing, 177–178
    See also Staffing
Just-In-Time Purchasing, 392, 397

K

Key Performance Indicators (KPIs), 211, 223, 347
Kosher, 23, 89
KPIs, 211, 223

L

Labor, 7, 25, 37, 43, 82–83, 87, 96–97, 133–143, 152–153, 160, 164, 175–177, 183–184, 186–188, 198, 208, 211, 217, 224, 244, 256, 265, 305, 337–342, 345, 347–351, 353, 357, 359, 362, 377, 413–414, 422–423, 425, 430–431, 434, 437–440
Labor Costs Per Meal, 350
Labor Unions, 208, 244, 351
Late Trays, 13–14
Lateral Communication, 229
Layout, 12, 18, 25, 41, 163, 302–304, 349, 361–379, 398, 416
Leftovers, 49, 72, 75, 84–85, 88, 138, 284, 288–289, 291, 298, 302, 305, 406, 440
Legal Implications, 91, 98, 130, 198
Likert Scale, 109–110

M

Management by Objectives, 194
MAP, 162–163, 263, 275, 277, 283, 304, 338
Marketing, 18, 37, 56, 103, 237, 386, 412–415, 418–419, 421–422
Master Schedule, 182, 184
MDS, 127
Meal Service, 1–4, 6, 10, 12, 17, 28–30, 84, 87, 97–98, 102–105, 123–125, 137–138, 177, 214, 335, 402, 415–416, 419, 438
Meals per Labor Hour, 183, 337
Measurements, 35, 40, 45–47, 51–52, 71, 89, 125, 303, 350
Meat, 11, 20–24, 26, 38, 48, 50, 58, 64–66, 71–74, 77–79, 86–87, 93, 121, 163, 250, 261, 272–275, 277–279, 284–287, 289–290, 293–295, 297–299, 304–305, 310, 319–320, 339–340, 356, 384–385, 388–389, 396–397, 399–400, 405, 418, 435
Medications, 77, 104, 264
Meetings, 29, 85, 102, 108, 204, 227–233, 236–237, 241, 244–245, 273, 352, 368, 425
Menu, 1–4, 6–14, 17–33, 35–37, 39, 41, 43–46, 49–50, 52–53, 55–59, 62–64, 66–67, 75, 77–78, 81–88, 90, 92–93, 103–104, 107–108, 116, 118–119, 121–122, 124–125, 129, 137, 142, 165, 169, 177, 213, 217, 238, 294, 300–301, 303–305, 313, 342, 346–349, 362, 368, 372, 375, 383–384, 386, 390, 392, 394–395, 397, 399, 401, 409, 411, 413, 416–428, 433–436, 438–440
Menu Planning, 17–20, 23–27, 55, 67, 87, 92–93, 125, 213, 347
Menu Substitutions, 18, 28, 57
Minimum Data Set, 127
Minutes per Meal, 183
Mission Statement, 103
Mold, 65, 276, 288–289, 370

Monthly Food Cost, 346
Monitoring, 18, 29–31, 57–58, 64, 75, 97, 115, 117, 136, 142, 186, 290, 292, 295–296, 300–305, 308, 319–320, 338, 349, 357, 377–378, 394, 403, 435–436
Motivation, 161, 164, 166, 173, 193, 205, 218–220, 222–223
MSDs, 266–267, 269, 323
MSG (Monosodium Glutamate), 289
Musculoskeletal Disorders, 266, 269
See also MSDs

National Sanitation Foundation, 318, 335
See also NSF
Natural Toxins, 283, 288
Norovirus, 254–255, 257, 284, 286
NSF, 261, 318, 335, 370–372
Nutrition Support, 91–93, 99

OJT, 167, 171, 230
On-the-job Training, 160–161, 167–168, 170, 218, 230
See also OJT
Open-Ended Question, 109–111
Operating Budget, 337–353, 356–357, 434
Operating Statement, 412, 430, 432–433
Organization Chart, 133, 138, 141–143, 191, 203, 213–214, 222–223
Orientation, 51, 90, 140, 145–146, 159–164, 170, 173, 191, 193, 195, 198, 203, 214, 260, 322, 331–332
OSHA (Occupational Safety and Hazard Administration), 164, 214, 237, 265–266, 268, 270, 331, 335
Overtime, 152, 155–156, 175, 182–183, 185–188, 200, 338–339, 349, 351, 434, 437

Packaging, 9, 271, 275–278, 294, 297–298, 300, 304, 384–385, 387, 414
Pad, 85–87, 392
Pantry, 6, 96, 260, 362, 399, 402
Par Levels, 394, 398
Parasite, 282–283, 286, 288, 294
Parenteral Nutrition, 93
Pasteurized, 59–61, 67, 72, 74, 274, 276, 279, 285, 287, 294
Pathogens, 251, 254, 277, 282–287, 292, 294, 302, 305, 314, 325, 330, 333
Payroll, 182–183, 185–186, 339, 407, 430
PDCA (Plan, Do, Check, Act), 115, 129
Performance Review, 165, 189, 192–198, 200
Performance Standard, 116–117, 165, 167, 188–192, 194, 197, 200, 203–204, 214, 222–223
Permit Holder, 250
Person In Charge, 142, 250, 254, 256–257, 308
Personal Hygiene, 170, 250, 285–286, 288, 291, 299, 302, 311
Personnel, 14, 88, 133–136, 146, 150–151, 159–161, 164, 176–178, 186, 189–210, 213, 216, 228, 231, 237, 249–270, 301, 313–314, 319, 322, 348, 351–352, 403–404, 407–408
Pest Management, 307, 334
Pesticides, 283, 289–290, 292, 310, 333
Physical Design, 3
Physical Hazards, 291
Physical Inventory, 346, 393–396, 399–400
Pilferage, 40, 403, 406
Plate Waste, 18, 55, 88–89, 107, 117, 121–122, 223
Plumbing, 322, 329–330
POD System, 4
Policy and Procedure, 3, 97, 180, 203, 212, 214, 237
Portion Control, 29, 35, 52–54, 75, 77, 165, 439
POS, 85, 339, 426–427, 435–436
Potable Water, 251, 292, 311, 329–330
Potentially Hazardous Foods, 275, 281
Preventative Maintenance, 327, 376
Prime Vendor, 274, 342, 382, 389–391, 425
Prions, 283
Profitability Analysis, 412–414
Progressive Discipline, 203–204, 206
Promotion, 151, 192–193, 198, 210, 219, 228, 415–416, 419, 422
Purchase Order, 64, 381, 388, 396–397, 403–404, 407, 439
Purchasing Decisions, 369, 372, 387, 404
Purchasing Practices, 311, 429, 435
Purchasing Specifications, 116, 274, 305, 381, 430
Purchasing Standards, 58, 72

QI, 97–98, 114–115, 127
See also Quality Indicators
Quality Assurance, 114–115, 130, 140–141, 266
Quality Improvement, 79, 97, 114–115, 140, 241
Quality Indicators, 113, 129–130, 276
Quality Standards, 57, 66–67, 69–74, 83, 116–119, 122–123, 129, 167, 272, 274

Ready-to-Eat Foods, 38, 43, 251, 261, 277–278, 297
Receiving, 58, 82, 84, 93–94, 102, 124, 137, 139, 152, 158, 173, 191, 194, 204, 261, 271–281, 288, 291, 299, 301, 304–305, 314, 332, 341, 347, 362, 366–369, 384, 389–390, 396–400, 402, 404–405, 408, 439
Recipe, 18–19, 27–29, 31, 35–56, 58, 61, 63–64, 66–67, 70, 73–78, 82–84, 86–90, 97, 116, 118–119, 138, 190, 217, 300–301, 346–347, 383–384, 386, 392, 396, 399, 402, 418–419, 421, 423, 426, 436, 438–440
Registered Dietitian Nutritionist (RDN), 25, 27, 43, 92–93, 98, 104, 128, 236, 386, 439
Regulations, 2, 10, 20–21, 23–25, 28, 58–59, 66, 98, 103, 122, 127–128, 130–131, 136, 146, 148, 150, 153, 164, 169, 182, 198, 211, 214, 216–217, 230, 237–239, 245–246, 249, 258, 265, 267, 278, 293, 307–310, 312, 316, 318, 321, 325, 329–331, 334–335, 366, 369–370

Reheating, 9, 25, 67, 72, 82, 250, 284, 291, 295, 297–298, 302, 305, 311, 320
Religious Practices, 23, 147
Reportable Health Information, 254
Reports, 6, 127, 139, 141–142, 182–183, 186, 218, 230, 241, 254–257, 265, 312, 349, 363, 411–412, 426, 429–440
Request for Proposal, 369
 See also RFP
Requisition, 35, 52–53, 138, 350, 381, 401–403, 425
Restaurant Style Dining, 8
Restricted Employee, 255
Rethermalize, 5
Revenue, 18, 106, 134, 224, 337–343, 345–346, 411–428, 430–431, 433–438
RFP, 369, 372
Risk, 41, 130, 152, 164, 170, 201, 237, 245, 249, 253–256, 258–260, 264, 267, 282, 285–286, 294, 297, 301, 303–305, 307–308, 311, 314, 317, 319, 334, 394, 418
Risk Management, 164, 237, 249, 256
Roux, 74, 89

S

S.M.A.R.T. Goals, 217, 225, 240
Safe Food Handling, 249–335
Safety, 4, 9–10, 14, 25, 28, 39–41, 59, 64–65, 67, 71–72, 83, 88–89, 105, 114–115, 120, 123, 126, 129, 161–167, 170–171, 174, 193, 201, 208, 218–219, 223, 230, 237, 245, 247, 249–250, 253–254, 256, 258–263, 265–267, 270–272, 274–275, 278–280, 282, 287–289, 291, 297, 299–300, 302–303, 305–310, 312, 314–316, 318, 320–324, 327, 329, 331–333, 335, 351, 360, 362, 365–366, 370–374, 377–378, 383–384, 391, 397–398, 406
Safety Data Sheet, 165, 249, 267, 270, 323, 331–332, 335
Salary Survey, 353
Salmonella, 59, 254–255, 283–285, 287, 292, 302, 333
Sanitary, 59, 249, 251, 253, 280, 321, 324–325, 330, 334–335
Sanitizers, 252, 311, 321, 325, 327, 329
Satisfaction, 18–19, 21, 36, 53, 60, 86, 90, 101–112, 114, 117, 121, 124, 170–172, 189, 209–210, 215, 219, 222–223, 237, 240, 409
Scaling, 41, 43–44, 46–47, 52
Scheduling, 71, 84, 86–87, 116, 136, 163, 175–188, 208, 213, 229, 338, 362, 391
Screening, 127, 140, 153–155, 159, 288
SDS, 165, 267, 331–332
Security, 106, 126, 129, 168, 202, 218–219, 246, 271, 282, 312, 315, 319, 334, 343, 352, 366, 401–402, 404–406, 427, 439
Selective Menu, 2, 10–13, 28, 32, 104, 124, 417
Self-Audit, 122–123, 263
Service Options, 3–4
Sexual Harassment, 150–152, 164, 201
Shellfish, 54, 64–65, 272–273, 276, 279, 284–286, 288–290, 293, 310, 375, 385
Shelving, 259, 277, 317, 368
Slacking, 293

Social Networking, 214
Software, 6, 32, 43, 50, 52, 85, 182–183, 238, 240, 346, 356–357, 376, 390, 402–403, 425, 434
SOP, 212–214, 237, 299, 305, 308
 See also Standard Operating Procedure
Specification, 18, 29, 36, 41, 57–59, 63–64, 79, 115–116, 272, 274, 305, 316, 329, 355, 358–359, 361, 369, 372–374, 381–386, 388–389, 397–398, 404–405, 407, 430, 435
Split Shift, 177
Staffing, 2–3, 9–10, 14, 18, 31, 36–37, 45, 85, 87, 111, 129–130, 133–143, 145, 173, 176–178, 180, 182–183, 188, 191, 206, 210, 213, 215, 313, 322, 349, 351, 362, 382, 396, 426, 439
Standard Operating Procedure, 140, 213, 237, 299, 301, 305, 308, 426
Standard Weights and Measures, 27–28
Standardized Recipe, 29, 35–56, 67, 75, 77–78, 82–83, 86, 88–89, 116, 118, 138, 190, 301, 346–347, 402, 423, 440
Staphylococcus Aureus, 284
Static Menu, 26
Storage, 25, 40, 59–60, 65, 90, 253, 262, 271–281, 283–284, 288, 291–292, 297–298, 300–302, 305, 311, 315–317, 320–321, 326, 332–334, 343, 357, 362–363, 365–366, 368–369, 378, 393–394, 396–403, 406, 439–440
Strategic Plan, 134
Stress Management, 240
Substitutions, 13, 15, 18, 28, 57, 75–76, 125, 129, 405
Succession Planning, 210
Sulfites, 289
Supplements, 32, 48, 91–99, 340, 386, 439
Suppliers, 58, 66, 75, 126–127, 171, 233, 245, 272, 369, 371–374, 377–378, 382–383, 386, 388–389, 404, 407
Surveys, 13, 18, 31, 55, 101, 107–108, 112, 114, 117, 121, 124, 126–127, 129, 209–210, 227

T

Table d Hote, 27
Taste Panel, 45, 88, 94, 117–118
Temperature, 4–7, 9–10, 24, 30, 38, 41, 52, 59, 61, 67–68, 70–72, 74, 83, 87, 107–108, 114–115, 117, 120–121, 170–171, 190, 194, 215, 224, 232, 250, 252, 259, 261, 264, 275, 277–279, 281, 284–285, 287–288, 291–299, 301–305, 308, 311, 317, 319–321, 325–327, 329–330, 359, 364–366, 377, 383, 439
Termination, 139, 200–202, 204–206
Terminology, 28–29, 66, 182, 272, 337, 339, 393
Test Tray, 30, 107, 114, 119–120
The Joint Commission, 9, 16, 122, 125–126, 131, 164, 238
Theft, 40, 201, 312, 366, 394–395, 398–399, 403–406, 439
Therapeutic Diet, 12, 14, 25, 103
Thermometer, 38, 70–71, 83, 261, 278, 293–294, 296, 319–320, 324, 326, 384, 398

Training, 3, 8–9, 14, 19, 25, 29, 31, 53, 67, 73, 76, 78, 83–84, 89–90, 102, 116–118, 123, 127, 131, 134–136, 143, 150, 159–174, 177–178, 186, 191–194, 196–197, 199–200, 203–205, 210, 218–220, 229–231, 233–235, 237, 241, 244, 250, 260, 263–265, 267, 269–270, 299, 303, 305, 308, 311, 322, 324, 327, 329, 332, 334–335, 344, 351, 359, 371, 373–374, 377–378, 390, 405, 425
Tray Accuracy, 114
Trayline Service, 4, 30, 53
Turnover Rate, 133, 135–136, 145, 164, 206–207

U

UHT (Ultra-High Temperature Process), 277, 279
UL (Underwriter's Laboratories), 318, 335, 370–372
Ultra-Pasteurized, 61
Unemployment, 153, 206, 237, 349
Unions, 208, 244, 351–352
United States Department of Agriculture, 171
Upward Communication, 228
USDA, 19–20, 24, 33, 43, 56, 58–59, 64, 66, 79, 125, 210, 272–273, 279–280, 310, 335, 339, 343–344, 383–384, 409

V

Vendor, 63, 65–66, 111, 137, 166, 171, 245, 247, 267, 271–274, 279, 322, 325, 342–344, 356, 358–359, 374, 378, 382, 384, 386–392, 399–401, 403–405, 408–409, 421, 423, 425, 435
Verification, 9, 272, 302, 304, 402
Virus, 257, 272, 284, 286, 288

W

Warewashing, 251, 261, 311, 317–318, 321, 325, 329, 367
Waste Management, 329–330
Water, 2, 26, 36, 44, 67–70, 73–74, 76–77, 96, 120, 218, 250–252, 256, 258–259, 262, 264, 271–272, 277, 282, 284–287, 292–293, 297–298, 310–313, 316, 321–326, 329–330, 357–359, 363–364, 372, 378
Weights and Measure, 17, 27–28, 40
Work Climate, 220–222
Work-Related Injury, 266
Workers Compensation, 153, 349

Y

Yeast, 21, 39, 62, 69–70, 119, 288
Yield, 35–41, 43–44, 46–50, 53, 64, 66, 76–77, 89, 346, 384, 387, 405, 436
Yield Percentage, 48–49